The Elderly with
Chronic Mental Illness

Enid Light, PhD, directs the psychosocial and family research program within the Mental Disorders of the Aging Research Branch, National Institute of Mental Health. She is a graduate of George Washington University and the University of Maryland. Dr. Light has contributed to the literature in evaluation studies, mental health service systems research, and psychosocial and family factors in aging and Alzheimer's disease.

Barry D. Lebowitz, PhD, is Chief of the Mental Disorders of the Aging Research Branch of the National Institute of Mental Health and a member of the adjunct faculty of the Department of Psychiatry of the Georgetown University School of Medicine. He is a graduate of McGill University and Cornell University and served on the faculties of Portland State University, the Catholic University of America, and George Washington University. Dr. Lebowitz is a Fellow of the Gerontological Society of America and was elected as a founding member of the Council on Aging of the American Sociological Association. A frequent participant in public and scientific forums, Dr. Lebowitz serves on the editorial boards of a number of professional scientific journals and has made many published contributions to the literature of gerontology and geriatrics. Along with Carl Salzman, MD, Dr. Lebowitz edited *Anxiety in the Elderly* (Springer Publishing Company, 1991).

The Elderly with Chronic Mental Illness

Enid Light, PhD
Barry D. Lebowitz, PhD
Editors

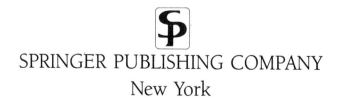

SPRINGER PUBLISHING COMPANY
New York

Springer Publishing Company, Inc.
536 Broadway
New York, NY 10012-3955

90 91 92 93 94 / 5 4 3 2 1

Library of Congress Cataloging-in-Publication Data

The Elderly with chronic mental illness / Enid Light, Barry D.
  Lebowitz, editors.
      p. cm.
  Includes bibliographical references and index.
  ISBN 0-8261-7280-6
  1. Geriatric psychiatry—Research.   2. Chronically ill—Research.
I. Light, Enid.   II. Lebowitz, Barry.
  [DNLM: 1. Chronic Disease—in old age.   2. Mental Disorders—in
old age.   3. Research.   WT 150 E374]
RC451.4.A5E43   1991
618.97′689′0072—dc20
DNLM/DLC
for Library of Congress   90-10421
                                                               CIP

Printed in the United States of America

Contents

Introduction

The United States is experiencing a dramatic increase in the number of individuals who reach old age. Significant in this large and growing population of older people is a substantial number with serious, persistent, and chronic mental disorder. In particular, those with early onset disease represent a new and challenging component of this patient population. Though in earlier times there was truth to the observation that the sick died younger than the well, we are now seeing patients with an array of chronic mental illnesses who survive into older age. This increased survival is the result of many factors; the general improvements in health and life circumstances have played a part, as have the proliferation of community based and institutional services appropriate to the needs of those with chronic mental disorder. The actual number of such individuals will continue increasing well into the 21st century as the general population ages. Yet, the research base essential to our knowledge about the nature, course, treatment, and outcome of mental illness with a chronic course is severely limited.

In this volume we attempt to encourage research in this area in two ways. First, the authors of the chapters address many of the complex theoretical and methodological issues that have hindered research in the past. In particular, the series of chapters by Toner and Stueve, McAdams and Jeste, and Schultz and Visintainer focus in great detail on some of the challenging methodological, measurement, and statistical aspects of conducting research on this population. Second, each of the contributors to this volume suggests and explores emerging lines of promising research and makes recommendations regarding the refinement and elaboration of research areas that have already been undertaken.

Several recurrent themes emerge. The most central and overarching theme running through all of the chapters is the need for careful multidisciplinary, longitudinal research that recognizes and addresses the relationship between brain, behavior, and environment, and for the support and training of researchers engaged in this difficult research. It is suggested that in order to understand some of the (incremental) changes in the course of illness over time, frequent follow-up interviews should be conducted and attention given to quality of life issues (Gurland & Toner).

The authors stress the importance of recognizing the heterogeneity of this population. Even with recent improvements to diagnostic classification systems, older adults with the same diagnosis are heterogeneous in significant aspects regarding their illness, for example, age of onset, treatment history and outcome, services required, and along psychosocial dimensions. Several chapters suggest the need to examine the chronically mentally ill population along specific dimensions such as sociocultural (Faulkner), social networks (Cutrona, Lenihan, Suhr, & Russell) including family caregivers (Cohler, Pickett, & Cook; Smyer & Birkel), homelessness (Cohen), as well as along biological dimensions such as gender (Yassa, Uhr, & Jeste), responsiveness to medication, and the influence of age on the disease process.

Another major theme cutting across this volume is the recognition of a high prevalence of coexisting mental and physical illness and substance abuse in this population. Issues of comorbidity are important for a fuller understanding of suicide and depression in the elderly (Conwell & Caine), medications, functional and social limitations, and a host of treatment delivery issues (Buckwalter; Gottesman, Peskin, & Kennedy; Burns).

Taken together, the chapters in this volume set forth a research agenda that can illuminate our understanding of the nature, consequences, and treatment of chronic mental illness in the elderly. Taken together, they also make a strong statement about the importance of considering the chronically mentally ill elderly within a developmental and family context.

We hope that this book will be an inspiration and an invitation to researchers to undertake the pressing challenge of conducting studies on the chronically mentally ill elderly.

We want to express our gratitude to each of the contributors to this volume; they have taken on a difficult task of thinking beyond the state of the art and in many cases have extended the scope of the knowledge base of the field far beyond present activities. Their creativity, commitment to the task, and excitement about this project have been an inspiration to us. We want to acknowledge, as well, the contribution of the Springer Publishing Company and of Dr. Ursula Springer and Kathleen O'Malley to this overall project—they have been innovative, helpful, and supportive throughout, and we are proud to have this book included in their groundbreaking list in the field of aging.

ENID LIGHT, PhD
BARRY D. LEBOWITZ, PhD

Contributors

Kathleen C. Buckwalter, PhD, RN
College of Nursing
University of Iowa
Iowa City, IA

Richard C. Birkel, PhD
College of Health and Human
  Development
The Penn State University
University Park, PA

Barbara J. Burns, PhD
Professor of Medical Psychology
Duke University Medical Center
Durham, NC

Eric D. Caine, MD
University of Rochester Medical
  Center
Director, NIMH Clinical Research
  Center for the Study of
  Psychopathology of the Elderly
University of Rochester School of
  Medicine and Dentistry
Rochester, NY

Carl I. Cohen, MD
Department of Psychiatry
SUNY Health Science Center at
  Brooklyn
Brooklyn, NY

Bertram J. Cohler, PhD
Department of Psychology
The University of Chicago
Chicago, IL

Yeates Conwell, MD
University of Rochester
NIMH Clinical Research Center for
  the Study of Psychopathology of
  the Elderly
University of Rochester School of
  Medicine
Rochester, NY

Judith A. Cook, PhD
Director
Thresholds Research Institute
Chicago, IL

Carolyn E. Cutrona, PhD
Department of Psychology
University of Iowa
Iowa City, IA

Audrey Olsen Faulkner, PhD, ACSW
School of Social Work
Rutgers, the State University
New Brunswick, NJ

Barry S. Fogel, MD
Associate Director
Center for Gerontology and Health
  Care Research
Brown University
Providence, RI

Mercedes M. Garcia, PhD
Department of Psychiatry and
  Behavioral Sciences
UCLA School of Medicine
Los Angeles, CA

Leonard E. Gottesman, PhD
President
Community Services Institute, Inc.
Naraberth, PA

Barry Gurland, FRCP (London), FRC
  Psych.
Director
Columbia University Center for
  Geriatrics and Gerontology
John E. Borne Professor of Clinical
  Psychiatry
Columbia University
New York, NY

Dilip V. Jeste, MD
Department of Psychiatry
University of California, San Diego
La Jolla, CA

Kathleen M. Kennedy, PhD
Community Services Institute, Inc.
Naraberth, PA

Andrew F. Leuchter, MD
Department of Psychiatry and
  Behavioral Sciences
UCLA School of Medicine
Los Angeles, CA

Lou Ann McAdams, PhD
Biostatistician
Harbor–UCLA Medical Center
Research and Education Institute Inc.
Population Research Center
Torrence, CA

Ellen Peskin, MA
Community Services Institute, Inc.
Naraberth, PA

Susan A. Pickett, PhD
Department of Psychology
The University of Chicago
Chicago, IL

Raymond Raschko, MSW
Director of Elder Services
Spokane Community Mental Health
  Center
Spokane, WA

Daniel Russell, PhD
Center for Health Services Research
College of Medicine
University of Iowa
Iowa City, IA

Richard Schulz, PhD
Director of Gerontology
University of Pittsburgh
UCSUR
Pittsburgh, PA

Kathleen Schutte, MA
Department of Psychology
University of Iowa
Iowa City, IA

Michael A. Smyer, PhD
College of Health and Human
   Development
Pennsylvania State University
University Park, PA

Anne Stueve, PhD
Center for Geriatrics and Gerontology
Columbia University
New York, NY

Julie A. Suhr, BA
Department of Psychology
University of Iowa
Iowa City, IA

John A. Toner, EdD
Department of Geriatric Research
Psychiatric Institute
Center for Geriatrics and Gerontology
Columbia University
New York, NY

Sarita Uhr, MD
Staff Psychiatrist
San Diego Senior Evaluation and
   Treatment Unit
Assistant Clinical Professor Psychiatry
University of California, San Diego
La Jolla, CA

Paul Visintainer, PhD
Department of Psychiatry and
   University Center for Social and
   Urban Research
University of Pittsburgh
Pittsburgh, PA

Ramzy Yassa, MD
Douglas Hospital Center
Verdun, Quebec, Canada

Steven H. Zarit, PhD
Assistant Director of Gerontology
   Center
College of Health and Human
   Development
The Pennsylvania State University
University Park, PA

PART I

Understanding and Defining the CMI Elderly Population

The Chronically Mentally Ill Elderly: Epidemiological Perspectives on the Nature of the Population

Barry Gurland, John A. Toner

ISSUES IN DEFINING
AND CHARACTERIZING CHRONICITY

Epidemiology is the study of disease, defects and disabilities in populations, and the various personal and environmental factors that affect how such conditions become manifest (Mechanic, 1970). The epidemiologist approaches the study of these conditions by delimiting, defining, locating, counting and characterizing them (Goldman, Gattozzi & Taube, 1981). The first step in applying these principles to chronic mental illness in the elderly is to clarify the characteristics of mental illness that justify the use of the term chronic.

The Random House dictionary defines chronic as inveterate, constant, habitual; continuing a long time or recurring frequently; having had a long disease. These defining terms do evoke aspects of chronic mental illness that distinguish it from acute mental illness, but are vague and also do not make explicit the usefulness of this distinction. Without knowing the relevance (value) of the concept of chronicity it is difficult to make the definition more precise. All the components of the definition are quantitative (e.g., length, frequency, constancy) but the numerical value of the quantity is not stated (e.g., how long, frequent or constant must a condition be to be chronic?). Similarly, there is no guidance from the dictionary definition as to when an acute mental condition should be deemed to have become chronic.

There clearly are important health care policy, service practice, and health science implications attached to the concept of chronicity of mental conditions: by use of the term chronicity, attention can be shifted from the more socially admired, straight forward, remunerative, and dramatically effective treatment of acute conditions to the challenges of caring for chronic disorders with their multidisciplinary, interactive consequences, need for continuity and coordination of prolonged complex services, and often small (but important) gains for therapy. This identifies the value of the concept of chronicity and points to the qualitative features of the clinical picture and appropriate treatment program that can be turned into indicators of chronicity which are not reliant on an arbitrary cut point on a quantitative dimension.

Another set of qualitative indicators of chronicity is the extent to which a condition alters the patient's life style. The processes associated with the acute condition (i.e., symptoms, dysfunction, treatment) are short term and for this reason need not involve substantial intrusion into the organization of the patient's life. In contrast, the corresponding processes of a chronic condition inevitably change the nature of the patient's life: life activities cannot be suspended and then resumed intact as in an acute condition but must go forward with adjustments for the ongoing chronic processes. This refers to decisions on jobs, career plans, interpersonal relations, living arrangements, and the like; to the level of life dissatisfaction and symptom intensity that must be accepted on a long term basis; and to the degree to which life must accommodate treatment as opposed to treatment accommodating life. Many of these issues adhering to the defining effects of chronicity can be assumed under the rubric of "quality of life"; which broadly refers to "a series of attributes among those definitely sick" (Spitzer, 1987) and, as Katz (1987) cautions, "is a concept that is subject to multiple viewpoints."

In other words, a mental illness is recognized to move from the acute to the chronic mode when certain changes occur in the organization of care and when quality of life issues become merged with quality of care. This shift is highly correlated with the length of illness but the lapse of time between onset of illness and the shift to chronicity may vary with the type of mental illness, historical and social context, patient characteristics, and treatment approach. Thus, any attempt to reach a single definition of chronicity in terms of duration of illness is likely to be arbitrary and often misleading.

There is a need for research to identify criteria for chronicity of mental illness that will serve better than duration of illness alone for the purposes of study of the determinants of chronicity, program evaluation, and the planning of appropriate care. Based on the considerations discussed above, the examination of candidate criteria should include:

1. Quality of life criteria: (a) impairments of functional status in the performance of the basic and instrumental activities of daily life; and in such areas as social relationships, morale and life satisfaction, intellectual processes (e.g., learning, memory), communication skills, work, use of leisure time, initiative, and access to environmental and material resources; (b) severity levels of symptomatic distress, or behaviors which are dangerous or disturbing to others because of the mental condition; (c) the extent to which current impairments of the sufferer's functional status are the basis for planning and decisions respecting the future. For example, where there exist impairments of functional status which by their nature are extended in time (e.g., being unemployed rather than on sick leave; having few potential social contacts rather than temporarily suspending visiting; or having realistically little expectation of satisfying activities); (d) the extent to which major options affecting quality of life, such as location of residence and degree of independence have been predicated on the illness effects; and (e) the extent to which there are areas of functional status which are not touched by the illness (i.e., the balance between affected and unaffected areas) or times (hours, days or periods) or activities which are free of impairments (not pervasively involved by the illness).

2. Quality (or organization) of care criteria: (a) the weight placed on stabilization, slowing decline or gaining limited improvement of function rather than attempting a cure in setting the goals of treatment; (b) the breadth of treatment and assistance to the patient in maintaining a community tenure or relocating to sheltered accommodation; or in otherwise adapting to a life restricted by the illness; as contrasted with treatment narrowly directed at relieving symptoms or reversing an illness process; (c) the intensity of consideration of possible long term side effects of treatment; or of the problems of delivering maintenance treatment; and (d) the limitations imposed on the range of treatment options by health care insurance with a cap on length or frequency of treatment or exclusion of personal assistance and environmental interventions.

It is notable that many of the criteria for defining chronicity are best understood as *continua* rather than categories; chronicity is a matter of degree. This renders it even more difficult to accept those definitions which depend on a particular duration of illness or a specific number of hospitalizations as validly reflecting the intensity and extensiveness of chronicity.

If it is true, as argued here, that the defining characteristic of chronicity in respect to mental disorder in old age is a blurring of the distinctions between quality of life, quality of care, and course of the disorder, then the criteria for chronicity may look something like this: (a) the patient's quality of life is presently and in prospect substantially determined by the course of his/her disorder, and/or the history of the patient's quality of life has been characterized by the history of his/her mental condition; (b) health care decisions are based on the expectation that active treatment will be needed for the foreseeable future and that some level of functional impairment will persist; (c) the patient has to spend considerable time each year and probably each day, in seeking or receiving health care; (d) the patient must make major choices in life style, such as residential location, on the basis of their impaired functioning and/or the need to accommodate treatment; and (e) the family or other caregiver finds their lives and plans altered by the course of the disorder.

A research agenda for defining and characterizing chronicity of mental illness should logically precede the epidemiological strategies and subject matter mentioned in the opening paragraph of this paper. However, it is impractical to approach urgent research issues in this orderly sequence. Interim definitions of chronicity must therefore continue to be based on criteria which are presently feasible and widely accepted (see Goldman & Manderscheid, 1987). These have generally been aimed at defining the chronic patient rather than chronic illnesses.

Some of the standard definitions of the chronic patient are:

1. Duration of hospitalization or other treatment greater than a stipulated amount: 1 year of continuous stay in mental hospital or nursing home; or longer than 90 days in a general hospital or private psychiatric hospital. The rationale for these quantitative criteria is presumably that the chances of release or recovery are diminished to a negligible level beyond these points of duration.
2. Previous hospitalization for more than a certain duration of illness. Any hospitalization of 6 months or longer in the last 5 years; or two or more hospitalizations in the last twelve months; or hospitalization followed by outpatient care.
3. At risk for institutional admission.
4. Impairments and disabilities (e.g., mentally disabled): variously quantified as prolonged; partial or total; moderate or severe; substantial; numbers of areas involved among self-care, interpersonal relationships, work, schooling, receptive or expressive communication, learning, mobility, independence, personal hygiene, self direction, recreation, economic self-sufficiency.
5. The presence of a diagnosis of severe mental illness or emotional disorder, especially schizophrenia.
6. Recipient of Social Security Disability Insurance or Supplemental Security Income; or unable to engage in gainful employment for 12 months.
7. In a supervised residence or sheltered work program.

These "practical" definitions do not directly address the chronicity in its essential nature as a function of the quality of life and care. Nor do symptoms without disability rate as chronic in these practical terms. A further conceptual problem is that hospitalization is invoked as a definition of chronicity rather than as one of its outcomes; patients with a chronic course to their disorder and their treatment may never be hospitalized; or at least not in the previous 5 years.

The practical definitions of chronicity have a heavy reliance on measures that focus on problems of occupational incapacity and hospitalization, both of which are costly to government (society). This is well reflected in indices of duration of incapacity and hospital stay; they do not capture the full importance of chronicity to the patient, the family and the health care professions.

Whatever definitions of chronicity are adopted, they might be variously applied to a disorder, an outcome, a patient or a treatment regimen. When used to describe a disorder it is implied that the disorder determines the chronic course; applied to the course of a disorder the implication is that this is one of a range of outcomes for that disorder and there are multiple potential determinants of the presence and degree of chronicity; chronic care refers to the features of quality of care previously listed; in theory, chronic treatment could outlast the chronic course of a disorder.

The use of the term chronic to apply to a disorder is very likely to be misleading since it suggests that the disorder is almost invariably chronic: this use has included organic mental disorders, schizophrenia, paranoid disorders, somatoform disorders, and personality disorders (all of above have been recognized as causes of disability by the Social Security Administration). Alcohol, drug abuse, and mental retardation are also candidates for this term. However, so-called chronic disorders may not follow a chronic course, while disorders that are typically acute (such as major depression and general anxiety) may assume a chronic course (Weissman & Klerman, 1977). Furthermore, some disorders may in some instances manifest only one or two acute episodes and never again relapse, yet require chronic care (e.g., maintenance treatment).

LONGITUDINAL STUDIES

The longitudinal dimension is integral to the defining characteristics of chronicity in relation to mental disorder. The different aspects of chronicity require longitudinal study in order to dissect and interrelate them. Particularly, longitudinal description will prevent the attribution of chronicity to disorders and patients rather than to phases of the course of the disorder or the nature of treatment. Moreover, the effect of aging on the inception, duration and outcome of chronicity can be best elucidated by longitudinal study.

Yet, there are relatively few studies which are sufficiently longitudinal in that they follow the course of a patient's disorder and treatment across the span of years from adulthood (or younger) to old age and death; with a frequency that fills in the events between the onset of the disorder and the period of old age; and with enough detail and scope to cover the elements of chronicity (e.g., quality of life and care indicators).

Table 1.1 lists twelve studies employing the longitudinal approach to the study of chronic mental illness. These selected studies come closer than most to meeting the design requirements outlined above and will serve to illustrate the present limitations of this field and the need to encourage new studies, or continue established studies, with improved methods.

In some studies, the selection of subjects into a cohort for follow-up is biased in such a way (e.g., taken from a particular practice setting, or from among those who have been hospitalized for a specified time, or have escaped hospitalization by a certain age) as to make the findings more contributive to the clinical practice of prognosis than an understanding of the degree to which the course of a disorder is chronic. It is certainly helpful to be able to anticipate which cases in commonly encountered clinical situations will become chronic, but the study of cohorts selected from particular clinical contexts will not provide a view of the extent to which the disorder under investigation is likely to be chronic; nor the determinants of chronicity across all cases of the defined disorder. Unselected (i.e., representative) samples of a defined disorder are required for fundamental and definitive studies of the chronicity of mental illness.

Some of the reports do not embrace a sufficient length of follow-up to be able to judge the persistence or development of chronicity in old age, or the effect of aging on chronicity; bearing in mind that we are here concentrating on mental conditions beginning before the period of old age. For example, the typical age of onset of schizophrenia is before 35 years and it would require a minimum follow up of 40 to 50 years to obtain a definitive picture of chronicity; not only does this exceed the patience, endurance and financing of most investigators and their successors but it also presupposes a large enough initial cohort to leave substantial numbers surviving and remaining under surveillance into old age. An alternative which allows quicker returns involves a cross-sequential analytic design, but this requires sampling of adequate numbers of cases of all ages from adulthood to old age. The studies which fulfill these criteria are scanty.

Mapping the chronic course of illness to old age does not necessarily provide information on the course of chronicity in old age; for that one needs to track cases through old age to death. It is entirely possible that even illnesses with a long standing chronic course may subside in old age; if so, this may be a valuable salvation of a life previously blighted by the chronic illness. Conversely, treatments which are successful at improving the quality of life during the adulthood of patients should not be finally judged until their impact and consequences have been evaluated during the later stages of life; the latter should weigh in the balance as heavily as the results earlier in life.

TABLE 1.1 Selected Longitudinal Studies of Chronic Mental Illness

Name and site of study	Setting/length of follow-up	Population characteristics	Outcome indicators	References
The Iowa 500 Study, University of Iowa Psychiatric Hospital, Iowa	Inpatient psych. hospital/30–40 year follow-up	525 consecutive admissions selected according to Feigner's research criteria for schizophrenia and affective disorders during the period from 1934–44. Four decade follow-up. The mean age at admission was 35 years old.	Successful community placement, marital status, residential placement, occupation, mortality, causes of death, diagnostic stability, psychiatric status	Coryell & Tsuang, 1986; Tsuang & Woolson, 1978; Tsuang & Dempsey, 1979; Tsuang, Woolson, & Fleming, 1980; Tsuang, Woolson, Winokur, & Crowe, 1981
Kings County Psychiatric Hospital Study of Schizophrenic Outpatients	Psychopharmacology Treatment and Research Clinic, Kings County Hospital, Center, New York, NY/15 year follow-up	646 chronic schizophrenic patients between the ages of 18–45, referred to clinic for maintenance pharmacotherapy, with DSM-III diagnoses of schizophrenia, and mental illness of 1 year or more. The mean age at admission was 30 years (range of 18–45).	Hospitalization, level of independence, public assistance	Englehardt et al, 1982
International Pilot Study of Schizophrenia (IPSS), Washington, D.C.	Two general hospitals with psychiatric wards and one state hospital/2 and 5 year follow-up	1,202 patients meeting research criteria, residing in catchment area for 6 months or more, with psychotic symptoms on admission. The mean age was 29 years (range = 15–45).	Unemployment, social relations, poor heterosexual relationships	Strauss & Carpenter, 1974, 1977

9

(continued)

TABLE 1.1 (continued)

Name and site of study	Setting/length of follow-up	Population characteristics	Outcome indicators	References
Massachusetts Mental Health Center Study of Remitting Schizophrenics	Inpatient psych. hospital/10 year follow-up	56 patients diagnosed on admission (1959–62) as schizophrenics and exhibiting Bleuler's primary symptoms and achieving full remission and hospitalized ≥ 2 years. The mean age at admission was 32 years.	Hospitalization, diagnostic stability, mortality, social impairment, marital status, use of phenothyazines, orientation in time, place and person	Vaillant, 1978
The Chestnut Lodge Follow-Up Study, Chestnut Lodge Hospital, Rockville, Maryland	Private inpatient Psychiatric Hospital/15 year follow-up	446 patients without organic brain syndrome discharged between 1950 and 1975 and hospitalized ≥ 90 and meeting rigorous research criteria. Median age at admission was 31.	% time in hospital, % time employed, diagnostic stability, continued treatment, social contacts and activities, global functioning	McGlashan, 1984a, 1984b, 1986
Alberta Hospital, Follow-up of First Admissions, Alberta, Canada	Inpatient Psychiatric Hospital/10 year follow-up	92 first admission schizophrenics with a first hospital admission in 1963 without alternative of secondary dx. The mean age on admission was 34 years (range = 14–66 years)	Marital status, psychiatric condition, economic productivity, social adjustment, employment	Bland, Parker, & Orn, 1976
Vermont Longitudinal Study, Vermont State Hospital	Inpatient Psychiatric Hospital/32 year follow-up	269 back-ward "hopeless" cases selected to participate in a drug placement program between 1955–1960. The mean age of the patients was 40 years.	Education, marital status, psychological and social functioning, hospitalization, income	Harding et al., 1987

10

Study	Setting/Follow-up	Sample	Variables	Reference
Course of Schizoaffective Illness Study, University Psychiatric Clinic, Zurich, Switzerland	Hospital based Psychiatric Unit/20 year follow-up	245 hospital admissions with affective or schizoaffective diagnoses admitted from 1959–1963. The mean age at admission was 31.8 years.	Age, mortality, cause of death, duration of illness, number and length of episodes, remission, type of treatment	Angst, Felder, & Lohmeyer, 1980
Geriatric Mental Illness, San Francisco Medical Center, California	General Hospital Psychiatric Observation Ward/ 3, 5, 8, and 11 year follow-up	534 patients not previously admitted to a psychiatric facility and aged 60 years or older.	Mortality, residential placement, physical and social self-maintenance, orientation	Epstein, Robinson, & Simon, 1971
Course of Schizophrenia Into Old Age, Lausanne, Switzerland	Inpatient Psychiatric Hospital/37 years catamnestic follow-up	1642 schizophrenics (using Kraepelin's diagnostic criteria) who were less than 65 years old at first hospitalization and reached 65 years or more and were hospital patients at the beginning of the study in 1963. The mean age at first hospitalization was 37 years.	Mortality, cause of death, marital status, social, familial, and professional adaptation, occupation, vocational training, global mental health, course of illness, intensive symptoms (stupor, anxiety), nonproductive symptoms (indifference, withdrawal, delusions, etc.)	Ciompi, 1976
The Lundby Cohort University of Lund, Lund, Sweden	Community study/25 year follow-up	2550 inhabitants living within a geographically defined area of southern Sweden	Environment, age, life expectancy, mortality, incidence and risk of depression	Hagnell et al, 1982
Geriatric Inpatient Study, Rockland Psychiatric Center, Orangeburg, New York	Public Inpatient Psychiatric Hospital/4 year follow-up	1515 mental hospital inpatients aged 65 years or older receiving care at the Center from 1/1972–12/1976	Length of stay, diagnosis, treatment effectiveness	Goodman & Siegel, 1986

In some longitudinal studies, the follow-up does not give much direct information on quality of life:

1. The emphasis may be on mortality, which is more salient for relatively acute illnesses than for chronic illnesses; in the latter it is the manner of living (and perhaps dying) more than the time of dying that counts.

2. The outcomes may be mainly administrative or fiscal in perspective; frequency and total duration of institutional stay, community placement, employment, marital status, and the like belong in this category. It may be argued that community tenure, employment and marriage are indicators of good quality of life but it seems equally plausible that there is substantial variance of the quality of life within these categories or their opposites.

The indicators of the type and location of treatment do fall within the domain of the quality of care definition of chronicity but are often not reported in enough detail to gauge whether the treatment regimen is reflective of, or imparts, to, the course of the disorder a chronic quality. Patients may be in an institution for reasons that are more social than determined by the need for treatment or by the effects of the disorder, institutional treatments may vary widely in the degree to which they restrict or enhance the patient's life, patients located in the community may or may not be considerably restricted or impaired by the treatment regimen they must follow.

3. The outcomes may be more in the nature of end points than interval status; that is to say that the information bears upon where the patient ended up at a particular point in time rather than the long period of time that it took to get to the endpoint. It is the slow and continuous evolution of the patient's history that contains the best information on the quality of that life and the chronicity of the course of the disorder; and which measurement requires frequent follow-up evaluations and appropriate methods to portray the consequences of the disorder.

The presence, type and severity of symptomatology is a follow-up measure that is fairly frequently reported in longitudinal studies of mental disorder and is well within the domain of quality of life. Nevertheless, the measures of symptomatology employed may (and often do) veer from being central to quality of life when they are directed at the activity of the illness rather than the degree to which the symptoms are distressing, disabling and intrusive.

There is a notable lack of studies fulfilling all the criteria discussed here but the few that come close to the ideal seem exclusively concentrated on the diagnosis of schizophrenia. Cases of depression and other diagnoses that are included in these exemplary studies appear to have crept in by virtue of their presence in settings from which total or random samples were taken and in which schizophrenia predominates (thus leaving only small numbers of cases with other diagnoses). Perhaps, preoccupation with administrative perspectives on chronicity, to the exclusion of quality of life and care considerations in defining chronicity, has led to the problems of chronicity in other diagnoses being relatively overlooked.

CONCLUSIONS

A critical review such as this runs the risk of lapsing into the counsel of perfection. We therefore should acknowledge the great importance of continuing the stream of studies on the chronicity of mental illness, that have already formed a basis for clinical, public health and basic research approaches to improving care and planning for the sufferers from chronic mental illness. However, we also urge that there be leadership, guidance and support for addressing the issues we have raised in this paper regarding epidemiological concepts and strategies for further study of the nature of chronicity of mental illness, with specific respect to the lifespan and old age.

There is a challenging and potentially productive opportunity for serious study of quality of life and care factors as they pertain to chronicity of mental illness. The scientific foundation for investigation of these issues is now being laid down, as related by Sidney Katz (a pioneer in this field) in his editorial preface (Katz, 1987) to the proceedings of *The Portugal Conference: Measuring Quality of Life and Functional Status in Clinical and Epidemiological Research*. Moreover, the necessity of supporting the laborious work entailed in longitudinal studies within a lifespan framework is becoming apparent and hopefully will attract a suitable amount of funding. A more precise and authentic view of chronicity of mental illness than presently obtains, may well open up new possibilities for management of care and of secondary or tertiary prevention for these patients and their conditions.

REFERENCES

Angst, J., Felder, W., & Lohmeyer, B. (1980). Course of schizoaffective psychoses: Results of a follow-up study. *Schizophrenia Bulletin, 6,* 579-585.

Bland, R. C., Parker, J. H., & Orn, H. (1976). Prognosis in schizophrenia: A ten-year follow-up of first admissions. *Archives of General Psychiatry, 33,* 949-954.

Ciompi, L. (1976). Catamnestic long-term study on the course of life and aging of schizophrenics. Translated by S. Clemens (1980). *Schizophrenia Bulletin, 6,* 606-618.

Coryell, W., & Tsuang, M. T. (1986). Outcome after 40 years in DSM-III schizophreniform disorder. *Archives of General Psychiatry, 43,* 324-328.

Engelhardt, D. M., Rosen, B., Feldman, J., Engelhardt, J. A. Z., & Cohen, P. (1982). A 15-year follow-up of 646 schizophrenic outpatients. *Schizophrenia Bulletin, 8*, 493–503.

Epstein, L. J., Robinson, B. C., & Simon, A. (1971). Predictors of survival in geriatric mental illness during the eleven years after initial hospital admission. *Journal of the American Geriatrics Society, 19*, 913–922.

Goldman, H. H., Gattozzi, A. A., & Taube, C. A. (1981). Defining and counting the chronically mentally ill. *Hospital & Community Psychiatry, 32*, 21–27.

Goldman, H. H., & Manderscheid, R. W. (1987). Chronic mental disorder in the United States. In R. W. Manderscheid & S. A. Barrett (Eds.), *Mental health, United States.* DHHS Pub. No. (ADM 87-1518). Washington, DC: Superintendent of Documents, U.S. Government Printing Office.

Goodman, A. B., & Siegel, C. (1986). Elderly schizophrenic inpatients in the wake of deinstitutionalization. *American Journal of Psychiatry, 143*, 204–207.

Hagnell, O., Lanke, J., Rorsman, B., & Ojesjo, L. (1982). Are we entering an age of melancholy? Depressive illnesses in a prospective epidemiological study over 25 years: The Lundby Study, Sweden. *Psychological Medicine, 12*, 279–289.

Harding, C. M., Brooks, G. W., Ashikaga, T., Strauss, J. S., & Breier, A. (1987). The Vermont longitudinal study of persons with severe mental illness, I: Methodology, study sample, and overall status 32 years later. *American Journal of Psychiatry, 144*, 718–826.

Katz, S. (1987). The science of quality of life. *Journal of Chronic Diseases, 40*, 459–463.

Mechanic, D. (1970). Problems and prospects in psychiatric epidemiology. In E. H. Hare & J. K. Wing (Eds.), *Psychiatric Epidemiology.* London: Oxford University Press.

McGlashan, T. H. (1984a). The Chestnut Lodge follow-up study. I. Follow-up methodology and study sample. *Archives of General Psychiatry, 41*, 573–585.

McGlashan, T. H. (1984b). The Chestnut Lodge follow-up study. II. Long-term outcome of schizophrenia and the affective disorders. *Archives of General Psychiatry, 41*, 586–601.

McGlashan, T. H. (1986). Schizotypal personality disorder. Chestnut Lodge follow-up study: VI. Long-term follow-up perspectives. *Archives of General Psychiatry, 43*, 329–334.

Spitzer, W. O. (1987). State of science 1986: Quality of life and functional status as target variables for research. *Journal of Chronic Diseases, 40*, 465–471.

Strauss, J. S., & Carpenter, W. T. (1974). The prediction of outcome in schizophrenia. II. Relationships between predictor and outcome variables: A report from the WHO international pilot study of schizophrenia. *Archives of General Psychiatry, 31*, 37–42.

Strauss, J. S., & Carpenter, W. T. (1977). Prediction of outcome in schizophrenia. III. Five-year outcome and its predictors. *Archives of General Psychiatry, 34*, 159–163.

Tsuang, M. T., & Woolson, R. F. (1978). Excess mortality in schizophrenia and affective disorders: Do suicides and accidental deaths solely account for this excess? *Archives of General Psychiatry, 35*, 1181–1185.

Tsuang, M. T., & Dempsey, M. (1979). Long-term outcome of major psychoses. II. Schizoaffective disorder compared with schizophrenia, affective disorders, and a surgical control group. *Archives of General Psychiatry, 36*, 1302–1304.

Tsuang, M. T., & Woolson, R. F., & Fleming, J. A. (1980). Causes of death in schizophrenia and manic-depression. *British Journal of Psychiatry, 136*, 239–242.

Tsuang, M. T., & Woolson, R. F., Winokur, G., & Crowe, R. R. (1981). Stability of psychiatric diagnosis: Schizophrenia and affective disorders followed up over a 30- to 40-year period. *Archives of General Psychiatry, 38,* 535–539.

Vaillant, G. E. (1978). A ten-year follow-up of remitting schizophrenics. *Schizophrenia Bulletin, 4,* 78–85.

Weissman, M. M., & Klerman, G. L. (1977). The chronic depressive in the community: Unrecognized and poorly treated. *Comparative Psychiatry, 18,* 523–532.

2

Gender Differences in Chronic Schizophrenia: Need for Further Research

Ramzy Yassa, Sarita Uhr, Dilip V. Jeste

Gender differences in schizophrenia were noted as early as the late 19th century with the publications by Kraepelin (1971) and Bleuler (1950). Yet, over the years, relatively few studies have dealt with these differences in detail. Indeed, as Goldstein (1988) states, much of the literature dealing with the subject assumes that the illness is similar in men and women, in spite of some rather consistent evidence to the contrary.

Gender differences have been found in different aspects of the schizophrenic syndrome. These include (1) age at onset of psychosis and first hospitalization, (2) symptom presentation and diagnosis, (3) biochemical and neuroradiological investigations, (4) neuroleptic response, and (5) prognosis.

We propose to present these aspects with a detailed review of the literature. This review primarily covers English and French language literature.

Dr. Jeste's work was supported, in part, by NIMH grant #1-R01-MH43693-01 and by the Veterans Administration.

AGE AT ONSET OF PSYCHOSIS
AND FIRST HOSPITALIZATION

Several studies have reported that the age at onset of schizophrenic symptoms is 2 to 6 years earlier in men than in women (Braatay, 1934; Malzberg, 1935; E. Bleuler, 1950; Brown, Bone, Dalison, & Wing, 1966; Achte, 1967; Novik & Odegaard, 1967; M. Blueler, 1968, 1974, 1978; Hartmann & Meyer, 1969; Kraepelin, 1971; Forrest & Hay, 1971, 1972; McCabe, 1975; Nystrup, 1976; Bland, 1977; Huber, Gross, Schuttler, & Linz, 1980; Ciompi, 1980; Lewine, Strauss, & Gift, 1981; Loranger, 1984; Sartorius et al., 1986; Stromgren, 1987; Shimizu, Kurachi, & Noda, 1988). In one study, men developed schizophrenia 10 years earlier than women (Watt & Szulecka, 1979). On the other hand, two studies (Locke, Kramer, & Timberlake, 1958; Bland & Orn, 1978) found no significant difference between men and women in age at onset. This latter study, which only included 43 patients with schizophrenia (22 men, 21 women), found that the mean age at onset of psychosis was lower in women (31 years) than in men (35 years).

First admissions among male patients with schizophrenia are more frequent before the age of 30 than among female patients (Brown, Bone, Dalison, & Wing, 1966; Nowik et al., 1967; M. Bleuler, 1968, 1974, 1978; Hartman & Meyer, 1969; Forrest & Hay, 1971, 1972; McCabe, 1975; Huber, Gross, Schuttler, & Linz, 1980; Stromgren, 1987). In some studies, the male:female ratio of first admissions was found to be as high as 4:1 before the age of 20 (McCabe, 1975).

On the other hand, studies dealing with late onset schizophrenia (i.e., schizophrenia with onset after age 44) found that women were affected more often than men (Jeste et al., 1988; Harris & Jeste, 1988). In this population, the male:female ratio was found to be 1:2 (Jeste et al., 1988).

These findings of an earlier onset of schizophrenia in men and later appearance of psychotic symptoms in women seem to be universal as they have been consistently reported in all the studies.

Is this gender difference specific for schizophrenia? To address this issue, several studies have been conducted. Leventhal, Shuck, and Rothstein (1984) compared 64 schizophrenic patients with 30 nonschizophrenic patients using DSM-III criteria and found that psychiatric symptoms appeared earlier in men (irrespective of diagnosis) than in women, with male schizophrenic patients exhibiting the earliest symptoms among all the subgroups. On the other hand, Fremming (1951) found that the mean age at onset of psychotic symptoms in male schizophrenic patients (29 years) was less than that of female schizophrenic patients (31 years). However, he also found that the mean age at onset of manic depressive symptoms was earlier in women (35 years) than in men (41 years). Helgason (1964) also noted that the mean age of male schizophrenic patients was less than that of the mean age of male manic depressives, and male patients with "functional" psychosis were older than women with this diagnosis (40.6 years versus 39.8 years, respectively). Analyzing data from the Canadian register for first admissions of psychosis, Bland (1977) found differences in mean age between men and women for schizophrenia, paranoid states, and reactive psychosis but not for bipolar disorder. He also reported that the catatonic and schizoaffective subgroups differed in gender ratio from schizophrenia as a whole, with an overrepresentation of women (similar to affective psychosis). McCabe (1975), comparing schizophrenic patients with those having reactive psychosis or bipolar disorder, found that there was a difference between men and women only in schizophrenia.

Thus, although relatively few studies have been conducted comparing different diagnostic categories with schizophrenia, there is consistency in the finding of a gender difference in onset of schizophrenic symptoms.

SYMPTOM PRESENTATION AND DIAGNOSIS

Several studies have indicated that male schizophrenic patients have more severe symptoms than female schizophrenic patients. Another replicated finding is that the stricter the diagnostic measure, the less the women are represented.

Lewine and associates (1981, 1984), using six diagnostic criteria for schizophrenia, found that the stronger the criteria, the more men than women were diagnosed as suffering from the illness (Research Diagnostic criteria, Feighner and Associates criteria, Taylor and Abrams's criteria, and "Flexible System"). With looser criteria, the ratio of men to women was considerably higher (New Haven Schizophrenia Index and First-rank symptoms criteria).

For example, Westermeyer and Harrow (1984), comparing DSM-II and DSM-III criteria in 141 patients, found that DSM-II criteria (which are more liberal) included more women schizophrenics than did DSM-III criteria.

If we use the process-reactive dichotomy, several studies have indicated that more men than women are diagnosed as having process schizophrenia than reactive schizophrenia (Becker, 1956; Lane, 1968; Allon, 1971; Harrow, Westermeyer, Silverstein, Strauss, & Cohler, 1986). Affleck, Burns, & Forrest (1976), using Schneiderian criteria, found that more men were given the diagnosis of schizophrenia/schizophreniform dimensions, while more women were diagnosed as paranoid psychosis/other dimension.

As for the symptom clusters, affective symptoms were described more commonly in women than in men (Bland, 1977; Lewine, 1981; Westermeyer & Harrow, 1984; Goldstein & Link, 1988). Tsuang, Dempsey, and Rauscher (1976), using Feighner criteria, found that among patients diagnosed as having "atypical schizophrenia" women were overrepresented (71% of the group), while of those diagnosed as suffering from schizophrenia, 48% were women.

Dangerous, asocial behavior was more common in men (Nystrup, 1976; Salokengas, 1983; Goldstein, 1988). Negative symptoms were described more frequently in men than in women in several studies (Huber, Gross, & Schuttler, 1975, 1980; Pogue-Geile & Harrow, 1984; Kolakowska et al., 1985; McCreadie et al., 1987; Goldstein & Link, 1988). McCreadie et al. (1987) also found more neurological signs in men than in women (50% versus 17%, respectively).

Suicide has also been reported to be more prevalent in men than in women (Seeman, 1982; Tsuang & Woolson, 1978; Tsuang, 1983; Breier & Astrachan, 1984). Furthermore, one study found that male relatives of schizophrenic patients were particularly subject to high suicide rates (Tsuang, 1983). Thus, men tend to be diagnosed more often than women as suffering from schizophrenia with stricter diagnostic criteria. This may be due to the fact that women present more often with atypical symptoms of schizophrenia (e.g., affective coloring, schizoaffective symptoms as well as less negative symptoms) than men. This is of great importance when dealing with the question of prognosis, as more men with better prognosis will be excluded with these stricter criteria. This point also raises the important question: Should we have different diagnostic criteria for schizophrenia for women than for men?

BIOCHEMICAL AND
NEURORADIOLOGICAL INVESTIGATIONS

There have been relatively few studies of gender differences relating to biochemical and neuroradiological abnormalities in schizophrenic patients. Baron, Gruen, Levitt, and Kane (1984) found that platelet monoamine oxidase (MAO) activity was lower in male than in female schizophrenic patients. Lewine (1985) reported a positive correlation between platelet MAO activity and negative symptoms in male schizophrenic patients but not in females. However, Males and Von Kammen (1983) found no gender differences in platelet MAO activity.

Ventricular brain ratio (VBR) has been studied extensively in CT scans of schizophrenic patients, yet only a few studies have compared VBR between men and women. Kolakowska et al., (1985) noted men to have larger VBR than women. However, three other studies found no significant gender difference (Reveley, Reveley, & Murray, 1984; Iacono, et al., 1988; Shelton et al., 1988).

The thickness of the corpus callosum has recently been the focus of one study (Nasrallah et al., 1986). These authors compared 38 schizophrenic patients with 41 healthy controls using Magnetic Resonance Imaging and found a significant increase in the mean callosal thickness in the middle and anterior but not the posterior parts of the callosal body. This difference was due to a significant increase in the callosal thickness in schizophrenic women but not in men. A thicker callosum implies that the two cerebral hemispheres have more interhemispheric fibers and may thus be less differentiated and less lateralized in cognitive task specialization.

Thus, as noted, very few studies have been carried out at the biochemical and neurological levels at present, and the few publications seem to be contradictory. We need longitudinal studies comparing different parameters in men and women as they relate to the prognosis of the illness.

NEUROLEPTIC RESPONSE

Very few systematic studies have been conducted to evaluate gender differences in the response to neuroleptic therapy (Awad, 1985).

Goldberg, Schooler, Davidson, and Kayce (1966) observed that with placebo, men improved more than women. With neuroleptics, however, women improved more than men. The authors postulated that placebo responders were those in whom the pathophysiology was more highly loaded with psychological stress factors, while drug improvers had greater genetic loading.

During the past two decades, several studies have appeared indicating that women respond better to neuroleptics than men do and also that women seem to survive longer in the community than men (Hogarty, Goldberg, & Schooler 1974; Seeman, 1982, 1985; Young & Meltzer, 1980). It has further been suggested that premenopausal women need lower neuroleptic doses than men while this is reversed with postmenopausal women (Marriott & Hiep, 1978). This finding was related to the possibility that estrogens, which have an antidopaminergic effect, may have a protective effect on premenopausal women, but not during menopause and thereafter. However, more recently Zito, Craig, Wanderling, and Siegel (1987) found that 46 schizophrenic women received a higher mean daily dose (1688 ± 1556 mg chlorpromazine equivalent) than 83 men receiving neuroleptic therapy (1284 ± 1044). Age was not found to be significantly correlated with the mean total daily dose. Another study by Merlis, Sheppard, Collins, and Fiorentino (1970) reported that when women were switched to placebo, they showed a greater increase in symptom intensity than men, who were able to survive the change. However, this study had several flaws. First, the diagnosis was not stated, and second, the women subjects had more psychotic symptoms before the switch than did the men.

Goldstein et al. (1978) compared patients treated with high (1 ml) versus low (0.25 ml) doses of fluphenazine enanthate with or without crisis-oriented family therapy. The investigators assessed relapses during the 6-week period and at 6-month follow-up of 104 young acute schizophrenic patients. Relapses were greatest in the low-dose no-family therapy group (48%) and lowest in the high-dose family-therapy group (0%). Men showed greater residual symptoms in high-dose rather than low-dose conditions. The reverse was true for women. Men with good premorbid histories showed a negligible rate of relapse and less symptoms while receiving low dose and family therapy. Those with poor premorbid histories were dose sensitive and had a short-term reduction in symptoms with family therapy that completely reversed in longer follow-up. Women with good and poor premorbid histories responded to high-dose fluphenazine with family therapy. However, both relapsed when the dose was lowered. This seems to confirm the study by Merlis, Sheppard, Collins, and Fiorentino (1970), who found that women show more psychotic symptoms when placed on placebo.

Another area that has been studied over the years is neuroleptic side effects, in particular, the extrapyramidal reactions. Dystonias, whether acute (Ayd, 1983; Arana, Goff, Baldessarini, & Kupers, 1988) or tardive (Yassa, Nair, & Dimity, 1986a) occur more commonly in young men. Tardive dyskinesia occurs more often in older women (Jeste & Wyatt, 1982; Smith & Baldessarini, 1980; Yassa, Nair, & Schwartz, 1986b).

The problem of gender differences in neuroleptic response is obviously complex. There are many contradictory statements in the literature. However, it seems that women respond better to neuroleptics in long-term follow-up, although they appear to require more sustained and higher-dose medication than men do. The problem of age differences and dosage level has, however, not been dealth with satisfactorily in the literature.

PROGNOSIS
Short-term Follow-up Studies (up to 5 years)

These are studies reporting follow-up of discharged patients for a period not exceeding 5 years following their first hospitalization. Measures of outcome have usually included ability to stay in the community during the period observed, symptom assessment, and social adaptability. In some studies, short-term outcome was found to be more favorable in ment than in women (Hogarty, Goldberg, & Schooler, 1974; Goldstein, Rodnick, Evans, May, & Steinberg, 1983; Watt & Szvlecka, 1979; Watt, Katz, & Shepherd, 1983; Westermeyer and Harrow, 1984; Goldstein, 1988). One study, using DSM-III criteria (1980), followed patients for up to 40 years, but also reported their observations 4 years after the first psychiatric hospitalization (Lloyd, Simpson, & Tsuang, 1985). The investigators observed no significant gender differences in schizophrenic patients after this 4-year follow-up. It is possible that with the restrictive diagnostic criteria of DSM-III (1980), women with better prognosis might have been excluded.

Intermediate-term Follow-up Studies (6 to 15 years)

Most of these studies (mean follow-up period 10.3 years, with range being 8 to 14 years) reported a better prognosis for women than for men (Affleck, Burns, &

Forrest, 1976; Nyman & Jonsson, 1983; Salokengas, 1983; Goldstein, 1988). Men were reported to fare worse in number of rehospitalizations, symptom-free state, interpersonal interaction, and social reintegration.

Long-term Follow-up Studies (longer than 15 years)

Here, the gender differences were not as impressive as those in studies with shorter-term follow-up. We should stress, however, that the issue of gender difference has not been the primary focus of longitudinal studies of schizophrenics. Although most studies of long-term course reported the ratio of male to female patients, only three of these studies mentioned gender differences in outcome. These studies were those of Bleuler (1968, 1974), Huber, Gross, and Schuttler (1975, 1980) and Ciompi (1980). Bleuler (1968) studied 208 schizophrenic patients over a period of 23 years in a prospective fashion: 100 men and 108 women. Bleuler followed their course personally and knew many of their relatives. The incidence of broken homes was higher than that in the general population and, furthermore, was higher in female schizophrenics than in male schizophrenics. Female schizophrenics had lived longer with schizophrenic parents and with stepparents (especially stepmothers) than did male schizophrenics. The worst relationship in the family had existed between female probands and their mothers. Bleuler concluded that early familial difficulties in the childhood of girls caused a predisposition to schizophrenia (Bleuler, 1968, 1974).

Huber, Gross, Schuttler, and Linz (1980) studied 502 schizophrenic patients (293 males and 209 females) over approximately a 22-year period. The investigators found that the only gender difference in outcome was a more favorable long-term social recovery of female schizophrenics. The investigators defined social recovery as being employed at one's previous occupational level. Sixty percent of women were considered socially recovered as compared to 51% of men. In addition, female patients from disrupted families had a less favorable long-term prognosis, whereas the males had a more favorable one. This finding supported Bleuler's hypothesis that early adverse family relationships might affect the disease course in women.

Ciompi (1980) followed 289 schizophrenic patients (92 males and 197 females) in a 37-year prospective study. At follow-up, the average age for men was 75.2 years and for women 75.8 years. In this population, women died at a higher rate (185%) than men (161%) if mortality was set at 100% for the "average" population. However, global overall evolution of symptoms did not reveal significant gender differences. Ciompi speculated that the aging process affected the course of schizophrenia. Florid, acute symptoms tended to disappear with age, whereas indifference, amotivation, and affective withdrawal tended to predominate. New symptoms rarely appeared with aging.

Two other major long-term studies of schizophrenic patients by Tsuang, Dempsey, and Rauscher (1976), who followed patients for an average of 35 years, and Harding, Brooks, Ashikaga, Strauss, and Breier (1987), who conducted a 32-year prospective study, did not report any significant gender differences in long-term outcome.

As noted from the above discussion, the short-term outcome of schizophrenia seems to favor women, who appear to respond better to neuroleptics, reintegrate easier into society, and need less rehospitalization than men. However, longer-term studies indicate that women do not fare better or worse than men. This, along with greater longevity of women, may explain the finding by Brown, Bone, Dalison, and Wing (1966) that women outnumbered men in long-term facilities in the age bracket 60 years and over.

TOWARD AN EXPLANATION OF GENDER DIFFERENCES IN SCHIZOPHRENIA

As the preceding discussions show, a number of studies have indicated gender differences in age at onset of symptoms, symptom presentation, neuroleptic response, as well as prognosis in schizophrenia. These investigations, although using different diagnostic criteria and conducted across cultures, have generally demonstrated that women tend to fare somewhat better than men.

Several possible theoretical explanations have been put forward to explain this gender difference. These fall into two basic categories: sociocultural and biological hypotheses.

Sociocultural

It has been suggested that because men are presumed to be the socially aggressive gender, schizophrenia might present itself at an earlier age in men than in women. Thus, in men, symptoms may manifest around the age of puberty when the social stresses are greater and may affect them more severely. Women, on the other hand, may be overprotected at home, and although early symptoms may appear at the same time as those in men, women might be sheltered by their parents or spouse. However, as noted earlier, studies in which the age at the first appearance of symptoms was reported, found that there was a later onset of symptoms in women (Lewine, 1981; Loranger, 1984). In this regard, it is of interest that despite changing roles of the genders, recent follow-up studies came to the same conclusion—that is, men start earlier in life to develop schizophrenic symptoms than women do. Thus, although psychosocial stress may be a factor in the development of schizophrenia, it is certainly not the only factor.

Biological

Some investigators have suggested that estrogen is a strong antidopaminergic agent (Seeman, 1982, 1985) and may in fact act as a neuroleptic in premenopausal women. This may explain why younger women do not need as much neuroleptic as younger men (Seeman, 1983). On the other hand, estrogens do not protect postmenopausal women; hence these patients need larger doses of neuroleptics than men in the same age groups.

There is an age-related fall in the number of D_2 receptors. It has been suggested that men may start with a relatively greater number of D_2 receptors but lose them at a greater rate with increasing age, leaving older women with a relative excess of D_2 receptors (Wong et al., 1984, 1986; Pearlson & Rabins, 1988). (D_2 receptors are implicated in the development of schizophrenic symptoms.)

Other exciting areas that have not been fully explored include gender differences in biological parameters such as platelet MAO activity (Baron, Gruen, Levitt, & Kane, 1984; Lewine, 1985) and variations in VBR size (Kolakowska et al., 1985) and corpus callosum thickness (Nasrallah et al., 1986).

Thus, several biochemical, neuroradiological, and sociocultural factors interacting together may lead to the vulnerability of men to develop a more severe type of schizophrenia. This has been dubbed by Lewine (1985) as the "amotivational syndrome" characteristic of schizophrenia in men. Seeman (1985) has even classified schizophrenia in men as the type II schizophrenia, which is characterized by flat affect, poor speech, poor response to neuroleptics, and a poor outcome (Crow, 1985). This contrasts with women, who seem to suffer more often from the type I syndrome, which is characterized mainly by positive symptoms, good response to neuroleptics, and a potentially reversible outcome.

MAJOR GAPS IN KNOWLEDGE AND NEED FOR FURTHER RESEARCH

Based on the literature reviewed in this chapter, it is clear that there are a number of important questions that need to be answered regarding gender differences. Such questions include

1. Why are schizophrenic females more susceptible to early adverse "psychosocial stimuli" than their male counterparts?
2. Why do schizophrenic women have more "atypical symptoms" than schizophrenic men?
3. Are "negative symptoms" less common in schizophrenic women because they have a later age of onset of illness and negative symptoms are uncommon in late-onset schizophrenia?

4. Does aging reduce the gender differences in outcome in schizophrenia since affective withdrawal and amotivation predominate with age? We raise this question because short-term studies show a more favorable outcome for schizophrenic women but long-term outcome studies do not support a gender difference.
5. Does menopause, with its endocrinologic changes, contribute to the long-term course of schizophrenic women not being more favorable than that of schizophrenic men in contrast to the short-term outcome?
6. Does noncompliance with neuroleptics differ between the sexes, and if so, how does this affect long-term outcome?

Further, a review of the literature suggests that it is important for any researcher in the field to consider the possibility of gender differences in schizophrenia. The importance of this issue lies in several areas of research.

First, the use of stricter criteria for schizophrenia may affect the clinical picture and outcome of schizophrenia. As suggested in our review, the more stringent the criteria for schizophrenia, the more women are excluded. This may mean that different sets of criteria may be needed for men and women, taking into consideration symptom clusters on which investigators agree. For example, a researcher may choose include some affective symptoms for diagnosing schizophrenia in women.

Second, few studies have been conducted on gender differences in the biochemical as well as brain-imaging indices of schizophrenia. This may give us some indications of pathophysiology as well as prognosis and response to treatment.

Third, few studies to date have concentrated on the differential response of men and women to neuroleptic medication. Although some authors have indicated that premenopausal and postmenopausal women differ in their response (Seeman, 1983), no extensive studies have tested this hypothesis.

Fourth, few studies have concentrated their efforts on chronic schizophrenic patients filling the psychogeriatric wards: course, response to neuroleptics, and psychosocial rehabilitation in relation to gender.

SUMMARY

Gender differences in the presentation, pathophysiology, course, and treatment of schizophrenia have not received adequate attention. Published studies suggest that women tend to have a later age of onset of illness, more "positive" symptoms, less severe psychopathology, better response to neuroleptics, and more favorable short-term outcome than men. There are, however, considerable gaps in our knowledge, and there is a clear need for further studies in this potentially exciting field of research.

REFERENCES

Achte, K. A. (1967). On prognosis and rehabilitation in schizophrenic and paranoid psychoses. *Acta Psychiatrica Scandinavica, 43* (Suppl. 196).

Affleck, J. W., Burns, J., & Forrest, A. D. (1976). Long-term follow-up of schizophrenic patients in Edinburgh. *Acta Psychiatrica Scandinavica, 53,* 227-237.

Allon, R. (1971). Sex, race, socioeconomic status, social mobility and process-reactive ratings of schizophrenics. *Journal of Nervous and Mental Disease, 153,* 343-350.

Arana, G. W., Goff, D. C., Baldessarini, R. J., & Kupers, G. A. (1988). Efficacy of anticholinergic prophylaxis for neuroleptic-induced acute dystonia. *American Journal of Psychiatric, 145,* 993-996.

Awad, A. G. (1985). Prediction of response to neuroleptic drug therapy in schizophrenia. *Canadian Journal of Psychiatry, 30,* 241-242.

Ayd, F. J. (1983). Early-onset neuroleptic-induced extrapyramidal reactions: A second survey, 1961-1981. In J. T. Coyle & S. J. Enna (Eds.), *Neuroleptics: Neurochemical, Behavioral and Clinical Perspectives* (pp. 75-92). New York: Raven Press.

Baron, M., Gruen, R., Levitt, M., & Kane, J. (1984). Platelet MAO and clinical phenomenology of schizophrenia. *Journal of Psychiatry Research, 11,* 205-209.

Becker, W. (1956). A genetic approach to the interpretation and evaluation of the process-reactive distinction in schizophrenia. *Journal of Abnormal Social Psychology, 53,* 229-236.

Bland, R. C. (1977). Demographic aspects of functional psychoses in Canada. *Acta Psychiatrica Scandinavica, 55,* 369-380.

Bland, R. C., & Orn, H. (1978). 14-year outcome in early schizophrenia. *Acta Psychiatrica Scandinavica, 58,* 327-338.

Bleuler, E. (1950). *Dementia Praecox or the Group of Schizophrenias* (Y. Zinkin, trans). New York: International Universities Press.

Bleuler, M. (1968). A 23-year longitudinal study of 208 schizophrenics and impressions in regard to the nature of schizophrenia. In D. Rosenthal & S. Kety (Eds.), *The Transmission of Schizophrenia* (pp. 3-12). New York: Pergamon Press.

Bleuler, M. (1974). The long-term course of the schizophrenic psychoses. *Psychological Medicine, 4,* 244-254.

Bleuler, M. (1978). *The schizophrenic disorders: Long-term patient and family studies.* New Haven, CT: Yale University Press.

Braatay, T. (1934). Manner zwischen 15 und 25 jahren; mental hygieinische unter suchungen mit besonderer berucksichtigung der schizophrenia fabritius und sonner. Oslo.

Breier, A., & Astrachan, B. M. (1984). Characterization of schizophrenic patients who commit suicide. *American Journal of Psychiatry, 141,* 206-209.

Brown, G. W., Bone, M., Dalison, B., & Wing, J. K. (1966). *Schizophrenia and Social Care.* London: Oxford University Press.

Ciompi, L. (1980). Catamnestic long-term study on the cause of life and aging of schizophrenics. *Schizophrenia Bulletin, 6,* 606-618.

Crow, T. Y. (1985). The two-syndrome concept: Origins and current status. *Schizophrenia Bulletin, 11,* 471-486.

Forrest, A. D., & Hay, A. J. (1971). Sex differences and the schizophrenic experience. *Acta Psychiatrica Scandinavica, 47,* 137-149.

Forrest, A. D., & Hay, A. J. (1972). The influence of sex on schizophrenia. *Acta Psychiatrica Scandinavica, 48,* 49-58.

Fremming, K. (1951). *The Expectation of Mental Infirmity in a Sample of the Danish Population.* London: Cassell.

Goldberg, S. C., Schooler, N. R., Davidson, E. M., & Kayce, M. M. (1966). Sex and race differences in response to drug treatment among schizophrenics. *Psychopharmacologia, 9,* 31-47.

Goldstein, J. M. (1988). Gender differences in the course of schizophrenia. *American Journal of Psychiatry, 145,* 684-689.

Goldstein, J. M., & Link, B. G. (1988). Gender and the expression of schizophrenia. *Journal of Psychiatry Research, 22,* 141-155.

Goldstein, M. J., Rodnick, E. H., Evans, J. R., May, P. R. A., & Steinberg, M. R. (1978). Drug and family therapy in the aftercare of acute schizophrenia. *Archives of General Psychiatry, 35,* 1169-1177.

Harding, C. M., Brooks, G. W., Ashikaga, T., Strauss, J. S., & Breier, A. (1987). The Vermont longitudinal study of persons with severe mental illness. II. Long-term outcome of subjects who retrospectively met DSM-III criteria in schizophrenia. *American Journal of Psychiatry, 144*(6), 727-735.

Harris, M. J., & Jeste, D. V. (1988). Late onset schizophrenia: An overview. *Schizophrenia Bulletin, 14,* 39-55.

Harrow, M., Westermeyer, J. F., Silverstein, M., Strauss, B. S., & Cohler, B. J. (1986). Predictors of outcome in schizophrenia: The process-reactive dimension. *Schizophrenia Bulletin, 12,* 195-207.

Hartmann, W., & Meyer, J. E. (1969). Long-term hospitalization of schizophrenic patients. *Comprehensive Psychiatry, 10,* 122-127.

Helgason, T. (1964). Epidemiology of mental disorders in Iceland. *Acta Psychiatrica Scandinavica, 40* (Suppl. 173).

Hogarty, G. E., Goldberg, S. C., & Schooler, N. R. (1974). Drug and sociotherapy in the aftercare of schizophrenic patients. *Archives of General Psychiatry, 31,* 609-618.

Huber, G., Gross, G., & Schuttler, R. (1975). A long-term follow-up study of schizophrenia: Psychiatric cause of illness and prognosis. *Acta Psychiatrica Scandinavica, 52,* 49-57.

Huber, G., Gross, G., Schuttler, R., & Linz, M. (1980). Longitudinal studies of schizophrenic patients. *Schizophrenia Bulletin, 6,* 592-605.

Iacono, W. G., Smith, G. N., Moreau, M., Beiser, M., Fleming, J. A. E., Lin, T-Y, & Flak, B. (1988). Ventricular and sulcal size at the onset of schizophrenia. *American Journal of Psychiatry, 145,* 820-824.

Jeste, D. V., Harris, M. J., Pearlson, G. D., Rabins, P., Lesser, I. M., Miller, B., Coles, C., & Yassa, R. (1988). Late-onset schizophrenia: Studying clinical validity. In D. V. Jeste & S. Zisook (Eds.), *Psychosis and depression in the elderly,* Vol. 11 (pp. 1-14). Psychiatric Clinics of North America. Philadelphia: W. B. Saunders.

Jeste, D. V., & Wyatt, R. J. (1982). *Understanding and treating tardive dyskinesia.* New York: Guilford Press.

Kolakowska, T., Williams, A. O., Ardern, M., Reveley, M. A., Jambor, K., Gelder, M. G., & Mandelbrote, B. M. (1985). Schizophrenia with good and poor outcome. *British Journal of Psychology, 146,* 229-246.

Kraepelin, E. (1971). *Dementia praecox and paraphrenia*. R. M. Barclay (trans), G. M. Robertson (Ed.). New York: Krieger.

Lane, E. (1968). The influence of sex and race on process-reactive ratings of schizophrenics. *Journal of Psychology, 68*, 15-20.

Leventhal, D. B., Schuck, J. R., & Rothstein, H. (1984). Gender differences in schizophrenia. *Journal of Nervous and Mental Disease, 172*, 464-467.

Lewine, R. (1980). Sex differences in the age of symptom onset and first hospitalization in typical schizophrenia, schizophreniform psychosis and paranoid psychosis. *American Journal of Orthopsychiatry, 50*, 316-322.

Lewine, R. (1981). Sex differences in schizophrenia: Timing or subtypes? *Psychological Bulletin, 90*, 432-444.

Lewine, R. (1985). Schizophrenia: An amotivational syndrome in men. *Canadian Journal of Psychiatry, 30*, 316-318.

Lewine, R., Burbach, D., & Meltzer, J. Y. (1984). Effect of diagnostic criteria on the ratio of male to female schizophrenic patients. *American Journal of Psychiatry, 141*, 84-87.

Lewine, R., Strauss, J., & Gift, T. (1981). Sex differences in age at first hospital admission for schizophrenia: Fact or artifact? *American Journal of Psychiatry, 138*, 440-444.

Locke, B., Kramer, M., & Timberlake, C. (1958). Problems in interpretation of patterns of first admissions to Ohio state public mental hospitals for patients with schizophrenic reactions. *Psychiatric Research Reports, 10*, 1722-1728.

Loranger, A. W. (1984). Sex differences in age at onset of schizophrenia. *Archives of General Psychiatry, 41*, 157-161.

Lloyd, D., Simpson, J. C., & Tsuang, M. T. (1985). Are there sex differences in the long-term outcome of schizophrenia? Comparisons with mania, depression and surgical controls. *Journal of Nervous and Mental Disease, 173*, 643-649.

McCabe, M. S. (1975). Demographic differences in functional psychoses. *British Journal of Psychiatry, 127*, 320-323.

McCreadie, R. G., Wiles, D. H., Moore, J. W., Grant, S. M., Crocket, G. T., Mahmood, Z., Livingston, M. G., Watt, J. A. G., Greene, J. G., Kershaw, P. W., Todd, N. A., Scott, A. M., London, J., Dyer, J. A. T., Philip, A. E., Bachelor, D., & Menzies, C. (1987). The Scottish first episode schizophrenia study. *British Journal of Psychiatry, 150*, 331-338.

Males, K. L., & Van Kammen, D. P. (1983). Platelet MAO activity and long-term outcome in schizophrenia and schizoaffective disorder. *American Journal of Psychiatry, 40*, 794-796.

Malzberg, B. (1935). A statistical study of age in relation to mental disease. *Mental Hygiene, 19*, 449-476.

Marriott, P., & Hiep, A. (1978). Drug monitoring at an Australian depot phenothiazine clinic. *Journal of Clinical Psychiatry, 39*, 206-212.

Merlis, S., Sheppard, C., Collins, L., & Fiorentino, D. (1970). Polypharmacy in psychiatry: Patterns of differential treatment. *American Journal of Psychiatry, 126*, 1647-1651.

Nasrallah, H. A. (1986). Cerebral Hemisphere Asymmetries and Interhemispheric Integration in Schizophrenia. In H. A. Nasrallah & D. R. Weinberger (Eds.), *Handbook of schizophrenia* (Vol. 1, pp. 157-174). New York: Elsevier.

Nasrallah, H. A., Andreason, N. C., Coffman, J. A., Olson, S. C., Dunn, V. D., Ehrhardt, J. C., & Chapman, S. C. (1986). A controlled magnetic resonance imaging study of copus callosum thickness in schizophrenia. *Biological Psychiatry, 21*, 274-282.

Noreik, K., Askrup, C., & Dalgard, O. S. (1967). Age at onset of schizophrenia in relation to socio-economic factors. *British Journal of Psychiatry, 43,* 432-443.

Nyman, A. K., & Jonsson, H. (1983). Differential evaluation of outcome in schizophrenia. *Acta Psychiatrica Scandinavica, 68,* 458-475.

Nystrup, J. (1976). A hospital population of schizophrenic patients undergoing change. *Acta Psychiatrica Scandinavica, 53,* 211-226.

Pearlson, G., & Rabins, P. (1988). The late-onset psychoses: Possible risk factors. In D. V. Jeste & S. Zisook (Eds.), *Psychosis and Depression in the Elderly* (Vol. 11. pp. 15-32). Psychiatric Clinics of North America. Philadelphia: W. B. Saunders.

Pogue-Geile, M. F., & Harrow, M. (1984). Negative and positive symptoms in schizophrenia and depression: A follow-up. *Schizophrenia Bulletin, 10,* 371-387.

Reveley, A. M., Reveley, M. A., & Murray, R. M. (1984). Cerebral ventricular enlargement in non-genetic schizophrenia: A controlled twin study. *British Journal of Psychiatry, 144,* 89-93.

Salokangas, R. K. R. (1983). Prognostic implications of the sex of schizophrenic patients. *British Journal of Psychiatry, 142,* 145-151.

Sartorius, N., Jablensky, A., Korten, G., Ernberg, G., Anker, M., & Cooper, J. E. (1986). Early manifestations and first-contact incidence of schizophrenia in different cultures. *Psychological Medicine, 16,* 909-928.

Sartorius, N., Jablensky, A., & Stromgren, E. (1978). Validity of diagnostic concepts across cultures. In L. C. Wynne, R. L. Cromwell, & S. Matthysse (Eds.), *The Nature of Schizophrenia—New Approaches to Research and Treatment* (pp. 657-669). New York: John Wiley and Sons.

Seeman, M. V. (1982). Gender differences in schizophrenia. *Canadian Journal of Psychiatry, 27,* 107-111.

Seeman, M. V. (1983). Interaction of sex, age and neuroleptic dose. *Comprehensive Psychiatry, 24,* 125-128.

Seeman, M. V. (1985). Clinical and demographic correlates of neuroleptic response. *Canadian Journal of Psychiatry, 30,* 243-245.

Shelton, R. C., Karson, C. N., Doran, A. R., Pickar, D., Bigelow, L. B., & Weinberger, D. R. (1988). Cerebral structural pathology in schizophrenia: Evidence for a selective prefrontal cortical defect. *American Journal of Psychiatry, 145,* 154-163.

Shimizu, A., Kurachi, M., & Noda, M. (1988). Influence of sex on age at onset of schizophrenia. *Japanese Journal of Psychiatry and Neurology, 42,* 35-40.

Smith, J. M., & Baldessarini, R. J. (1980). Changes in prevalence severity and recovery in tardive dyskinesia with age. *Archives of General Psychiatry, 37,* 1368-1373.

Stromgren, E. (1987). Changes in the incidence of schizophrenia? *British Journal of Psychiatry, 150,* 1-7.

Tsuang, M. T. (1983). Risk of suicide in the relatives of schizophrenics, manics, depressives, and controls. *Archives of General Psychiatry, 44,* 396-400.

Tsuang, M. T., Dempsey, M., & Rauscher, F. (1976). A study of "atypical schizophrenia." *Archives of General Psychiatry, 33,* 1157-1160.

Tsuang, M. T., & Woolson, R. F. (1978). Excess mortality in schizophrenia and affective disorders. *Archives of General Psychiatry, 35,* 1181-1185.

Watt, D. C., & Szulecka, T. K. (1979). The effect of sex, marriage and age at first admission on the hospitalization of schizophrenia during 2 years following discharge. *Psychological Medicine, 9,* 529-539.

Watt, D. C., Katz, K., & Shepherd, M. (1983). The natural history of schizophrenia: A 5-year prospective follow-up of a representative sample of schizophrenics by means of a standardized clinical and social assessment. *Psychological Medicine, 13,* 663-670.

Westermeyer, J. F., & Harrow, M. (1984). Prognosis and outcome using broad (DSM-II) and narrow (DSM-III) concepts of schizophrenia. *Schizophrenia Bulletin, 10,* 624-637.

Wong, D. F., Wagner, H. N., Dannals, R. F., & Pearlson, G. D. (1984). Effects of age on dopamine and serotonin receptors measured by positron tomography in the living human brain. *Science, 226,* 1393-1396.

Wong, D. F., Wagner, H. N., Tune, L. E., Dannals, R. F., Pearlson, G. D., Links, J. M., & Tamminga, C. A. (1986). Positron emission tomography reveals elevated D2 dopamine receptors in drug-naive schizophrenics. *Science, 234,* 1558-1563.

Yassa, R., Nair, V., & Dimitry, R. (1986a). The prevalence of tardive dystonia. *Acta Psychiatrica Scandinavica, 73,* 629-633.

Yassa, R., Nair, V., & Schwartz, G. (1986b). Early versus late onset psychosis and tardive dyskinesia. *Biological Psychiatry, 21,* 1291-1297.

Young, M. A., & Meltzer, H. Y. (1980). The relationship of demographic, clinical and outcome variables to neuroleptic treatment requirements. *Schizophrenia Bulletin, 6,* 88-101.

Zito, J. M., Craig, T. J., Wanderling, J., & Siegel, C. (1987). Pharmaco-epidemiology in 136 hospitalized schizophrenic patients. *American Journal of Psychiatry, 144,* 778-782.

3

Suicide in the Elderly Chronic Patient Population

Yeates Conwell, Eric D. Caine

In the popular mind, psychiatric conditions are not commonly associated with death. However, it is well established that mortality rates in psychiatric patients exceed those of the general population. Martin, Cloninger, Guze, and Clayton (1985a, 1985b), for example, found that death from all causes occurred more than twice as often in psychiatric outpatients followed for a mean of seven years than among controls, and Black, Warrack, and Winokur (1985a, 1985b, 1985c) found excessive mortality for most psychiatric diagnoses in both sexes within 2 years of discharge in the Iowa Record Linkage Study. A closer look at causes of death reveals that suicide is a major factor in this excess mortality, seen at rates 15 times greater than expected by Martin et al. (1985b) and up to 80 times as often in the diagnostic subgroups of the populations studied by Black and colleagues (1985a). Indeed, psychiatric illness can be fatal, with the cause of death most commonly being suicide.

Although suicide is an outcome of psychiatric illness more often associated with young populations than old, this conclusion is not one based on extensive research findings. The data available on suicidal behavior in the elderly are scarce, and those concerning the chronically mentally ill in late life even more rare. Following a review of the demography of suicide and its known risk factors, we will examine what is known about suicide in chronic psychiatric patient populations. Having demonstrated that the elderly are poorly represented in such studies, we will consider the complementary issue—what are the psychiatric conditions suffered by populations of suicide victims? Again, we find the elderly poorly described. With that background, we will outline questions for future research in the suicidal behavior of chronically ill elderly psychiatric patients and consider methods with which to answer them, drawing on our experience at the University of Rochester's Laboratory of Suicide Studies.

THE DEMOGRAPHY OF SUICIDAL BEHAVIOR

In the United States in 1985, 29,453 people died by suicide, making it the eighth leadings cause of death that year. The annual rate in the general population was 12.3 per 100,000 (National Center for Health Statistics, 1987). Although based on official death certificates, these figures are likely to be underestimates of the true prevalence because of the lack of a standard definition of suicide by coroners and medical examiners (Rosenberg et al., 1988) and a reluctance to attach the label of suicide in equivocal circumstances, given the commonly perceived stigma for victims and their families.

Figure 3.1 demonstrates striking differences in suicide rates by age, sex, and race. Because of the threefold rise in rates for adolescents and young adults during the past three decades, there has been a justifiable concern and focus in the academic and popular press on youth suicide (Brent et al., 1988; Shafii, Carrigan, Whittinghil, & Derrick, 1985). Nonetheless, it is the elderly who have the highest suicide rates of any age group.

Although suicide is only the thirteenth most common cause of death in those 65 years and older, it accounted for 5,788 deaths nationwide in 1985, compared to 5,121 for 15–24-year-olds (National Center for Health Statistics, 1987). As the elderly are the fastest growing segment of the population, the absolute number of their suicides will continue to rise. Haas and Hendin (1983) project that the number of suicides being committed by older people will double by the year 2030 as a function of this demographic shift alone. Furthermore, epidemiologic studies show that younger adults now have generally higher suicide rates than did their grandparents at that age. As younger adults move into late life, their suicide rates will rise above those of our current elderly cohort (Blazer, Bachar, & Manton, 1986; Manton, Blazer, & Woodbury, 1987). There is, therefore, a demographic imperative to the study of suicide among the elderly.

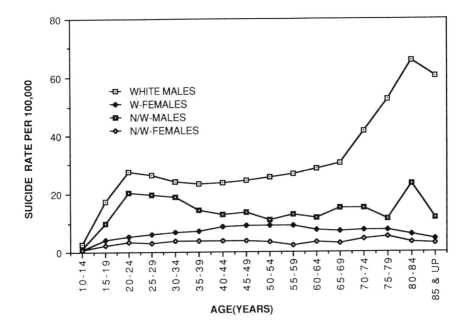

FIGURE 3.1 Suicides—by age, race, and sex—1985.

Source: National Center for Health Statistics, 1987.

MAJOR DETERMINANTS OF SUICIDAL BEHAVIOR

Gender is a major determinant of suicide risk. Reference to Figure 3.1 shows that suicide rates are higher throughout the lifespan for males than females, with the difference most pronounced in late life. This discrepancy reflects the fact that men use more violent means to kill themselves than do women (McIntosh & Santos, 1982). Although many more women attempt suicide than men, many fewer complete it. Rich, Ricketts, Fowler, and Young (1988) conclude that males who attempt suicide do so with higher lethal intent than do women.

The gender difference also reflects the underlying psychopathologies to which men and women are prone. Alcohol and drug abuse are significantly more common in men than women and are highly prevalent in populations of completed suicides, as we will further discuss below.

Another determinant of suicidal behavior highlighted in Figure 3.1 is *race.* Nonwhites, especially blacks, have generally lower suicide rates than same-sex whites across the lifespan. However, Manton, Blazer, and Woodbury (1987) have found, using cohort and life table analyses, a striking rise in suicide rates for nonwhite males between 1962 and 1981. The increase has been particularly pronounced in late life, implying that although racial differences remain, the gap is narrowing. Nonwhite racial status is becoming less protective against suicide in late life.

Many investigators have suggested that one's *living situation* is related to suicide risk. Sainsbury (1955, 1978), for example, stressed that social isolation may increase the tendency to suicide in the general population, while Roy (1982a, 1984) made a similar observation in controlled studies of psychiatric patients. Barraclough (1971) reported in detail the circumstances of 30 suicides over the age of 65 years. Fifty percent of his sample lived alone, compared to 20% of the general community from which they were drawn. He found that suicide in this elderly population was more highly correlated with living alone than with any other social variable measured in this, the only comprehensive psychological autopsy study of elderly suiciders. Of course, living alone is not synonomous with being lonely and/or socially isolated. To assess the role of living situation in suicidality better, we must learn more about the social support networks, both real and perceived, of elderly populations, suicidal and nonsuicidal, patient and nonpatient (see Curtrone, Henikon, Suhr, & Russell, this volume).

Marital status is another frequently cited factor determining suicide risk. It is generally accepted that individuals who are separated and divorced are at highest risk, followed in order by those who are widowed, single, and married. Kreitman (1988), however, has recently shown that widowhood may be under-estimated as a precipitant to suicide. The young widow may be at especially high risk, possibly because the loss is so often unexpected and the spouse ill prepared. While elderly widows may be at relatively lower risk, the frequency of the loss of spouse in later life makes it a pressing issue for future research.

Other types of *loss* and stressful life events are associated with suicide risk as well. Retirement, deaths of friends and family, and loss of status and economic security are common examples in late life. Luscomb, Clum, and Patsiokas (1980) found that older suicide attempters experienced more stress prior to their attempt than did nonsuicidal psychiatric controls, whereas no such difference was evident between younger attempters and controls. Even losses sustained early in life are known to be associated with suicide in later years (Bunch, Barraclough, Nelson, & Sainsbury, 1971; Zilboorg, 1936). However, the extent and nature of both recent and remote life events have not been systematically explored in suicidal elderly.

Physical illness is the most commonly cited precipitant stressor in elderly suicide (Mackenzie & Popkin, 1987). Sainsbury (1955) estimated that while physical illness contributed to suicide in 10% of younger cases, the figure rose to 27% in middle age and 35% of elderly suicides. Robins, Murphy, Wilkinson, Gassner, and Kayes (1959) and Chynoweth, Tonge, and Armstrong (1980) made similar observations, while Dorpat, Anderson, and Ripley (1968) found an even higher rate. Seventy percent of their cases studied retrospectively had indications of medical illness, nearly all of which were chronic. The illness was felt to have directly contributed to the suicide in 51% of cases, with the proportion in which a medical illness was involved increasing from 13% in those less than 39 years of age to almost 70% in suicides over 60 years.

Psychiatric Illness

Of all the risk factors for completed suicide, however, the most powerful is a prior history of psychiatric illness or suicide attempt. The implications of this fact for the study of suicide in elderly chronic patient populations are self-evident. Yet psychiatric patient populations in late life remain largely unstudied.

Pokorny (1983) followed 4,800 Veterans Administration (VA) psychiatric inpatients prospectively for 5 years, finding a suicide rate 12 times that of other veterans. Of patients admitted after suicide attempt, 2% completed the act for each year of follow-up. Generalization of these findings to an older population is made difficult by the fact that only 5% of patients admitted to the study were over the age of 60 years, and only 1 percent of suicides committed were in this group.

Gardner, Bahn, and Mack (1964) employed a useful technique for the study of suicide in psychiatric patient populations—cross-linkage of medical examiner records with a psychiatric case register (PCR). Of 180 suicides committed between 1960 and 1962, they found that 36% had prior psychiatric contacts with the Monroe County, N.Y., PCR. Data provided with regard to age, sex, and diagnosis supported the following conclusions: With increasing age, a higher percentage of female suiciders had been in psychiatric treatment at some point prior to death than had male suiciders; with increasing age, suiciders were more likely to have been last seen in inpatient settings; and patients over the age of 55 years had higher suicide rates than did patients under the age of 55 (251 per 100,000 versus 144 per 100,000). The lethality of suicidal behavior in elderly psychiatric patients was further supported by the observation that while 2% of the entire patient population who attempted suicide went on to complete within one year, 6% of attempters over the age of 55 completed suicide during the same time interval. We are aware of no studies which have reported follow-up of elderly suicide attempters for longer periods to determine whether this enormous mortality persists.

A more recent cross-linkage study was conducted by Evenson, Wood, Nuttall, and Cho (1982) using the Missouri Department of Mental Health Case Registry for the years 1972–1974. Within the group of 207 white patient suicides, males had rates six times higher and females ten times higher than those of the general population. In further contrast to general population statistics, they found no increase in suicide rates with increasing age among psychiatric outpatients and, surprisingly, a trend for rates to drop with increasing age for former psychiatric inpatients. This finding was supported by Barner-Rasmussen, Dupont, and Bille (1986), who also found a disproportionately small number of suicides older than

65 years among almost 4,000 Danish psychiatric patients who suicided while hospitalized or within 1 year of discharge. They ascribed this result to the high proportion of dements in their elderly inpatient sample, for which the diagnosis-specific suicide rate was low.

One implication of these findings is that patient populations may be different from nonpatient samples with regard to suicidal behaviors. Babigian, Lehman, and Reed (1986) directly addressed this issue using the Monroe County PCR to study 776 completed suicides between the years 1966 and 1975. They found that 43% had had psychiatric contact. Comparing patient and nonpatient samples, they found that psychiatric patients who suicided had a lower male-to-female ratio than nonpatient suicides and that rates did not increase with age for those who had prior psychiatric contacts. They concluded that profiles of suicide risk developed from general population samples may be misleading for clinicians working in psychiatric settings. There is a need, therefore, to better characterize suicide behaviors specific to psychiatric patients and to distinguish them from those aspects of the behavior typical of general or nonpatient populations.

DIAGNOSIS IN PSYCHIATRIC PATIENT SUICIDES

The most common psychopathologies associated with suicide behavior in patient populations are affective disorders, schizophrenia, and substance abuse. Representative diagnostic distributions from four studies of psychiatric patient suicides are provided in Table 3.1. Differences between studies are accounted for by variations in the diagnostic methodologies, patient populations, and study sites.

What conclusions can one draw from these disparate studies of psychiatric patient populations about the association of age, diagnosis and suicide risk?

TABLE 3.1 Primary Diagnoses by Percent of Psychiatric Patient Suicides

Diagnoses	Kraft & Babigian (1976) (n = 81)	Roy (1982a) (n = 90)	Pokorny (1983) (n = 67)	Babigian, Lehman, & Reed (1986) (n = 334)
Affective Disorder	33	46	27	30
Schizophrenia	27	38	28	22
Alcohol & Drug Abuse	11	1	32	10
Personality Disorder	16	13	6	14
Organic Brain Syndrome	5	*	1	*
Other Dx	8	*	4	23

*Not separately reported.

One consistent finding is that "organic brain syndrome," although a diagnosis in large part of late life, is associated with a relatively low suicide rate. Pokorny (1983), for example, found only one suicide with the diagnosis of organic brain syndrome in follow-up of 4,800 VA patients. Evenson et al. (1982) also found a lower age-adjusted rate for organic brain syndrome patients than any other diagnostic group, although still higher than the general population. Gardner et al. (1964) found the same for patients with a known diagnosis of chronic brain syndrome.

One can speculate that demented and brain-damaged individuals are less able to orchestrate a lethal suicide attempt, or perhaps are too well supervised to carry it through. Alternatively, neurobiologic changes associated with some central nervous system (CNS) pathologies might be protective. However, disorders such as multiple sclerosis and Huntington's disease may be associated with elevated suicide rates, presumably through the frequent co-occurrence of significant affective disturbances. There is clearly a need to specify for clinical purposes which CNS disorders are associated with low and which with high suicide risk. More far-reaching is the hope that through correlation of risk profile and anatomic deficit we may draw conclusions about the neurological substrates of suicidal behavior. In addition, the prevalence and nature of other aggressive or self-destructive behaviors in these patients are poorly documented and offer a potential area of fruitful research.

Reference to Table 3.1 shows that a significant percentage of patients who suicide are suffering from *schizophrenia*. The study of this patient population is especially relevant to the question of chronic mental illness in suicide with increasing age. Indications to this point, however, are that suicide is more common in younger schizophrenics. Several groups have shown that schizophrenics who commit suicide generally die in early adulthood (Breier & Astrachan, 1984; Roy, 1982b; Virkhunen, 1974), with a duration of illness of from 5 to 10 years (Breier & Astrachan, 1984; Roy, 1982b; Wilkinson & Bacon, 1984).

Furthermore, Gardner et al. (1964) found that the suicide rate for younger schizophrenics tended to be higher than for schizophrenics in later life. There exists the possibility, therefore, that suicide rates drop for schizophrenics as they age. Why? The question remains unanswered but reflects the clinical and/or neurobiological heterogeneity of schizophrenic conditions. In addition, we are not aware of any data on the prevalence of suicide in later onset schizophrenia, paraphrenia, or delusional disorder.

Alcohol and drug abuse are disorders commonly associated with suicidal behavior. Up to 15% of alcoholics commit suicide, most commonly as a late sequela of the illness (Hirschfeld & Davidson, 1988). With regard to age, Murphy (1986) stated that suicide is a phenomenon of alcoholics in midlife and that it is less common in young adulthood and for alcoholics over the age of 60 years. Gardner et al. (1964) calculated a suicide rate for alcoholics over the age of 55 of over 600/100,000 compared to a rate for those under 55 of 255/100,000; Pokorny (1983) found alcoholism to be more common in patient suicides over 40 years of age (42%) than in those under 40 (6%). The older group, however, was not further divided to investigate whether the diagnosis again became less common in late-life suicide. While there is no doubt that alcoholism greatly increases the risk for suicidal behavior at any age, it remains unclear how that risk changes across the life cycle.

Affective diagnoses, in general, are the most prevalent disorders among psychiatric patient suicides. Furthermore, unlike schizophrenic and substance abuse diagnoses, the few data available imply that risk for suicide among patients with affective disorders increases with age. Roy (1982a), for example, found that affectively disordered suicides were significantly older than sex-matched non-suicidal patient controls. Gardner et al. (1964) calculated that the suicide rate for patients over the age of 55 years with the diagnosis of affective psychosis was 475/100,000 compared to those under 55 with a rate of 207/100,000. Although Pokorny (1983) found affective disorder diagnoses in a lower proportion of patients over 40 than under 40, this discrepancy may be explained in part by the very high prevalence of alcoholism in his older VA patient group, possibly obscuring primary affective diagnoses.

Controversy exists regarding when suicidal behavior most commonly occurs in the course of affective psychopathology. Some investigators conclude that because suicide frequently occurs during hospitalization for depression, or shortly after discharge (Fawcett et al., 1987), it is a behavior associated with recent onset affective illness (Hirschfeld & Davidson, 1988). However, Barraclough and Pallis (1975) found a longer duration of illness in depressives who suicided than those who did not. Again, although affective disorder is clearly a major factor in late-life psychiatric patient suicides, insufficient data exist with which to confidently characterize suicidal behavior in elderly chronic patients.

PSYCHIATRIC ILLNESS IN POPULATIONS OF ELDERLY SUICIDERS

Because psychiatric services are underutilized by the elderly, access to the relevant data is often not available to those best equipped to study and treat suicidal behaviors in late life. Whereas people age 65 years and over constituted 12% of the population in 1985, they accounted for only 6.5% of ambulatory psychiatric visits (National Institute on Aging, 1987). This pattern of utilization contrasts sharply with that of other medical services. That same 12% of the population accounted for over 20% of ambulatory visits to all medical specialties. Therefore, a necessary alternative to considering suicide in psychiatric patients is to study the psychopathology of those who have attempted or completed suicide, regardless of patient status. Again, however, insufficient data pertinent to the elderly have been collected.

The *psychological autopsy* provides the most detailed means to document the psychiatric histories, diagnoses, and premorbid behaviors of a subject after suicide. Originally developed by Shneidman and Farberow (1961) for the investigation of the cause of undetermined deaths, it has subsequently been used to make postmortem diagnoses and describe symptoms of suicide victims in childhood and adolescence (Shafii et al., 1985; Brent et al., 1988), hospitalized patients (Neill, Benensohn, Farber, & Resnik, 1974), and the general population (Barraclough, Bunch, Nelson, & Sainsbury, 1974; Chynoweth et al., 1980; Dorpat & Ripley, 1960; Rich, Young, & Fowler, 1986; Robins et al., 1959). Typically, relatives, friends, caregivers, and others familiar with victims' symptomatology, background, and family circumstances are interviewed to elicit information relevant for study.

The array of psychiatric diagnoses made in four psychological autopsy studies (Table 3.2) is similar to that for psychiatric patient populations (Table 3.1). Notably, diagnosable psychiatric illness is found to be present in virtually all cases, with affective disorder and substance abuse most common.

With regard to the interaction between age and diagnosis, Dorpat and Ripley (1960) found schizophrenia to be the most common diagnosis in completed suicides under the age of 40, alcoholism most common between the ages of 40 and 60, and psychotic depression most common in suicides over the age of 60.

TABLE 3.2 Primary Psychiatric Diagnoses by Percent in Completed Suicide—Psychological Autopsy Studies

Diagnoses	Robins et al. (1959) (n = 134)	Dorpat & Ripley (1960) (n = 108)	Barraclough et al. (1974) (n = 100)	Chynoweth et al. (1980) (n = 135)
Affective Disorder	55	30	70	33
Schizophrenia	3	12	3	4
Alcohol & Drug Abuse	30	27	16	22
Personality Disorder	*	9	*	3
Organic Brain Syndrome	5	4	*	*
Other Dx	*	18	4	12
No Dx	3	0	7	1
Physical Illness	5	0	*	25

*Not separately recorded.

Similarly, Carlson (1984) reanalyzed Robins's detailed case histories (1981) to show that affective disorder diagnoses were more common and alcoholism less frequent in those over 65 compared to younger suicide victims. In their study of 183 completed suicides in the San Diego area, Rich, Young, and Fowler (1986) found significantly more affective disorders in those over the age of 30 than under, and significantly more drug abuse in the younger group.

Only one study has looked in detail at suicides age 65 years and over. Barraclough (1971) studied 30 suicides in this age group. He found that four patients (13%) did not meet criteria for a mental illness, one (3%) had a possible confusional state, and one had preexisting chronic alcoholism. The remainder had a depressive syndrome. The most prominent symptoms were insomnia, weight loss, and withdrawal from usual activities, noted in at least 75% of cases, with 50% showing hypochrondriasis, guilt, difficulty concentrating, and anxiety. He further noted that 63% had an affective syndrome with a duration of less than 1 year. Only four subjects had the onset of diagnosable psychopathology before the age of 55 years, and over 75% had had no prior psychiatric contact at all. Fifty percent had died within 1 week of seeing their general practitioner.

Although we must exercise caution in generalizing results from a study conducted in Great Britain 20 years ago to our current age and an American population, its potential implications are profound. They include the observation that suicide in late life is most commonly associated with affective psychopathology of recent onset, a condition we ordinarily associate with good prognosis for recovery. Furthermore, these victims are rarely seen in psychiatric settings. They more commonly present to primary care providers with acute or chronic somatic complaints typically associated with depression but inadequately treated as such. These observations further reinforce the need to differentiate between the suicides of elderly psychiatric patients and nonpatients; it seems ever more likely that their presentation and underlying psychopathologies may differ significantly.

ATTEMPTED SUICIDE IN LATE LIFE

Those who attempt suicide represent a larger population, for whom data are more accessible to many researchers than victims of completed suicide. However, while there is clearly overlap of the two populations, there is ongoing debate about the nature and extent of that overlap (Linehan, 1986). The question is equally unresolved in the elderly and could be approached through the comparison of suicide attempters and completers in late life.

Paykel, Myers, Lindenthal, and Tanner (1974) found that 0.6% of a general population sample had attempted suicide in the last year, while 3% reported to Schwab, Warheit, and Holzer (1972) that they had made such attempts at some point in their lives. Estimates of the ratio of attempts to completed suicide range from 8:1 to as high as 20:1 for the general population but are lower for the elderly. Parkin and Stengel (1965) found, for example, only four attempters for each completed suicide victim in those over 60 years of age, and Schmid and VanArsdol (1955) found that, whereas 5% of attempts were fatal among 20–29-year-olds, those over the age of 60 years died over 60% of the time they attempted. This discrepancy with the younger population may be explained in part by increasing frailty in the elderly, making any attempt more damaging, or by greater social isolation with a lower chance of rescue. However, the observation by McIntosh and Santos (1985) that for white males and blacks of both sexes older victims used more violent means than the young supports the view that the elderly also have higher lethal intent.

Elderly attempters, therefore, constitute a population at especially high risk for going on to complete suicide. They represent a useful group for prospective study in the hope of identifying, in those whose outcome is death by suicide, both long- and short-term predictors. Because of the relative rarity of the event, of course, populations for follow-up by necessity need to be very large. One example is the sample of depressives enlisted in the NIMH Collaborative Program on the Psychobiology of Depression, the suicides of which were described by Fawcett et al. (1987). However, longitudinal follow-ups of large groups of chronic elderly patient populations cannot be expected to yield data productively until retrospective studies, in particular psychological autopsy designs, better define the groups at highest risk and the questions most amenable to prospective study.

THE PSYCHOBIOLOGY OF SUICIDE

Suicide is a multidimensional behavior, the understanding of which may be enhanced by considering cultural, sociological, and psychological perspectives. With rapid advances in the neurobiological sciences over the last two decades, provocative findings are being reported that may ultimately provide a pathophysiological perspective as well. In generally mixed or younger samples, changes of central serotonin (5-HT) function have consistently been shown to correlate with suicidal behaviors. Measures of 5-hydroxy-indoleacetic acid (5-HIAA) in cerebrospinal fluid (CSF) have been found to be lower in suicide attempters than nonattempters (Asberg, Traskman, & Thoren, 1976), especially if the attempt was a violent one (Banki, Arato, Papp, & Kurcz, 1984); in prisoners who had committed impulsive violent crimes (Linnoila et al., 1983); and in alcoholics, even while abstinent (Ballenger, Goodwin, Major, & Brown, 1979). In affective disorders, low CSF 5-HIAA may be a trait marker related to increased risk of suicide, although the relationship between low 5-HIAA and suicide attempts has also been found in schizophrenia (Ninan et al., 1984) and personality disorders (Brown et al., 1982).

Postmortem studies have found reduced 5-HT and 5-HIAA levels in the brains of depressives and suicides compared to controls (Shaw, Camps, & Eccleston, 1967; Bourne et al., 1968), as well as changes in imipramine and 5-HT-2 receptor binding sites in the hippocampus (Perry, Marshall, Blessed, Tomlinson, & Perry, 1983), frontal (Stanley, Virgilio, & Gerschon, 1982), and occipital cortex (Perry et al., 1983) of suicide victims.

Despite the extent and consistency of these neurochemical findings, changes in structure and function of the serotonin system in late-life suicides have gone essentially unexplored. This fact is due in part to the lack of data on changes of 5-HT in the normal aging process and to the confounds of physical illness and medications that are so often present in elderly populations. Additionally, there have been no morphologically oriented studies to assess the integrity of 5-HT neuronal structures and how they may change with increasing age.

RESEARCH METHODOLOGIES AND POPULATIONS FROM WHICH TO DRAW

While the data on suicide in the elderly are scarce, those concerning elderly psychiatric patients are rarer still. There is a need, therefore, for a broad range of well-designed research focusing on both older populations in general and elderly psychiatric patients in particular.

Record Reviews

An immediately accessible source of data concerning completed suicides is reports compiled by medical examiners (ME) and coroners in the course of their investigations. A principal advantage of these records is that they should include all cases in a particular geographic area from which consecutive series or random samples can be easily drawn. The dates of death are generally well defined, and in many instances associated toxicologic and tissue autopsy data are available. Major disadvantages of ME case reports include their lack of standardization and vast differences from site to site and investigator to investigator in the quality and quantity of data collected. As a rule, the records do not include past psychiatric, personal, and social histories in any organized way, although these problems can be minimized through education of willing investigators.

The Office of the Medical Examiner of Monroe County has maintained a standard over many years of thorough documentation and investigation of suicide and questionable deaths. Our own efforts in the Laboratory of Suicide Studies to define better the nature of late-life suicide began with a review of these records. The reports of 246 completed suicides aged 50 years and older revealed the trends listed in Table 3.3 (Conwell, Rotenberg, & Caine, 1990). Supporting the literature cited above, we found that physical illness and loss became the most common precipitants to suicide with increasing age, whereas job, financial, and family or interpersonal problems became less common. Both men and women used increasingly violent means to kill themselves with increasing age, and alcohol was less commonly a factor. The expected demographic features of late-life suicide were present in our sample, with age-adjusted suicide rates rising for men and falling for women after the age of 50. Because completed suicide is a relatively infrequent event, case-record review is a helpful exercise for the young investigator quickly to familiarize him or her with the clinical context of late-life suicide.

Database Linkage Studies

Despite their clinical utility, record reviews cannot provide extensive information on the psychopathologies of the victims. As noted previously, a valuable method with which to address this question in a retrospective fashion is through linkage of medical examiner records with psychiatric case registers (PCR). Although the Monroe County PCR used to such advantage by Gardner et al., (1964) and Kraft and Babigian (1976) ceased data collection in 1976, it provides a good example of the utility of such data. Between 1973 and 1976, there were 128 completed suicides aged 50 years and over investigated by the Monroe County Medical Examiner's Office. Having reviewed those records, we searched the PCR for any psychiatric service contacts made by these victims in the 13–16

TABLE 3.3 Trends with Increasing Age at Death in Completed Suicide (N = 246 Suicides > 50 years of age)

Stressors	
↑	medical illness
↑	loss
↓	job, financial issues
↓	family/interpersonal discord
Method	
↑	violent method used
Psychopathology	
↓	alcohol use/abuse
↓	prior psychiatric contacts (males only)

Source: Conwell, Rotenberg, & Caine (1990).

years prior to death. Fifty-three subjects (41.4%) had prior psychiatric histories, with the DSM-II diagnoses on last contact listed in Table 3.4. With increasing age there was a significant linear trend for the proportion with such histories to decrease, the change being much more robust for male than female suicide victims. Only 13.8% of males over age 74 were PCR registrants.

Table 3.5 shows the comparison of the 53 patient suicides age 50 and over with the 75 victims who had no prior psychiatric contacts documented by the PCR. The nonpatients were older, and more often male, married, and living with family. Physical illness was the most common stressor in nonpatient suicides in this age group, present significantly more often than in the patients who committed suicide. Psychiatric illness, of course, was significantly more common in the patient suicides for whom social isolation tended also to be a more common stressor.

Case registers provide a means for retrospectively answering questions about chronic elderly patient populations. They may be used, if sample sizes permit, to establish diagnosis and age-specific suicide rates to verify, for example, that risk for suicide in schizophrenia decreases with age, while that for affective disorders and alcoholism increases. Rates of suicide in patients with organic brain syndrome could also be established, as could the psychosocial correlates to suicidal behavior in these well-defined patient groups. Comparative rates for diagnostic subgroups of elderly patients could be calculated for hospitalized, institutionalized individuals versus noninstitutionalized outpatient samples, and the relationship explored between suicidal behavior, duration of illness, and psychiatric comorbidity.

Although cross-linkage studies have the advantage of establishing psychiatric diagnoses and symptom profiles antemortem, they rarely are suitable for establishing a subject's psychiatric status immediately prior to the suicidal act. Fur-

TABLE 3.4 Primary Diagnoses (DSM-II) of 53 Suicide Victims Age 50+ Years Having Prior Psychiatric Contacts

Diagnoses	N	%
Affective Psychosis	12	22.6
Neurotic Depression	12	22.6
Schizophrenia	9	19.0
Alcoholism	7	13.2
Adjustment Reaction	4	7.5
Organic Brain Syndrome	3	5.7
Personality Disorder	3	5.7
Other Diagnoses	2	3.8
No Diagnosis	1	1.9

TABLE 3.5 Characteristics of Completed Suicides, Age > 50 years, with and without Psychiatric Contacts

	Patient	Nonpatient	p^*
$N =$	53	75	
Age (mean ± SD)	60.5 ± 8.9	65.0 ± 11.4	.020
% Male	50.9	77.3	.003
% Marital Status			
Single	18.9	4.1	.016
Married	32.1	64.9	.0005
Separated & Divorced	20.8	12.2	NS
Widowed	28.3	18.9	NS
% Living Alone	45.3	20.0	.004
% With Family	47.2	72.1	.008
% With Precipitant Stressor			
Job/Financial	20.8	18.9	NS
Family Discord	28.3	22.7	NS
Physical Illness	18.9	41.3	.013
Psychiatric Illness	47.2	6.7	< .0001
Loss	36.4	26.7	NS
Isolation	13.2	2.7	.052

*p values were derived by chi square analyses for all variables except age, which is analyzed by t-test.

thermore, they provide no information on the psychopathology of victims who escaped recognition and treatment by the mental health system.

Psychological Autopsy Studies

Because the vast majority of suicide victims in late life were not in psychiatric care, and hence inaccessible for database linkage studies, the psychological autopsy methodology is particularly well suited to the elderly. Although the method suffers from the disadvantage of not having access to the subject, the data obtained from reliable informants allow detailed description of the victim's behavior, both remotely and immediately before death. Brent, Perper, Kolko, et al. (1988) have recently shown that neither the affective symptomatology of informants nor the amount of time since death interferes with reliable data collection. Although this early work is encouraging, additional study is needed to assure the reliability and validity of this approach.

A major difficulty with psychological autopsy studies to date has been that appropriate control groups for suicide victims are hard to define. Many studies have used none, and the value of the data is diminished. It is crucial that future studies clearly delineate comparison groups appropriate to the particular question under consideration and address the methodological issues which consequently arise. For example, in making the comparison of attempted and completed suicides, one must provide that the data sources are "parallel"—that the same types of information are gathered for both samples—and that information obtained from a living patient not be considered equivalent to an informant's data regarding a suicide victim's state of mind at the time of death. To raise these issues is simply to acknowledge the additional work needed to assure reliability and validity of the psychological autopsy methodology.

Descriptive Psychopathology

Given the lack of data concerning late-life suicide, the first level of inquiry to address with the psychological autopsy is clinical descriptive psychopathology. What is the distribution of psychiatric diagnoses among a consecutive series of elderly completed suicides? Then, beyond documentation of diagnoses, we need to test more rigorously in larger samples the observations made by Barraclough (1971) that the depressive illness of elderly suicides is often of short duration and mild severity, with prominent anxiety and hypochondriasis. What had been the course of that illness preceding death? Did they give warning of their intent? How did they behave, and what symptoms were most commonly displayed? A detailed account of events will have educational value for clinicians, and great heuristic value as well. Provided with an adequate description of the psychopathology of elderly suicide victims, we can better define hypotheses for future research.

Contributory Factors

In addition to descriptive and comparative studies of psychopathology in elderly suicide victims, there is pressing need to clarify the factors which contribute differentially, or uniquely, to the behavior in late life. Considerations include the life events associated with suicidal behavior in late life and the social networks of the victims. What are the stressful life events that occur in the lives of the elderly who attempt or complete suicide? How do they differ between the two groups, and how do they differ as a function of age? What constitutes the social network of elderly suicide victims, and how do they differ from nonsuicidal comparison groups? Psychological autopsy methodology can again help us move beyond the relatively coarse and unreliable assessments of investigators' reports to test further hypotheses suggested by the record review and existing literature. For example, did late-life suicide victims experience disproportionate amounts of physical illness in comparison to a control population? Do the elderly who commit suicide indeed experience more loss than age- and sex-matched normals? What is the temporal relationship between stressful events, the development of psychiatric symptoms, and suicide in the elderly? And how do these relationships change as a function of sex and age?

Physical Illness

Having established that physical illness is the most common precipitant to late-life suicidal behavior, we can use information obtained from records and caregivers to reconstruct the health status, as well as lifelong illness burden, of subjects. What are the medical conditions and medications most commonly associated with late-life suicide, and how might they contribute to the development of psychopathology or to the expression of suicidal behavior? Furthermore, data available for analysis in each case of completed suicide might include tissue autopsy and toxicology results, yielding, in combination, the opportunity for classical clinical-pathological correlation.

The role played by medications and alcohol in suicidal behavior is complex. Substance use, for example, may lead to disinhibition and release of overt aggressive feelings, induce depressive states, and elicit aggressive suicidal behavior directly through its neurochemical influence. It also may represent self-treatment for depressive states, in the case of alcohol or sedative-hypnotic drugs. We must ask, what are the patterns of drug and alcohol use of the elderly who attempt or complete suicide? Although alcohol seems less commonly to be a factor in elderly than young completed suicides, does the same observation hold for elderly psychiatric patients who take their own lives? Does the impact of substances of abuse on self-destructive behavior change with age or chronicity? What medications are most commonly prescribed to suicide victims, and how might they be related to the behaviors in question?

A comparison group for these clinical-pathological studies is difficult to define, beyond the requirements that subjects be age- and sex-matched and come to autopsy without any suspicion of suicide. Individuals who come to autopsy, in any case, are a select population for which the sources of bias regarding their medical backgrounds must be specified.

Personality and Coping Styles

Methods for the reliable assessment of personality style and Axis II psychopathology through retrospective informant interviews have yet to be developed. They are crucial, along with a means for studying coping skills of suicide victims and controls, to measure and understand better why some individuals suicide, while others with similar life circumstances do not. Following a psychological autopsy interview, one is frequently left with a strong impression of the victim's premorbid character configuration. The challenge remains how to quantify and validate these observations. Recurrent themes in psychological autopsy interviews of late-life victims include conflict over dependency, the personal meaning of loss and physical illness, the influence of early life loss in shaping that response, and the increasing inadequacy of coping strategies in late life that may have been successful and adaptive in earlier years.

Psychobiological Studies

Of the multiple determinants of suicidal behavior, biological factors have been least adequately studied in the elderly. As previously reviewed, a remarkably consistent body of research has established a link between suicide and central 5-HT dysfunction. Given the observations that suicide rates are so much higher with advancing age for males and that the elderly are more deliberate and lethal in their self-destruction, it is important to investigate whether changes in the 5-HT system with normal or pathological aging are involved. However, changes in the 5-HT system with normal aging have not been investigated adequately, and the brains from elderly suicide victims have not been studied at all. Clinical-pathological correlation, therefore, should be extended to include neurochemical and morphologic examination of brain tissue of suicide victims in late life for comparison with younger suicide victims and age- and sex-matched deceased controls.

Problems with this approach include the need rigorously to establish changes in the central 5-HT system with normal aging. Further complicating matters are the frequent concurrent medical illnesses and use of psychoactive medications by elderly individuals. These confounds are so frequent in clinical practice as to be virtually always present. Research designs, therefore, must be developed that do not exclude subjects on these bases but rather include them with these confounds identified as variables for study. Large and sophisticated brain acquisition projects will be necessary to gather these data, which should be coupled with the psychological autopsy investigations outlined above to offer maximal opportunity for clinical-pathological correlation.

CONCLUSIONS

Despite the fact that the elderly are as a group at highest risk for suicide, little is known about suicidal behavior in this population. Furthermore, even though suicide is too often the terminal outcome of functional psychiatric illness, its relative significance in the chronic psychiatric disorders of late life has gone virtually unexplored. There is a pressing need, therefore, for basic descriptive research to provide a meaningful clinical database and to define specific testable hypotheses. Assessment of completed suicides in late life should take full advantage of existing databases, as well as information systematically and sensitively obtained from informants through psychological autopsy methodologies. A major effort is needed to develop valid and reliable retrospective measures of premorbid character configuration, coping strategies, life events, and psychopathology. We must then develop close and comfortable working relationships with pathologists and neurobiologists to achieve a more complete picture of pathophysiologic and neurobiologic determinants of this fatal behavior.

A parallel effort should be conducted with suicide attempters in late life, as well as nonsuicidal comparison groups, to distinguish those features of elderly patients and nonpatients that place them at highest risk. Neurobiological studies and comparisons of elderly suicides with younger cohorts will help delineate the features of the behaviors unique to late life.

Ultimately, prevention is the goal of suicide research. Elderly chronic psychiatric patients, although potentially at high risk, may be more accessible to intervention than other populations. In any event, the design of effective treatment programs must be built upon a comprehensive understanding of the multiple determinants of suicidal behavior in late life.

REFERENCES

Asberg, M., Traskman, L., & Thoren, P. (1976). 5-HIAA in the cerebrospinal fluid: A biochemical suicide predictor. *Archives of General Psychiatry, 33,* 93–97.

Babigian, H. M., Lehman, A., & Reed, S. (1986). Suicide in psychiatric and non-psychiatric populations. *Acta Psychiatrica Belgica, 86,* 528–532.

Ballenger, J., Goodwin, F., Major, L., & Brown, H. (1979). Alcohol and central serotonin metabolism in man. *Archives of General Psychiatry, 36,* 224–227.

Banki, C., Arato, M., Papp, Z., & Kurcz, M. (1984). Biochemical markers in suicidal patients: Investigations with CSF amine metabolites and neuroendocrine tests. *Journal of Affective Disorders, 6,* 341–350.

Barner-Rasmussen, P., Dupont, A., & Bille, H. (1986). Suicide in psychiatric patients in Denmark 1971–81. I. Demographic and diagnostic description. *Acta Psychiatrica Scandinavica, 73,* 441–448.

Barraclough, B. M. (1971). Suicide in the elderly. *British Journal of Psychiatry* (Spec. Suppl. 6, Recent Developments in Psychogeriatrics), 87–97.

Barraclough, B. M., Bunch, J., Nelson, B., & Sainsbury, P. (1974). 100 cases of suicide-clinical aspects. *British Journal of Psychiatry, 125,* 355–373.

Barraclough, B. M., Pallis, D. J. (1975). Depression followed by suicide: A comparison of depressed suicides with living depressives. *Psychology Medicine, 5,* 55–61.

Black, D. W. G., Warrack, G., & Winokur, G. (1985a). Excess mortality among psychiatric patients: The Iowa Record Linkage Study. *Journal of the American Medical Association, 253,* 58–61.

Black, D. W. G., Warrack, G., & Winokur, G. (1985b). The Iowa Record Linkage Study I. Suicides and accidental deaths among psychiatric patients. *Archives of General Psychiatry, 42,* 71–77.

Black, D. W. G., Warrack, G., & Winokur, G. (1985c). The Iowa Record Linkage Study II. Excess mortality among patients with organic mental disorders. *Archives of General Psychiatry, 42,* 78-81.

Blazer, D. G., Bachar, J. R., & Manton, K. G. (1986). Suicide in late life: Review and commentary. *Journal of American Geriatric Society, 34,* 519-525.

Bourne, H. R., Bunney, W. E., Colburn, R. W., Davis, J. M., Shaw, D. M., & Coppen, A. J. (1968). Nonadrenaline, 5-hydroxytryptamine, and 5-hydroxyindoleacetic acid in hind brains of suicidal patients. *Lancet, ii,* 805-808.

Breier, A., & Astrachan, B. (1984). Characterization of schizophrenic patients who commit suicide. *American Journal of Psychiatry, 141,* 206-209.

Brent, D. A., Perper, J. A., Goldstein, C. E., Kolko, D. J., Allan, M. J., Allman, C. J., & Zelenak, J. P. (1988). Risk factors for adolescent suicide. *Archives of General Psychiatry, 45,* 581-588.

Brent, D. A., Perper, J. A., Kolko, D. J., & Zelenak, J. P. (1988). The psychological autopsy: Methodological considerations for the study of adolescent suicide. *Journal of the American Academy of Child and Adolescent Psychiatry, 27,* 362-366.

Brown, G. L., Ebert, M. H., Goyer, P. F., Jimerson, D. C., Klein, W. J., Bunney, W. E., & Goodwin, F. K. (1982). Aggression, suicide and serotonin: Relationships to CSF amine metabolites. *American Journal of Psychiatry, 139,* 741-746.

Bunch, J., Barraclough, B., Nelson, B., Sainsbury, P. (1971). Suicide following bereavement of parents. *Social Psychiatry, 6,* 193-199.

Carlson, G. A. (1984). More analysis of Eli Robins' data. *American Journal of Psychiatry, 141,* 323.

Chynoweth, R., Tonge, J. I., & Armstrong, J. (1980). Suicide in Brisbane: A restrospective psychological study. *Australia and New Zealand Journal of Psychiatry, 14,* 37-45.

Conwell, Y., Rotenberg, M. W., & Caine, E. D. (1990). Completed suicide at age 50 and over. *Journal of the American Geriatrics Society, 38,* 640-644.

Dorpat, T. L., Anderson, W. F., Ripley, H. S. (1968). The relationship of physical illness to suicide. In H. P. L. Resnik (Ed.), *Suicidal behaviors: Diagnosis and management.* Boston: Little Brown.

Dorpat, T. L., & Ripley, H. S. (1960). A study of suicide in the Seattle area. *Comprehensive Psychiatry, 1,* 349-359.

Evenson, R. C., Wood, J. B., Nuttall, E. A., & Cho, D. W. (1982). Suicide rates among public mental health patients. *Acta Psychiatrica Scandinavica, 66,* 254-264.

Fawcett, J., Scheftner, W., Clark, D., Hedeker, D., Gibbons, R., & Coryell, W. (1987). Clinical predictors of suicide in patients with major affective disorders: A controlled prospective study. *American Journal of Psychiatry, 144,* 35-40.

Gardner, E. A., Bahn, A. K., & Mack, M. (1964). Suicide and psychiatric care in the aging. *Archives of General Psychiatry, 10,* 544-553.

Haas, A. P., & Hendin, H. (1983). Suicide among older people: Projections for the future. *Suicide and Life Threatening Behavior, 13,* 147-154.

Hirschfeld, R. M. A., & Davidson, L. Clinical risk factors for suicide. *Psychiatric Annals, 18,* 628-635.

Kraft, D. P., & Babigian, H. M. (1976). Suicide by persons with and without psychiatric contacts. *Archives of General Psychiatry, 33,* 209-215.

Kreitman, N. (1988). Suicide, age, and marital status. *Psychological Medicine, 18,* 121-128.

Linehan, M. M. (1986). Suicidal people: One population or two? *Annals of the New York Academy of Sciences, 487,* 16–33.

Linnoila, M., Virkhunen, M., Scheinin, M., Nuutila, R., Rimon, R., & Goodwin, F. K. (1983). Low CSF 5-HIAA concentration differentiates impulsive from non-impulsive violent behavior. *Life Science, 33,* 2609–2614.

Luscomb, R. L., Clum, G. A., & Patsiokas, A. T. (1980). Mediating factors in the relationship between life stress and suicide attempting. *Journal of Nervous and Mental Disorders, 168,* 644–650.

Mackenzie, T. B., & Popkin, M. K. (1987). Suicide in the medical patient. *International Journal of Psychiatry in Medicine, 17,* 3–22.

Manton, K. G., Blazer, D. G., & Woodbury, M. A. (1987). Suicide in middle age and later life. Sex and race specific life table and cohort analyses. *Journal of Gerontology, 42,* 219–227.

Martin, R. L., Cloninger, C. R., Guze, S. B., & Clayton, P. J. (1985a). Mortality in a follow-up of 500 psychiatric outpatients. I. Total mortality. *Archives of General Psychiatry, 42,* 47–54.

Martin, R. L., Cloninger, C. R., Guze, S. B., & Clayton, P. J. (1985b). Mortality in a follow-up of 500 psychiatric outpatients. II. Cause-specific mortality. *Archives of General Psychiatry, 42,* 58–66.

McIntosh, J. L., & Santos, J. F. (1982). Changing patterns in methods of suicide by race and sex. *Suicide and Life Threatening Behavior, 12,* 221–223.

McIntosh, J. L., & Santos, J. F. (1985–1986). Methods of suicide by age: Sex and race differences among the young and old. *International Journal of Aging and Human Development, 22,* 123–139.

Murphy, G. E. (1986). Suicide in alcoholism. In A. Roy (Ed.), *Suicide* (pp. 89–96). Baltimore: Williams & Wilkins.

National Center for Health Statistics, Health Statistics for Older Persons, United States, 1986. (1987, June). Washington, DC: Vital and Health Statistics, Series 3, No. 25, PHS.

National Institute on Aging. (1987). Personal health needs of the elderly through the year 2020. Washington, DC: Public Health Service.

Neill, K., Benensohn, H. S., Farber, A. N., & Resnick, H. L. P. (1974). The psychological autopsy: A technique for investigating a hospital suicide. *Hospital and Community Psychiatry, 25,* 33–36.

Ninan, P. T., VanKammen, D. P., Scheinen, M., Linnoila, M., Bunney, W. E., & Goodwin, F. K. (1984). CSF 5-hydroxyindoleacetic acid levels in suicidal schizophrenic patients. *American Journal of Psychiatry, 141,* 566–569.

Parkin, D., & Stengel, E. (1965). Incidence of suicidal attempts in an urban community. *British Medical Journal, 2,* 133–138.

Paykel, E. S., Myers, J. R., Lindenthal, J. J., & Tanner, J. (1974). Suicidal feelings in the general population: A prevalence study. *British Journal of Psychiatry, 124,* 460–469.

Perry, E. K., Marshall, E. F., Blessed, G., Tomlinson, B. E., & Perry, R. H. (1983). Decreased imipramine binding in the brains of patients with depressive illness. *British Journal of Psychiatry, 142,* 188–192.

Pokorny, A. D. (1983). Prediction of suicide in psychiatric patients. *Archives of General Psychiatry, 40,* 249–257.

Rich, C. L., Ricketts, J. E., Fowler, R. C., & Young, D. (1988). Some differences between men and women who commit suicide. *American Journal of Psychiatry, 145,* 718-722.

Rich, C. L., Young, D., & Fowler, R. C. (1986). San Diego suicide study I. Young vs. old subjects. *Archives of General Psychiatry, 43* 577-582.

Robins, E. (1981). *The Final Months.* New York: Oxford University Press.

Robins, E., Murphy, G. E., Wilkinson, R. H., Gassner, S., & Kayes, J. (1959). Some clinical considerations in the prevention of suicide based on a study of 134 successful suicides. *American Journal of Public Health, 49,* 888-899.

Rosenberg, M. L., Davidson, L. E., Smith, J. C., Berman, A. L., Buzbee, H., Gantner, G., Gay, G. A., Moore-Lewis, B., Mills, D. H., Murray, D., O'Carroll, P. W., & Jobes, D. (1988). Operational criteria for the determination of suicide. *Journal of Forensic Science, 33,* 1445-1456.

Roy, A. (1982a). Risk factors for suicide in psychiatric patients. *Archives of General Psychiatry, 39,* 1089-1095.

Roy, A. (1982b). Suicide in chronic schizophrenia. *British Journal of Psychiatry, 141,* 171-177.

Roy, A. (1984). Suicide in recurrent affective disorder patients. *Canadian Journal of Psychiatry, 29,* 319-322.

Sainsbury, P. (1955). *Suicide in London.* Maudsley Monographs, No. 1. London: Chapman & Hall.

Sainsbury, P. (1968). Suicide and depression. *British Journal of Psychiatry* (Special Supplement 2), 1-13.

Sainsbury, P. (1978). Clinical aspects of suicide and its prevention. *British Journal of Hospital Medicine, 19,* 156-164.

Schmid, C. F., & VanArsdol, M. D. (1955). Completed and attempted suicides. A comparative analysis. *American Sociology Review, 20,* 273-283.

Schwab, J. J., Warheit, G. J., & Holzer, C. E. (1972). Suicidal ideation and behavior in a general population. *Diseases of the Nervous System, 33,* 745-748.

Shafii, M., Carrigan, S., Whittinghill, J. R., & Derrick, A. (1985). Psychological autopsy of completed suicide in children and adolescents. *American Journal of Psychiatry, 142,* 1061-1064.

Shaw, D. M., Camps, F. E., & Eccleston, E. G. (1967). 5-hydroxytryptamine in the hind brain of depressive suicides. *British Journal of Psychiatry, 113,* 1407-1411.

Shneidman, E. S., & Farberow, N. L. (1961). Sample investigations for equivocal deaths. In N. L. Farberow & E. S. Shneidman (Eds.), *Cry for Help* (pp. 118-129). New York: McGraw-Hill.

Stanley, M., Virgilio, J., & Gershon, S. (1982). Tritiated imiprimine binding sites are decreased in the frontal cortex of suicides. *Science, 216,* 1337-1339.

Virkhunen, M. (1974). Suicide in schizophrenia and paranoid psychosis. *Acta Psychiatrica Scandinavica, 250* (Suppl), 1-305.

Wilkinson, G., & Bacon, N. (1984). A clinical and epidemiological survey of parasuicide and suicide in Edinburgh schizophrenics. *Psychological Medicine, 14,* 899-912.

Zilboorg, G. (1936). Suicide among primitive and civilized races. *American Journal of Psychiatry, 92,* 1346-1369.

4

Culture, Chronic Mental Illness, and the Aged: Research Issues and Directions

Audrey Olsen Faulkner

With the current fiscal constraints on governmental spending for health and welfare has come a shift toward providing support only for the most urgent crises of the society. Research in mental health has been no exception; as funds have diminished, the thrust of the National Institute of Mental Health's (NIMH) research on aging has moved from health to illness.

The purpose of this chapter is to discuss cultural issues of concern in research about chronic mental illness in the elderly, and to set forth some recommendations for NIMH's future research directions related to this topic.

RESEARCH BACKGROUND

Age, mental illness and culture have not been systematically treated as an interactive triad of variables by most contemporary investigators working in the field of mental health and aging.

Since Leighton and associates (Hughes, Tremblay, Rapoport, & Leighton, 1960; Leighton, 1959; Leighton, Harding, Macklin, MacMillan, & Leighton, 1963) carried out the Stirling County Study of Psychiatric Disorder and Sociocultural Environment, and Srole et al. (1962) and Langner and Michael (1963) investigated the total prevalence of mental disorder among adults in Manhattan, sociocultural factors related to mental illness have not received concentrated attention. The Stirling County study focused on differences between English and Acadian culture, and the connection between environment and psychiatric disorder; the midtown Manhattan study related mental disorder to factors in the social environment. Hollingshead and Redlich (1958) had already made a significant contribution to the understanding of cultural factors and mental illness through their attention to the relationship between socioeconomic status and psychiatric illness. None of these studies dealt with old age as a major variable, but in Stirling County, data were collected on all age groups, thus providing a comprehensive look at "true and treated prevalence" among the aged of both cultures; the midtown Manhattan study included adults up to 59, and Hollingshead and Redlich included age as a standard demographic variable.

In the early and mid-1970s, investigators interested in the relationship between cultural factors and mental status of the aged began to explore the cultural milieux of minority aged and their contribution to mental *health* (Faulkner, Heisel, & Sims, 1975; Jackson, 1972; Kent, 1971; Maldonado, 1975), rather than mental *illness*. Sterne, Phillips, and Rabushka (1974) looked at the effects of the physical and social environment on the lives of both black and white urban elderly poor, without specific attention to mental health issues.

From the late 1970s to the present, ethnicity and aging, rather than the more general concept of culture and aging, has been a recognized subfield for gerontological investigation (Gelfend & Kutzik, 1979; Manuel, 1982; McNeely & Colen, 1983). This line of investigation has tended to be concerned with mental health and issues of social service need, access and delivery, rather than with mental illness as such. Where mental health has been a variable receiving attention, it has usually been broadly defined in terms of such concepts as life satisfaction, morale, and adjustment to aging. When mental status as a measure of impairment has been a variable for investigation, there have been some limited comparisons between racial groups, but with the more general concept of culture only occasionally addressed (Sokolovsky & Cohen, 1978). Jones and Korchin (1982) and Owan (1985) gathered a variety of perspectives on minority mental health, with some attention to relationships between culture and mental illness, but none of the contributors to their volumes addressed minority aging. Jones and Korchin did address methodological issues in carrying out research on mental health in minority communities.

The 1980s saw anthropologists (Fry et al., 1980, 1981; Keith, 1982; Strange et al. 1987) join investigators from the many other disciplines working in the field of gerontology.[1] The result was a resurgence of interest in culture and aging, but with the parameters determined more by the discipline's traditional interest in in-depth studies of the totality of life in more exotic cultures than in mental health or mental illness issues as such.

CULTURE

Culture is an ephemeral concept, often considered to encompass everything tangible and intangible that humankind has fashioned physically, psychologically and socially. The artifacts of day to day existence, as well as the norms and prescriptions for behavior and social interaction, rest under the cultural umbrella. Social structure, social status and social roles are included. So is the notion of an enclave—a physical or social space with recognized boundaries, where all persons share certain characteristics and all of them interact with the rest of the world in the same way. It can probably be agreed that when gerontologists interested in mental health and mental illness use the term "culture," it subsumes races, skin color, primary language, ethnicity (if claimed by the individual or if the individual is identified with an ethnic group by others), religion, socioeconomic status, age-gender role expectations, family structure and custom, and rural-suburban-urban and institution/community place of residence.

Markides and Mindel (1987) distinguish between cultural differences based on national origin, race and religion, and minority status and its resulting subordination and exclusion, and suggest that both have their separate influences on patterns of aging. In the United States, all of the aged, in the broadest sense, can be said to be members of the common national culture. Many belong to at least one additional subculture, which differs more or less from the overall culture. The perceived difference is generally related to how much or how little the subculture incorporates the characteristics of the dominant culture. Race and primary language are the most definitive cultural components when considering what is known and unknown about chronic mental illness of the aged. They are closely related to income, education, family composition and relationships, and place of residence, factors which in turn influence how mental illness is defined and how medical and social services will be deployed to deal with it. In this chapter, research questions that will be identified and research initiatives that will be proposed will focus on those components, with a primary emphasis on minority status.

CHRONIC MENTAL ILLNESS

The author will use the definition of chronic mental illness from the report *Toward a National Plan for the Chronically Mentally Ill* (DHHS, 1981). This definition, which is not specific to the elderly, builds on Minkoff's (1978) conceptualization of chronic mental illness as including diagnosis, level of disability, and duration of hospitalization. Organic brain syndrome, schizophrenia, recurrent depressive and manic-depressive disorders, paranoid and other psychoses, plus other disorders that may be chronic, are included. The basis for inclusion is the effect these disorders have in eroding or preventing the development of individuals' capacities in relation to three or more of such primary aspects of daily life as personal hygiene and self-care, self-direction, interpersonal relationships, social transactions, learning, and recreation, as well as the development of economic self-sufficiency. The definition includes those who have required institutional care of extended duration (including nursing home care) or out-patient care, as well as those who have received no treatment. Persons who are or were formerly residents of institutions (public and private psychiatric hospitals and nursing homes), and persons who are at high risk of institutionalization because of persistent mental disability are covered by the report's definition.

CULTURAL FACTORS AND CHRONIC MENTAL ILLNESS OF THE AGED

Persons in distinct subcultures generally are bicultural in that they must study and learn the ways of the majority culture in order to survive in it. The same expectation for bicultural knowledge does not universally apply to persons in the dominant culture. Since the majority of mental health practitioners are white, anglo, English speaking, and middle class, they must depend upon the literature and their own personal and professional contacts to determine if and how their professional behavior should be altered with persons whose color, language and social class may differ from theirs. Professionals from subcultural groups may be more attuned to the questions, but they, too, must depend on sources outside their own experience for the information they need in their practice.

Montgomery and Borgatta (1986) have called attention to the fact that myths about aging are drawn from the general culture and are carried on by professions and scientific disciplines. They point out that one of the difficulties in dispelling myths is that researchers often have not critically reviewed prior research and have cited the opinion of others, assuming it was fact. Theories about chronic mental illness of the aged in cultural subgroups are subject to these same limitations; in the absence of documented information, of which there is relatively little, often-cited opinion may become the mental health professional's "fact." The heterogeneity of subcultural populations further compounds the problems.

Issues of Definition of Chronic Mental Illness of the Aged

The DHHS report, whose definition of chronic mental illness was discussed earlier in this paper, calls attention to the fact that judgments about each of the dimensions of chronic mental illness are influenced by psychosocial factors such as poverty and racism.

Practice wisdom in the mental health professions suggests that the perception of mental illness in the elderly varies in racial, ethnic and income subgroups, perhaps because of different norms and standards for behavior, as well as different levels of tolerance for unusual behavior. We have little information about how these different groups view behavior to which mental health professionals would attach a clinical label (Liu, 1986). It may, however, be less a matter of differing perceptions about what constitutes emotional illness than a matter of perception about the availability and effectiveness of resources to deal with it. If those in the subculture who observe the behavior do not believe that a diagnosis will lead to help, they may not see defining the problem as a relevant exercise. In addition, if their experience has been that existing treatment methods are in conflict with cultural norms for appropriate behavior by individuals, families or the community, they are likely to avoid labeling the behavior, and are unlikely to urge their members to seek help.

Issues of Incidence and Prevalence

Closely related to definition are the issues of incidence and prevalence. Planners and providers are handicapped by a lack of either intragroup or intergroup comparative studies of the onset and the presence of chronic mental illness of the aged in cultural subgroups. Neither the scope nor the depth of the problem faced by these groups in their communities are adequately documented. The numbers of minority group aged in even large data sets, for example, are so small as to make questionable any generalizations about the characteristics of the larger groups to which they belong. Meaningful clinical data cannot readily be collected by survey methods, especially when language, class and color issues plague the research at all stages from conceptualization to interpretation. Treatment site case records provide data only on those chronically mentally ill aged who have been found; they tell us nothing about those who have not made their way through the treatment door, nor why they are missing.

ISSUES OF LOCATION OF THE CHRONICALLY ILL AGED

Most of the data available about the aged from cultural subgroups has been obtained in urban settings, where population concentrations are greater. Rural mental illness, like rural mental health, is a neglected area.

Watson (1986) has documented that minority group elderly are substantially underrepresented in nursing home and personal care residences relative to their proportions in the general population, and poses the need for research to explain the reason for this. Speculation that families in these cultural subgroups prefer to care for the impaired elderly at home to a greater degree than white anglo families do has not been subjected to even modest empirical test.

Issues of Treatment Methods and Outcomes in Cultural Subgroups

There is little systematic knowledge about the treatment outcomes for chronic mental illness among aged members of cultural subgroups. Hollingshead and Redlich (1958) documented that social class determined treatment in that era; no similar data provide current information about whether treatment methods for the several categories of chronic mental illness differ for the aged by cultural subgroup. Even less is known about the compatibility of treatment methods with the culture of racial and language groups, and the effect treatment method has on outcome for such individuals.

Issues of Interaction of Formal and Informal Support Systems

A pervasive popular conception is that families of racial, language, and ethnic minorities are closer-knit, and more supportive of their elderly than families of the majority culture. Whether this structure and ethos exists in fact, or whether the lack of available social resources for these groups is the determinant of behavior, awaits careful empirical investigation. Less attention has been paid to the quality of care provided to the elderly in these settings; the effect of caregiving on subcultural group families is only now beginning to claim researchers' attention (Taylor & Chatters, 1986). Given the high incidence of poverty in minority group families, the impact on family resources of caring for the chronically ill elderly member is an important area for research.

A critical issue in care for all elderly residing in the community is the interaction of the formal and informal support systems in their care. There is a beginning inventory of information about the informal support systems in some minority group communities (Vega & Miranda, 1985); there is almost no data about their interaction with the majority community's formal support system. Thus the opportunity for data-based correction of shortcomings and expansion of effective activity is unavailable.

Issues of Research Methodology

Since the late 1960s, minority groups have been vocal about the intrusion of social scientists into their communities. Fear of exploitation and damage to community and group image have served to limit collaboration with the scientific establishment (Jones & Korchin, 1982). While the training of minority researchers has helped to dispel some of the former antagonism toward data gathering, skepticism about the utility of research still exists. It can be assumed that these community attitudes will need attention if accurate data about the chronically mentally ill aged are to be collected for use by the mental health professions.

RECOMMENDATIONS

1. The National Institute of Mental Health should support a long term program of epidemiological studies of chronic mental illness of the aged in the nation's major racial and language groups. These studies should work to resolve the problem of potentially conflicting definitions of mental illness behavior held by the scientific community and cultural subcommunities. These studies should be adequate in scale to capture the heterogeneity as well as the homogeneity of populations. Where sampling rather than census methods are used, the sampling should yield adequate cases of population and economic subgroups to permit meaningful intragroup and intergroup comparisons.

2. In the short term, NIMH should support an initiative to pilot the adaptation of current data collection methodology and available instruments, and means for securing community cooperation, to yield a beginning data base on the chronically mentally ill elderly through small studies of subcultural populations. Carefully identified groupings of subpopulations that differ from the majority culture in race and language, in a variety of geographic locations throughout the nation, should be located and utilized in this initiative. A national committee of scholars and researchers, representative of the groups so identified, should be constituted and utilized for policy direction and problem solving.

3. NIMH should encourage potential investigators to include participants from cultural subgroups in research samples. Inclusion would need to be of sufficient magnitude to make meaningful intragroup and intergroup contrasts and comparisons possible.

4. NIMH should maintain, or facilitate the maintenance of, a national data bank of information about the chronically mentally ill aged in cultural subgroups. Relevant data sets should be solicited, and strategies for making them available to the research community should be developed.

5. NIMH should consider initiatives in the following areas: (1) Studies of the treatment of the chronically mentally ill elderly in subcultural populations. Attention should be given to types of treatment utilized for the various disorders, and to their outcomes; (2) Descriptive studies of the informal support systems for the chronically mentally ill aged in cultural subpopulations; (3) Descriptive studies of functioning of the formal support systems in relation to the chronically mentally ill aged in cultural subpopulations; and (4) Descriptive studies of the interaction of the informal and formal support systems in the detection, treatment and long-

term social support of the chronically mentally ill elderly in cultural subpopulations. Qualitative as well as quantitative methods should be utilized, to maximize insights and appropriate analysis in new research domains.

6. NIMH should sponsor a national conference to identify promising culturally-sensitive treatment programs for the chronically mentally ill elderly. This conference should be followed with an initiative to encourage investigators to submit proposals to test the more promising models.

CONCLUSION

The National Institute of Mental Health has been a major source of encouragement for investigators concerned with cultural factors in mental health. The time has come to focus attention on the chronically mentally ill elderly in culturally identifiable subpopulations. Such an effort will not only address concerns of equity and justice, but will contribute to the knowledge base that will permit the mental health professions to serve all elderly.

NOTE

1. Margaret Clark and Barbara Anderson had preceded them, with their publication of *Culture and Aging: An Anthropological Study of Older Americans* in 1967, but theirs remained the most substantial anthropological work for many years.

REFERENCES

Clark, M., & Anderson, B. (1967). *Culture and aging: An anthropological study of older Americans.* Springfield, IL: Charles C. Thomas.

Department of Health and Human Services, U.S. Public Health Service. (1981). *Toward a national plan for the chronically mentally ill.* Washington, DC: U.S. Government Printing Office.

Faulkner, A. O., et al. (1975). Life strengths and life stresses: Explorations in the measurement of the mental health of the Black aged. *American Journal of Orthopsychiatry*, 45(1), 102–110.

Fry, C. L., et al. (1980). *Aging in culture and society: Comparative viewpoints and strategies.* Brooklyn: J. F. Bergin Publishers, Inc.

Fry, C. L., et al. (1981). *Dimensions: Aging, culture and health.* New York: Praeger.

Gelfand, D. E., & Kutzik, A. J. (Eds.). (1979). *Ethnicity and aging: Theory, research, and policy.* New York: Springer Publishing Company.

Hollingshead, A., & Redlich, F. (1958). *Social class and mental illness.* New York: John F. Wiley and Sons.

Hughes, C. H., Tremblay, M-A., Rapoport, R. N., & Leighton, A. H. (1960). *People of Cove and Woodlot.* New York: Basic Books.

Jackson, J. J. (1972). Negro aged: Toward needed research in social gerontology. *The Gerontologist, 11*(1), 52–57.

Jones, E. E., & Korchin, S. J. (Eds.). (1982). *Minority mental health.* New York: Praeger.

Keith, J. (1982). *Old people as people: Social and cultural influences on aging and old age.* Boston: Little, Brown and Company.

Kent, D. P. (1971). The elderly in minority groups: Variant patterns of aging. *The Gerontologist, 11*(1), 26–29.

Langer, T. S., & Michael, S. T. (1963). *Life stress and mental health: The Midtown Manhattan Study.* New York: The Free Press of Glencoe.

Leighton, A. H. (1959). *My name is Legion.* New York: Basic Books.

Leighton, D. C., Harding, J. S., Macklin, D. B., MacMillan, A. M., & Leighton, A. H. (1963). *The character of danger: Psychiatric symptoms in selected communities.* New York: Basic Books.

Liu, W. T. (1986). Culture and social support. *Research on Aging, 8*(1), 57–83.

Maldonado, D. (1975). The Chicano aged. *Social Work, 20*(8), 213–216.

Manuel, R. C. (Ed.). (1982). *Minority aging: Sociological and social psychological issues.* Westport, CT: Greenwood Press.

Markides, K. S., & Mindel, C. H. (1987). *Aging and ethnicity.* Newbury Park, CA: Sage Publications, Inc.

McNeely, R. L., & Colen, J. L. (Eds.). (1983). *Aging in minority groups.* Beverly Hills: Sage Publications.

Minkoff, K. (1978). A map of chronic mental patients. In J. A. Talbott (Ed.), *The chronic mental patient* (pp. 11–37). Washington, DC: American Psychiatric Association.

Montgomery, R. J. V., & Borgatta, E. F. (1986). Plausible theories and the development of scientific theory: The case of aging research. *Research on Aging, 8*(4), 586–608.

Owan, T. C. (Ed.). (1985). *Southeast Asian mental health: Treatment, prevention, services, training and research.* Washington, DC: U.S. Government Printing Office.

Sokolovsky, J., & Cohen, C. (1978). The cultural meaning of personal networks for the inner-city elderly. *Urban Anthropology, 7,* 323–343.

Srole, L., Langner, T. S., Michael, S. T., Opler, M. K., Rennie, T. A. C. (1962). *Mental health in the metropolis: The Midtown Manhattan Study, vol. I.* New York: McGraw Hill Book Company, Inc.

Sterne, R. S., Phillips, J. E., & Rabushka, A. (1974). *The urban elderly poor.* Lexington, MA: D. C. Heath and Company.

Strange, H., Teitelbaum, M., et al. (1987). *Aging and cultural diversity: New directions and annotated bibliography.* South Hadley, MA: Bergin & Garvey Publishers, Inc.

Taylor, R. J., & Chatters, L. M. (1986). Church-based informal support among elderly blacks. *The Gerontologist, 26*(6), 637–642.

Vega, W. A., & Miranda, M. R. (Eds.). (1985). *Stress and hispanic mental health: Relating research to service delivery.* Washington, DC: U.S. Government Printing Office.

Watson, W. H. (1986). Nursing homes and the mental health of minority residents: Some problems and needed research. In M. S. Harper & B. D. Lebowitz (Eds.), *Mental illness in nursing homes: Agenda for research* (pp. 267–279). Washington, DC: U.S. Government Printing Office.

PART II
Family and Social Research Issues

5

Social Support and Chronic Mental Illness among the Elderly

Carolyn E. Cutrona, Kathleen Schutte,
Julie A. Suhr, Daniel Russell

Although advocacy groups for the elderly have become increasingly visible in recent years, one group of older adults has been largely ignored. Older adults who are afflicted with mental illness have received very little attention from either researchers or policymakers, and as a result, their special needs are not well understood.

Psychosocial factors, including both stress and social support, have been implicated among younger adult populations as playing an influential role in the etiology, course, and response to treatment of some kinds of mental illness (see reviews by Leavy, 1983; Wethington & Kessler, 1986). Although stress reduction is frequently advocated as an antidote to psychological distress, many of the stressors associated with aging are tangible realities that cannot be eliminated (e.g., bereavement, fixed income, physical frailty). Thus, enhancing social support has been proposed as an alternative means to protect those who are vulnerable to mental illness.

What is Social Support?

Social support refers to the psychological and tangible resources that are available to individuals through their relationships with family, friends, neighbors, work associates, and other nonprofessionals with whom individuals have contact. Although social support is often viewed as primarily beneficial during times of stress, research shows that those with rich support resources have better mental and physical health than those low in support, even in the absence of significant life stress (Cohen & Wills, 1985).

Although a number of different types of social support have been described, researchers appear to have converged on a set of five specific interpersonal qualities and behaviors that constitute support. These five support types can be classified into those that directly promote problem solving (instrumental support) and those that primarily promote emotional adjustment (emotional support). Included among instrumental support components are tangible aid and informational support. *Tangible aid* refers to concrete assistance, wherein goods or services are provided (e.g., financial assistance, transportation). *Informational support* involves information, advice, or guidance concerning possible solutions to a problem. Included among emotional support components are expressions of caring or attachment, network support, and esteem support. *Attachment* represents love and comfort that provide security in times of stress. *Social integration*, or *network support*, refers to feeling part of a group where members share common interests and concerns. *Esteem support* consists of bolstering the person's sense of competence or self-esteem. Providing the individual with positive feedback on skills and abilities and indicating a belief that the person is capable of coping with a stressful event are examples of this type of support.

Measuring Social Resources

Two approaches to assessing social resources have emerged. As described above, the social support approach involves assessing the extent to which family, friends, and other acquaintances provide instrumental and emotional support. Measures include items that ask direct questions about whether support is available from others (e.g., "Are there people you can rely on for help if you really need it?"). A second approach involves the assessment of more quantitative aspects of the person's social relationships and is termed the *social network* approach. It is assumed that structural aspects of the set or network of relationships that one has affects the type and availability of resources that are available. Some of the most commonly assessed network variables include number of people with whom the person interacts (network size), frequency of contact with others, and the extent to which individuals in the person's network know each other (density). In this chapter, we make the assumption that social support and social network variables overlap to some degree and that both affect the well-being of mentally ill individuals. Thus, both social support and social network studies are included in this review.

Psychopathology and Social Support

By far the greatest number of studies on psychosocial factors and mental health have focused on depressive disorders. Much less is known about the role of social support in other psychiatric disorders. Relevant research regarding the role of social support (or its absence) in the onset, presentation, course, and treatment of depressive disorders, schizophrenia, and alcohol abuse will be summarized here. For most disorders, studies of exclusively elderly patients are lacking, so conclusions must be extrapolated from studies of mixed-age adult samples.

For different disorders, social support appears to play a different role. For example, the absence of social support is probably of true etiological significance for relatively few disorders, most notably unipolar depression. However, social support may influence adherence to treatment regimens, probability of hospitalization, and capacity for functioning in the community. The most important potential function of social support will be highlighted for each disorder that is discussed.

Depressive Disorders

Network and Support Characteristics of Depressed Elderly

Descriptive information on the social network and social support resources of depressed versus nondepressed elderly is available from a number of different sources. Cross-sectional data of this type is useful in generating hypotheses about the specific social deficits that contribute to depression, but it must be borne in mind that one manifestation of depression is social withdrawal and a loss of interest in others. Thus, social deficits found to characterize depressed elders may be the result rather than the cause of depression.

Lower frequency of contact with others has been found in several studies that compared depressed to nondepressed elderly adults (Arling, 1987; Blazer, 1983; Essex, Klein, Lohr, & Benjamin, 1985). In a study of 200 men and women over age 80, frequency of social interaction was the strongest predictor of psychological well-being in a multiple regression analysis that included physical health and socioeconomic variables as predictors (Luke, Norton, & Denbigh, 1981). Regarding number of individuals with whom the older adult has regular contact, one study found that only number of network members similar to the target individual was associated with depression (Goldberg, VanNatta, & Comstock, 1985). In this large sample of elderly women, depressed women reported regular contact with a smaller number of individuals who were similar to themselves in age, religion, and gender. Availability of a confidant is another social resource that discriminates between depressed and nondepressed elders. Murphy (1982) found that lack of a confidant was a key factor in the onset of depression among elderly individuals of both sexes. Similarly, Blazer (1983) found lack of a confidant to characterize individuals suffering from major depression in a community sample of elderly adults. By contrast, only a lack of casual relationships distinguished depressed from nondepressed elderly persons in a study by Henderson et al. (1986). Regarding more qualitative aspects of relationships, in a study of elderly urban blacks, low perceived support from friends was associated with depressive symptoms (Smith-Ruiz, 1985). Finally, perceived consistency, predictability, and reciprocity of relationships with friends were found to be lower among depressed compared to nondepressed elderly women in a study by Essex et al. (1985).

Social Support Predicting the Onset of Depression

Only a small number of prospective studies have tested the extent to which poor social support predicts the onset of depressive symptoms among the elderly. Prospective longitudinal studies are particularly valuable because they allow statistical controls for initial level of psychopathology. When individuals are depressed, they may underestimate the quantity and quality of social support available to them. Because social support and depression are typically correlated (negatively) when assessed at the same point in time, a pattern of unremitting depression can give the appearance of a causal relationship between social support and depression unless appropriate statistical controls are employed. That is, low social support at time 1 may indeed be correlated with high depression at time 2, but this pattern may reflect nothing more than continuing depression from time 1 to time 2. Longitudinal studies in which statistical controls for the effects of concurrent depression can be employed in tests of social support's predictive power are one solution to this problem.

In a longitudinal study of 351 elderly community residents, Krause, Liang, and Yatomi (1989) tested both the extent to which changes in social support predicted changes in depression and the extent to which changes in depression predicted changes in social support (i.e., alienating others after symptom onset). Analysis of the data, using structural equation modeling techniques, clearly supported the primacy of change in social support. That is, although decreased satisfaction with social support significantly predicted increases in depressive symptoms 18 months later, increased depression did not significantly predict a drop in social support satisfaction.

In another longitudinal study of elderly adults, social support predicted depression and number of daily hassles over a 12-month period, controlling for initial level of depression using structural equation techniques (Russell & Cutrona, in press). Those individuals who reported high levels of instrumental support, esteem support, and attachment were less likely to report depressive symptoms and experienced a smaller number of hassles 12 months after the initial assessment.

Finally, Holahan and Holahan (1987) found that self-confidence in the domain of acquiring and managing social support was a significant predictor of both quality of social support and level of depressive symptoms 12 months later among the elderly. These results suggest the importance of attitudinal variables in the acquisition and maintenance of social resources.

Social Support as a Buffer against Negative Life Events

Social support was originally conceptualized as a protective factor or "buffer" against the deleterious effects of stressful life events (e.g., Cassel, 1976; Cobb, 1976). Several studies have examined the extent to which social support can protect elderly individuals against depressive reactions to various kinds of negative life events. In these studies, the *interaction* between social support and life stress is evaluated to test whether the strength of the relation between stress and depression is weaker among individuals who have high levels of social support than among individuals who have low levels of social support. The majority of the studies are cross-sectional, although a few employ more powerful longitudinal designs.

Arling (1987) found that instrumental social support (assistance, resources) protected elderly individuals who suffered from physical infirmity against depressive symptoms. A significant interaction was found between ADL score (an index of ability to perform activities required for independent daily living) and social support in the prediction of depressive symptoms, so that individuals who had limited functional capacity were less depressed if they also had high levels of social support. Krause (1986, 1987) found that the emotional impact of bereavement was buffered by several components of social support. Fewer somatic depressive symptoms (sleeplessness, loss of appetite) occurred among bereaved elders who reported high levels of emotional, informational, and tangible support. Emotional support buffered the effects of crime (Krause, 1986), and informational support and the provision of support to others buffered the effects of financial strain (Krause, 1987). In a longitudinal study, Cutrona, Russell, and Rose (1986) found that both information and tangible support buffered the effects of stressful life events in an elderly population. Individuals who reported a large number of stressful life events in the previous 6 months were less likely to be depressed, anxious, and lonely if they had high levels of these two forms of instrumental support.

To summarize, instrumental support that involves assistance and/or advice was effective in protecting elderly adults from depression in the context of physical infirmity and financial strain. In addition, instrumental support was beneficial in preventing emotional distress among individuals who suffered from an accumulation of multiple recent negative life events. All of these circumstances involve loss or depletion of resources. Thus, support that compensates in some way for the deficiencies experienced by the elderly adult is protective against depression. This is not to underestimate the importance of emotional support. Individuals who had suffered bereavement or victimization by crime benefited from emotional support. It has been hypothesized by Cutrona and Russell (1990) that different components of social support are important depending on the controllability of the stressful event and the life domain that it affects. In our model, controllable events (those that can be prevented or their impact diminished through instrumental behavior) lead to a need for instrumental support, whereas uncontrollable events (those that cannot be prevented or their impact diminished) lead to a need for emotional support. The results summarized above are consistent with our predictions in that bereavement and victimization by crime are clearly uncontrollable events, whereas the effects of illness and financial strain can be eased to some extent by an influx of resources and assistance. More research with elderly populations is needed to develop an understanding of the specific types of social support that are most beneficial to elderly individuals in the context of different kinds of stressful circumstances.

Social Support and the Severity and Course of Depressive Illness

Because depression is caused by multiple factors, including biochemical, environmental, and personality variables, it is possible that even the most supportive network cannot prevent the onset of depression. However, it is of great clinical importance to determine whether the severity and course of depressive illness can be affected by social support resources. Social support has been tested as a determinant of the severity and course of depressive illness by a number of researchers. However, a single study was located in which elderly patients were the exclusive focus. Thus, suggestive findings from studies of nonelderly adult clinical populations will also be summarized for comparison.

In the only study that dealt with recovery among elderly patients, Murphy (1983) followed for 12 months a sample of 103 elderly patients, all of whom had been diagnosed with major depression using either DSM-III or Feighner criteria. All subjects received antidepressant medication, and many received additional treatments as well. Approximately half of the sample was hospitalized at some point over the course of the study. At the time of entry into the study, patients were assessed with respect to the availability of a close confidant. Subjects received the highest intimacy rating if they lived with a close confidant, medium ratings if they reported having a confidant with whom they did not live, and the lowest rating if they reported no confidant. Contrary to prediction, these intimacy ratings did not predict which patients made a good recovery and which made a poor recovery by the time of the 12-month follow-up.

Most of the recent studies of nonelderly adult clinical populations have found social support to predict improvement and/or recovery from various types of depression, including unipolar depression (Billings & Moos, 1985), reactive depression (Brugha et al., 1987), neurotic depression (Mann, Jenkins, & Belsy, 1981), and bipolar depression (O'Connell, Mayo, Eng, Jones, & Gabel, 1985). In a study of nonpsychotic patients (primarily affectively disordered) who were followed after an index psychiatric hospitalization, the only variable that distinguished those who were readmitted from those who were not was the availability of social support (Goering, Wasylenki, Lancee, & Freeman, 1983). However, two studies yielded negative results in which social support did not predict the symptomatic outcomes of nonelderly depressed patients (Hirschfeld, Klerman, Andreason, Clayton, & Keller, 1986; Surtees, 1980).

The most serious potential consequence of depression is suicide. Although no studies of social support and suicide among the elderly were located, there is evidence that low social support is a factor that increases suicide risk (Balon, 1987; Roy, 1982; Stallone, Dunner, & Aheern, 1980). Further research is needed to determine whether low social support interacts with other risk factors (e.g., medical illness) or whether it should be conceptualized as an independent predictor. Also, it is important to determine whether social isolation is the only predictor of suicidal behavior or if perceived lack of support without actual isolation is also a significant predictor. (See chapter by Conwell & Caine, this volume, for a fuller discussion of suicide in the elderly.)

Taken together, the literature reviewed above suggests that those who have more abundant and higher-quality social support resources experience somewhat less severe symptoms and recover more quickly from depressive illness. This pattern was less consistent in studies that selected more severely depressed patients (e.g., Hirschfeld et al., 1986; Murphy, 1983). Thus, it may be that social support's effects are more pronounced among individuals suffering from less severe depressions. This suggests the importance of early support-based interventions, since their effectiveness may be greatest in the earlier stages of depression before a full-blown affective syndrome has developed. More research is needed on the effects of support on recovery from depression among the elderly, since the only study that followed a sample of elderly depressives (Murphy, 1983) did not show superior outcomes for those with higher levels of emotional support.

Schizophrenia and Social Support

If psychiatric disorders were placed on a continuum regarding the importance of psychosocial factors in their etiology, schizophrenia would be relatively far from the pole representing psychosocial factors as the primary causative agents. Other kinds of personal vulnerability factors (e.g., structural, biochemical) must be present for the disease to be manifested. However, a relatively large body of literature has accumulated that indicates a significant role for both stressful life circumstances and interpersonal resources in the course of the disorder among personally vulnerable individuals (see review by Goldstein, 1987). Most researchers conceptualize schizophrenia within the context of a vulnerability-stress model, in which the interaction of personal physiological vulnerability with external conditions and events determines whether and how severely symptoms will be manifested (Zubin & Spring, 1977).

Social Networks and Schizophrenia

A number of researchers have examined quantitative aspects of the social networks of individuals suffering from psychotic illnesses. One consistent finding is that schizophrenics tend to have relatively small social networks (Crotty & Kulys, 1985; Pattison, DeFrancisco, Wood, Frazier, & Crowder, 1975; Sokolovsky, Cohen, Berger, & Greiger, 1978). In one study, the average network size for schizophrenic patients was 6.4, compared to normals, who typically report 20 to 30 people in their social networks (Crotty & Kulys, 1985). Furthermore, it has been found that symptom severity correlates negatively with number of network members (Crotty & Kulys, 1985; Sokolovsky et al., 1978). Sokolovsky et al. (1978) compared the social networks of three groups of residents (many elderly) of single-room-occupancy hotels in New York City. These included schizophrenics with moderate to severe symptoms, schizophrenics with mild or no symptoms, and residents with no psychotic history. They found that the schizophrenics with more severe symptoms had an average network size of 10.2 persons, schizophrenics with less severe or no symptoms had an average network size of 14.7, and residents with no psychosis had an average network size of 22.6.

Not only severity of symptoms but age has been shown to correlate with network size among community dwelling schizophrenics. Elderly community-dwelling schizophrenics report smaller networks than do younger adults afflicted with this disorder (Grusky, Tierney, Manderscheid, & Grusky, 1985). Thus, a particular need for social integration may exist among deinstitutionalized elderly mentally ill.

Regarding the composition of the social network, degree of involvement of schizophrenic individuals with their families has received considerable research attention. Two studies have found the social networks of schizophrenics to be composed primarily of family members (Pattison et al., 1975; Tolsdorf, 1976). However, contact with family appears to decrease as a function of symptom severity and chronicity. In a study by Garrison (1978) of Puerto Rican–born schizophrenic women (some of whom were elderly), the less disturbed schizophrenic women relied heavily on family members, but the most disturbed relied almost solely on nonfamily members. A similar negative correlation between severity of symptoms and family involvement was found by Cohen and Sokolovsky (1979). Duration and frequency of hospitalization also has a negative effect on family contact. Patients who have had many and/or long hospitalizations tend to live alone, rather than with a spouse or family (Grusky et al., 1985). Thus, elderly schizophrenic patients may have little support from their families, who may have "given up" on them.

In a prospective study of 133 elderly individuals (mean age = 72.3 years) living in single-room-occupancy hotels, social network characteristics (number of transactions, frequency of contact, multiplex relationships, size, density, number of clusters, homogeneity) were significant predictors of individuals' ability to meet their daily needs independently (Cohen, Teresi, & Holmes, 1985). These network variables showed a dramatic increase in importance in the context of stress or poor health. Elders who faced traumatic life events or illness benefited more from social relationships than those not taxed by such circumstances.

Ambiguity exists concerning the direction of causality in studies on the effects of network and support resources on the course of psychotic illnesses. One symptom of schizophrenia is social withdrawal, and it may be that those with more severe symptoms are unable to build relationships with others and require more frequent hospitalization, both as a consequence of severity of illness. The direction of causality cannot be implied from correlational studies alone. However, the research of Sokolovsky and his colleagues provides particularly persuasive evidence that community-dwelling schizophrenics do form significant bonds with other people and that these bonds may serve important functions, especially if at least one member of the social network is relatively competent (e.g., Cohen & Sokolovsky, 1978). Thus, programs that promote contact between individuals with varying degrees of disturbance may be particularly beneficial to those who are more severely impaired.

Support-Based Treatment of Schizophrenia

Based on their review of the literature on psychosocial treatment of schizophrenia (all age groups), Mosher and Keith (1980) concluded that family and community-based therapies are consistently positive. In particular, behavioral treatments that improve social competence and family problem solving appear to reduce the risk of schizophrenic relapse (e.g., Falloon et al., 1982; Hogarty & Goldberg, 1973). However, Gallant (1983) suggested that just as the efficacy of neuroleptics may vary for different subtypes of schizophrenics, certain schizophrenic subtypes may benefit maximally from psychosocial therapy. He further suggests that although there are disagreements concerning the effect of such therapy on the course of schizophrenia (cf. Klein, 1980), there is widespread agreement that such treatment helps to decrease the secondary psychological, financial, and social consequences of schizophrenia and may also help to maintain treatment compliance.

Alcohol Abuse and Social Support

Etiology

Although no evidence unequivocally supports a causal role of social support in the etiology of alcoholism, some research suggests that it may be a factor. Crossman (1984) suggests that since about one-third of elderly alcoholics develop their drinking problems later in life, social environments and social problems faced by the elderly such as loss of social support may be precipitating events. According to Brown (1982), this is a common explanation for alcohol abuse in the elderly. He interviewed 30 chief administrators of midwestern health and social service agencies and found that 43% of them mentioned loss of social roles, 57% of them mentioned loneliness, and 27% of them mentioned absence of supportive social relationships as precipitants of alcohol abuse in their elderly clients.

Social Networks and Alcohol Abuse

Several studies have documented lower levels of social support and smaller social networks among alcohol abusers. The social networks of later-life-onset alcohol abusers were judged to be "relatively poor" at the time of admission in terms of both size and density in a study by Dupree, Broskowski, and Schonfeld (1984). The elderly alcohol abusers in this study had been successful in life and did not begin abusing alcohol until late life, often following stresses such as losses and reductions in their social networks. However, Giordano and Beckham (1985) reviewed studies relating social variables such as loneliness and bereavement to late-life-onset alcoholism and concluded that the evidence that does exist cannot clearly delineate a causal role for social support. The relationships between loss, bereavement, loneliness, lack of social support and alcoholism could be explained through mediating factors such as a negative perception of life. However, as for all of the disorders, more prospective longitudinal studies are required to disentangle the sequence of events that lead to late-life alcohol abuse.

Social-Support-Based Treatment

Crossman (1984) and Rathbone-McCuan and Bland (1975) suggest that increasing social support may be a particularly useful treatment for elderly alcoholics who began their problem drinking in response to interpersonal losses. Few empirical studies have incorporated social support components into the treatment of elderly alcoholics. Dupree et al. (1984) created a treatment program that included help in reestablishing viable social support networks for later-life-onset alcohol abusers. However, participation and continued involvement in treatment were major problems. Only half of those who began treatment completed the program. However, for those who did stay in the program, none returned to the abusive pattern.

Research on alcoholism treatment programs that strive to improve social support among younger adults are suggestive of a role for social support in intervention (e.g., Rosenberg, 1983), but better-controlled empirical research is needed before such social support intervention programs can be considered successful. Future studies might focus on more specific forms of support rather than the general supportiveness of the alcoholic's social network. For example, support that focuses on maintaining sobriety may be more beneficial than other forms of support.

PREVENTIVE SUPPORT-BASED INTERVENTIONS FOR THE ELDERLY

Although many researchers stress the importance of improving the social support available to elderly adults, little empirical research has been conducted on the efficacy of social-support-based intervention programs. Studies reviewed above indicate that elderly persons with higher-quality social support are less likely to manifest symptoms of mental illness, but we still do not know whether social support that is intentionally provided through community-based programs is effective in preventing mental illness. In this section, examples of support-based interventions for the elderly will be described and evaluation results summarized.

The Neighborhood Family Program (NF) (Ross, 1983) was a successful primary prevention program for the elderly in which a kinlike supportive community and a service and activities center were provided. The NF program allowed elderly adults to create a self-managed social support network. The dropout rate was unusually low, and participants reported a high degree of satisfaction with the program. A significant improvement in reported well-being among participants was noted at a 1-year follow-up.

Andersson (1985) reported a successful intervention to prevent loneliness in elderly women. Elderly women were randomly chosen to participate from a waiting list for admission to senior citizen apartments. The intervention consisted of strengthening the social networks of the women by making confidants available and allowing for social comparison through group discussions. Small neighborhood groups of 3–5 persons were formed that met to discuss concerns relevant to older adults, such as medical care, social services, and leisure activities. Subjects were interviewed before participation and 6 months' postintervention. Measures of loneliness, social contacts, alienation, self-esteem, trust, physical health, and activity level were taken. At the 6-month follow-up interview, subjects reported less loneliness and meaninglessness, and more self-esteem and social contact.

In a secondary prevention program, Heller and Thompson (1989) tested a support-based intervention for elderly, low-income, socially isolated women. The intervention consisted of providing each participant with a randomly matched peer with whom telephone contact was encouraged for a 6-month period. However, results did not indicate decreases in loneliness or increases in perceived social support as a result of the intervention. Because telephone partners were randomly matched, it may be that participants had little in common with one another and thus found it difficult to build a genuine friendship. Alternatively, the social isolation of these women may have reflected long-standing difficulties with interpersonal relationships (e.g., poor social skills, mistrust, a tendency to evaluate others negatively).

A network-enhancement program to prevent relapse among community-dwelling former psychiatric patients was reported by Cohen and Sokolovsky (1981). Participants were 156 residents of a single-room-occupancy hotel in Manhattan, half of whom were over age 60. The residents reported a wide range of problems (e.g., physical health, finances). They were given opportunities to form relationships with other residents, who could potentially offer various kinds of assistance to them. Only 19% of the residents required no services beyond the network intervention. The authors concluded that such interventions do not appear to be adequate substitutes for direct professional services.

A similar conclusion was reached by Chapman and Pancoast (1985), who described and evaluated several intervention programs focusing on improving the social support networks of elderly clients. Their evaluation of these three programs led them to conclude that a policy of replacing conventional formal services with informal social networks is not likely to be easy or cost-effective.

Evaluations of social support intervention programs for the elderly do not form a consistently positive picture of their effectiveness. Several researchers have suggested that the limited effectiveness of such programs is due to their simplification of the diverse needs of the elderly. Without attention to the complexity of the situation which the elderly person faces, interventions may be ineffective or even harmful (Rook, 1984). It is important to pay attention to health status, ethnicity, lifestyle, age, social class, gender, and type of stress in designing appropriate interventions for the elderly (Heller, Price, & Hoggs, 1990; Pelisuk & Minkler, 1980). In general, programs appear to be less successful with more disturbed populations (e.g., former psychiatric patients, social isolates). For these individuals, a combination of network and traditional professional interventions are probably required.

GENERAL SUMMARY AND IMPLICATIONS

Evidence suggests that elderly individuals who are chronically mentally ill have especially impoverished social support resources. Both age and number and duration of hospitalizations predict smaller social networks. Contact with family is especially likely to diminish with age and chronicity. After long years of dealing with a mentally ill spouse or parent, it has been hypothesized that "burnout" results (Grusky et al., 1985). Thus, for the chronically mentally ill elderly, interventions may have to focus on building social bonds with nonfamily members.

Findings are equivocal regarding the extent to which supportive relationships with others can modify the course of mental illness. In general, less severely afflicted individuals appear to benefit more from larger social networks and accessible social support. However, the data on social support and institutionalization suggests that individuals with better social support resources are able to avoid hospitalization for longer periods of time than those with less supportive relationships. It must be noted once again, however, that this association is stronger among those with less severe symptoms. The most severely disturbed individuals appear to require periodic inpatient care, regardless of the support available to them. Thus, it is important that traditional professional mental health services are readily accessible to these individuals and that they understand how to make use of such services.

Support-based interventions, both preventive and ameliorative, yield mixed results. Some appear to be highly successful, and others appear to have little effect. One reason for inconsistent results may be different levels of severity of disturbance across client populations, with the most severely disturbed individuals responding least well. A second explanation for inconsistent results of support-based interventions is our current lack of understanding of the specific support needs that result from different stressful life circumstances, stages in the life cycle, and psychiatric conditions. Relatively few studies have analyzed the specific support components that most benefit various patient populations. Suggestive findings from a few studies in which individual support components were analyzed were summarized, although conclusions must be viewed as tentative because of the small number of studies. Type of stressful event is one factor that may affect the type of social support that is needed. For example, instrumental support was shown to protect against depression among elderly individuals in the context of financial strain and physical infirmity (Arling, 1987; Krause, 1987). By contrast, emotional support was uniquely beneficial in preventing depressive reactions to bereavement and crime victimization (Krause, 1986, 1987). We have hypothesized that controllable events (those in which the actions of the self or others can prevent or lessen adverse consequences) require instrumental social support to promote optimal coping. Uncontrollable events (those in which the actions of self or others cannot prevent or lessen adverse consequences) require emotional support to facilitate acceptance and management of aversive emotions (Cutrona & Russell, 1990).

The specific social support needs of the elderly who suffer from chronic mental illness are not well understood. As noted previously, the social resources of elderly patients are more limited than those of younger psychiatric patients. However, the few social support interventions that have been tested for elderly adults have shown mixed results. It may be that such interventions ignore the fact that elderly adults who suffer from mental illness also experience all of the adverse consequences of aging, such as poor physical health, limited income, role loss, and loss of valued others through death or relocation. Thus, multiple services are frequently required. It is unreasonable to expect that support-based interventions alone will meet the multiple service needs of the aged mentally ill.

Finally, it should be noted that many of the studies reviewed in this chapter suffer from significant methodological weaknesses. More studies that use well-validated measures are needed. Standard diagnostic criteria should be utilized, and detailed information regarding severity of disorder should be included in research reports. Random assignment to treatment groups should be employed whenever ethically possible. Appropriate comparison groups or pre-post analyses should be included in the design of all intervention studies. Multidimensional measures of social support and social network variables should be administered in studies of support as a predictor of outcome. Finally, in studies of mixed age groups, analyses should be reported regarding differential effects for elderly adults.

REFERENCES

Andersson, L. (1985). Intervention against loneliness in a group of elderly women: An impact evaluation. *Social Science and Medicine, 20,* 355–364.

Arling, G. (1987). Strain, social support, and distress in old age. *Journal of Gerontology, 42,* 107–113.

Balon, R. (1987). Suicide: Can we predict it? *Comprehensive Psychiatry, 28,* 236–241.

Billings, A. G., & Moos, R. H. (1985). Life stressors and social resources affecting post-treatment outcomes among depressed patients. *Journal of Abnormal Psychology, 94,* 140–153.

Blazer, D. G. (1983). Impact of late-life depression on the social network. *American Journal of Psychiatry, 140,* 162–166.

Brown, B. B. (1982). Professionals' perceptions of drug and alcohol abuse among the elderly. *The Gerontologist, 22,* 519–531.

Brugha, T., Bebbington, P. E., MacCarthy, B., Potter, J., Stuart, E., & Wykes, T. (1987). Social networks, social support and type of depressive illness. *Acta Psychiatrica Scandinavica, 76,* 664–673.

Cassel, J. (1976). The contribution of the social environment to host resistance. *American Journal of Epidemiology, 104,* 107–123.

Chapman, N. J., & Pancoust, D. L. (1985). Working with the informal helping networks of the elderly: The experiences of three programs. *Journal of Social Issues, 415,* 47–63.

Cobb, S. (1976). Social support as a moderator of life stress. *Psychosomatic Medicine, 38,* 300–304.

Cohen, C. F., & Sokolovsky, J. (1978). Schizophrenia and social networks: Expatients in the inner city. *Schizophrenia Bulletin, 4,* 546–560.

Cohen, C. I., & Sokolovsky, J. (1979). Health-seeking behavior and social networks of the aged living in single room occupancy hotels. *Journal of the American Geriatrics Society, 27,* 270–277.

Cohen, C. I., & Sokolovsky, J. (1981). Social networks and the elderly: Clinical techniques. *International Journal of Family Therapy, 3,* 281–294.

Cohen, C. I., Teresi, J., & Holmes, D. (1985). Social networks and adaptation. *The Gerontologist, 25,* 297–304.

Cohen, S., & Willis, T. A. (1985). Stress, social support, and the buffering hypothesis. *Psychological Bulletin, 98,* 310–357.

Crossman, L. H. (1984). Alcohol abuse in the elderly. Implications for educational and human service programming. *Journal of Alcohol and Drug Education, 29,* 31–34.

Crotty, P., & Kulys, R. (1985, July-August). Social networks: The views of schizophrenic clients and their significant others. *Social Work,* 301–309.

Cutrona, C. E., & Russell, D. W. (1990). Type of social support and specific stress: Toward a theory of optimal matching. In I. G. Sarason, B. R. Sarason, & G. R. Pierce (Eds.), *Social support: An interactional view* (pp. 319–366). New York: Wiley.

Cutrona, C. E., & Russell, D. W., & Rose, J. (1986). Social support and adaptation to stress by the elderly. *Journal of Psychology and Aging, 1,* 47–54.

Dupree, L. W., Broskowski, H., & Schonfeld, L. (1984). The gerontology alcohol project: A behavioral treatment program for elderly alcohol abusers. *The Gerontologist, 24,* 510–516.

Essex, M. J., Klein, M. H., Lohr, M. J., & Benjamin, L. S. (1985). Intimacy and depression in older women. *Psychiatry, 48,* 159–178.

Falloon, I. R. H., Boyd, J. G., McGill, C. W., Razani, J., Moss, H., & Gilderman, A. M. (1982). Family management in the prevention of exacerbation of schizophrenia. *New England Journal of Medicine, 306,* 1437–1440.

Gallant, D. M. (1983). Outpatient treatment: Community and private practice support systems. *Journal of Clinical Psychiatry, 44,* 15–22.

Garrison, V. (1978). Social support of schizophrenic and non-schizophrenic Puerto Rican women in New York City. *Schizophrenia Bulletin, 4,* 561–596.

Giordano, J. A., & Beckham, K. (1985). Alcohol use and abuse in old age: An examination of type II alcoholism. *Journal of Gerontological Social Work, 9,* 65–83.

Goering, P., Wasylenki, D., Lancee, W., & Freeman, S. J. (1983). Social support and post-hospital outcome for depressed women. *Canadian Journal of Psychiatry, 28,* 612–617.

Goldberg, E. L., VanNatta, P., & Comstock, G. (1985). Depressive symptoms, social networks, and social support of elderly women. *American Journal of Epidemiology, 121,* 448–455.

Goldstein, M. J. (1987). Psychosocial issues. *Schizophrenia Bulletin, 13,* 157–171.

Grusky, O., Teirney, K., Manderscheid, R. W., & Grusky, D. B. (1985). Social bonding and community adjustment of chronically mentally ill adults. *Journal of Health and Social Behavior, 26,* 49–63.

Heller, K., Price, R. H., & Hoggs, J. R. (1990). The role of social support in community and clinical intervention. In I. G. Sarason, B. R. Sarason, & G. R. Pierce (Eds.), *Social support: An interactional view.* New York: Wiley.

Heller, K., & Thompson, M. (1989, May). *The structure of supportive ties among elderly women.* Paper presented at the Second Iowa Conference of Personal Relationships, Iowa City, IA.

Henderson, A. S., Grayson, D. A., Scott, R., Wilson, J., Rickwood, D., & Kay, D. W. K. (1986). Social support, dementia and depression among the elderly in the Hobart community. *Psychological Medicine, 16,* 379–390.

Hirschfeld, R. M. A., Klerman, G. L., Andreasen, N. C., Clayton, P. J., & Keller, M. B. (1986). Psycho-social predictors of chronicity in depressed patients. *British Journal of Psychiatry, 148,* 648–654.

Hogarty, G. E., Goldberg, S. C., & the Collaborative Study Group (1973). Drug and sociotherapy in the after care of schizophrenic patients. *Archives of General Psychiatry, 28,* 54–64.

Holahan, C. K., & Holahan, C. J. (1987). Self-efficacy, social support, and depression in aging: A longitudinal analysis. *Journal of Gerontology, 42,* 65–68.

Klein, D. F. (1980). Psychosocial treatment of schizophrenia, or psychosocial help for people with schizophrenia? *Schizophrenia Bulletin, 6,* 122–130.

Krause, N. (1986). Stress and sex differences in depressive symptoms among older adults. *Journal of Gerontology, 41,* 617–622.

Krause, N. (1987). Chronic financial strain, social support, and depressive symptoms among older adults. *Psychology and Aging, 2,* 185–192.

Krause, N., Liang, J., & Yatomi, N. (1989). Satisfaction with social support and depressive symptoms: A panel analysis. *Psychology and Aging, 4,* 88–97.

Leavy, R. L. (1983). Social support and psychological disorder: A review. *Journal of Community Psychology, 11,* 3–21.

Luke, E., Norton, W., Denbigh (1981). Medical and social factors associated with psychological distress in a sample of community aged. *Canadian Journal of Psychiatry, 26,* 244–250.

Mann, A. H., Jenkins, R., & Belsey, E. (1981). The twelve-month outcome of patients with neurotic illness in general practice. *Psychological Medicine, 11,* 535–550.

Mosher, L. R., & Keith, S. J. (1980). Psychosocial treatment: Individual, group, family, and community support approaches. *Schizophrenia Bulletin, 6,* 10–41.

Murphy, E. (1983). The prognosis of depression in old age. *British Journal of Psychiatry, 142,* 111–119.

Murphy, E. (1982). Social origins of depression in old age. *British Journal of Psychiatry, 141,* 135–142.

O'Connell, R. A., Mayo, J. A., Eng, L. K., Jones, J. S., & Gabel, R. H. (1985). Social support and long-term lithium outcome. *British Journal of Psychiatry, 147,* 272–275.

Pattison, E. M., DeFrancisco, D., Wood, P., Frazier, H., & Crowder, J. (1975). A psychosocial kinship model for family therapy. *American Journal of Psychiatry, 132,* 1246–1251.

Pelisuk, M., & Minkler, M. (1980). Supportive networks: Life ties for the elderly. *Journal of Social Issues, 36,* 96–116.

Rathbone-McCuan, E., & Bland, J. (1975). A treatment typology for the elderly alcohol abuser. *Journal of the American Geriatrics Society, 23,* 553–557.

Rook, K. S. (1984). The negative side of social interaction: Impact on psychological well-being. *Journal of Personality and Social Psychology, 46,* 1097–1108.

Rosenberg, H. (1983). Relapsed versus non-relapsed alcohol abusers: Coping skills, life events, and social support. *Addictive Behaviors, 8,* 183-186.

Ross, H. K. (1983). The neighborhood family: Community mental health for the elderly. *The Gerontologist, 23,* 243-247.

Roy, A. (1982). Risk factors for suicide in psychiatric patients. *Archives of General Psychiatry, 39,* 1089-1095.

Russell, D., & Cutrona, C. E. (in press). A longitudinal panel model of depression and social support among the elderly. *Psychology and Aging.*

Smith-Ruiz, D. (1985). Relationship between depression, social support, and physical illness among elderly blacks: Research notes. *Journal of the National Medical Association, 77,* 1017-1019.

Sokolovsky, J., Cohen, C., Berger, D., & Geiger, J. (1978). Personal networks of ex-mental patients in a Manhattan SRO hotel. *Human Organization, 37,* 5-15.

Stallone, F., Dunner, D. L., Aheern, J., et al. (1980). Statistical prediction of suicide in depressives. *Comprehensive Psychiatry, 21,* 381-387.

Surtees, P. G. (1980). Social support, residual adversity and depressive outcome. *Social Psychiatry, 15,* 71-80.

Tolsdorf, C. C. (1976). Social networks, support, and coping: An exploratory study. *Family Process, 15,* 407-417.

Wethington, E., & Kessler, R. C. (1986). Perceived support, received support and adjustment to stressful life events. *Journal of Health and Social Behavior, 27,* 78-89.

Zubin, J., & Spring, B. T. (1977). Vulnerability: A new view of schizophrenia. *Journal of Abnormal Psychology, 86,* 103-126.

6

The Psychiatric Patient Grows Older: Issues in Family Care

Bertram J. Cohler, Susan A. Pickett, Judith A. Cook

Among problematic aspects of family caregiving, none presents greater difficulties than care for the psychiatrically ill family member. Particularly where the ill family member is an adult offspring, the burden and role strain involved in caregiving may be compounded by feelings of embarrassment and resentment regarding the often intrusive and disruptive nature of the adult child's continuing impact upon the large family system. Belief that things will get better and that adult offspring will be able to resume the expectable course of adult life yields over time to feelings of disappointment and resignation regarding the future, together with concern for the offspring's well-being later in the course of life when both parents have died. To date, while there are a number of phenomenological reports by family members regarding the nature of caregiving for older mentally ill offspring, there has been little systematic study of the problem related to provision of such continuing care into later life.

Much available study has focused on schizophrenia and the impact of patterns of communication as determinants of the transactions thought disorder manifest as the illness or "expressed emotion" of resentment and hostility among family members as a factor determining rehospitalization. There has been much less discussion of the longer-term relationship between the psychiatric patient and family members responsible for providing care. Indeed, systematic study of this problem has been limited largely to cross-sectional studies of younger psychiatric patients, and if their parents live to older ages, there is increased likelihood of an older adult offspring requiring care from very old parents who also require care. This dilemma poses two interrelated problems: the presumed provider of care for older parents is able to provide very limited caregiving, and, at a time when parents are less able to provide support and assistance, these older parents confront the problem of continuing care of a troubled middle-aged or older offspring.

The present chapter considers this problem of reciprocal caregiving within the family of later life confronted by the need for providing care for an older adult offspring who is recurrently and severely mentally ill. Reflecting constitutionally determined vulnerability, translated into symptomatic distress as a consequence of often idiosyncratically defined life changes, episodic, recurring, psychiatric illness has an impact on a circle of relatives as well, often disrupting family functioning. Periods of symptomatic distress characterized by bizarre and so-cially unacceptable behavior alternate with periods of more effective functioning within family and community.

While, in the past, most psychiatric patients received long-term care as state hospital residents, with the movement toward deinstitutionalization over the past two decades, these patients spend ever larger amounts of time in the community, even during times of exacerbation of symptoms. Little is known regarding the course of the disturbance across the second half of life, and even less is known of the impact of deinstitutionalization upon patient and family as both grow older. The profound symptomatology of chronic mental illness evokes strong feelings on the part of family members attempting to provide such continuing care and support. In the following discussion, we shall be concerned with the psychiatrically disabled person and caregiving family members across the second half of life.

CAREGIVING, CRISIS AND LIFE COURSE

The dimension of time is often missing in models formulated to understand familial response to crisis; family structure and process vary as a consequence both of point in the course of life of family members and also those particular sociohistorical events that determine the outlook of a particular cohort of persons. Following Sorokin and Merton (1937), Roth (1963), and Neugarten, Moore, and Lowe (1965), the course of human life may be understood as a socially constructed, shared timetable regarding ages at which expected transitions might occur. Therefore, age and place in the life course of family members may be relevant in understanding both family resources for recognizing and dealing with problems, determining experience of burden and role strain experienced by family members in response to particular adversity and in understanding adjustment of family members to adversity.

Schizophrenia and the Need for Family Care

One area in which there has been study of caregiving for younger adult offspring (i.e., children in their early twenties to midthirties) concerns parents whose offspring develop major psychopathology such as schizophrenia. This illness represents an "ideal type" (Weber, 1905) of psychiatric impairment among adult offspring, providing an important source of information in understanding problems of caregiving of severely disabled adult offspring.

Severe psychiatric disturbances often occur first in late adolescence or young adulthood: symptoms of recurrent mental illness are particularly disruptive of the lives of other family members. Further, because of the impact of this disturbance upon the family, aspects of family structure and process have been studied in association with both *origin* and *course* of the illness. At the same time, much of the study of schizophrenia and family caregiving has been limited to the family of young adulthood. However, not only is the occurrence of first episodes of this illness possible across the course of adulthood (Kay & Bergman, 1980; Neugebauer, 1980; Cohler & Ferrono, 1987) through oldest age, but also the illness is one in which expression of symptoms may change across the adult life course: changes in symptom expression acorss the second half of life have been reported by Lawton (1972) and Bridge, Cannon, and Wyatt (1978), suggesting that quite different demands are made upon family caregivers over time. Indeed, viewed from a developmental perspective, the significance of this illness for consociates varies markedly with time since initial episode and present point in the course of life.

"Family Blaming," Etiology, and Reciprocal Socialization

Several decades of detailed empirical study (Mishler & Waxler, 1965, 1968; Waxler, 1974; Liem, 1974, 1980) have raised serious questions regarding perspectives on origins of schizophrenia emphasizing a simple model of forward socialization of prospective schizophrenic patients into communication deviance or maladaptive thinking by parents themselves showing such transactional nonrationality (Lidz, 1973; Singer & Wynne, 1963). In the first place, there have been problems in replicating findings across studies. Further, many of the findings have subsequently been attributed to such problems of methods as testing parents of schizophrenic patients at the time of offspring hospitalization when parental anxiety level is likely to be greatest, administering research protocols to target families at the psychiatric hospital while testing comparison families at home, selection of only particular data from projective techniques used in these studies, and attribution of causality to group differences. This latter problem is among the most serious for the family approach to understanding the origins and course of schizophrenia. As a consequence of reciprocal socialization within the family, the thought disorder and other positive symptoms characteristic of the illness may be learned by sympathetic parents who attempt to enter the troubled offspring's world in order to maintain the solidarity of the parent-offspring relationship, leading to appearance of parental transactional thought disorder (Cook & Cohler, 1986).

Similar problems are posed by recent study of the impact of family expression of hostile and critical feelings upon the course of the former patient's posthospital adjustment. Some studies, finding high levels of such "expressed emotion" (EE) associated with rehospitalization (Brown, Birely, & Wing, 1972; Brown, Monck, Carstairs, & Wing, 1962; Leff & Vaughn, 1980, 1985; Vaughn, 1986; Vaughn & Leff, 1976), implicitly support a model of "forward socialization" similar to that represented by studies of schizogenic parents in which attributes of parental characteristics are now associated not necessarily with onset of disturbance but with its subsequent course. This approach overlooks the concept of reciprocal socialization within the family, defined by Burgess (1926) as a "unity of interacting personalities." From the first studies of Kreisman and Joy (1976), to detailed accounts of life in families with a recurrently psychiatrically ill offspring (Sheehan, 1982), to the most recent work in the area (Hatfield, 1987b), study of issues of caretaking and burden have provided an important new perspective on problems of living with such patients. Rather than attributing blame of cause, we need more detailed study of the sources of such burden, means for changing perspectives from blame and attribution to understanding the problems of the whole family, and continuing, longitudinal research regarding life over time within these families as contrasted with those with a chronically physically ill offspring and families not facing such continuing distress.

Structural Response to Caregiving Issues: Formation of NAMI

Partially in reaction to this study of family psychopathology and offspring outcome, as well as an effort to provide a more effective lobbying organization for the rights of psychiatric patients, the National Alliance for The Mentally Ill (NAMI) was formed over the past decade. Focusing largely on problems posed for families of the severely and recurrently mentally ill, NAMI has been instrumental in a shift of emphasis in scholarly study of schizophrenia away from faulty socialization processes toward a more balanced view of problems inherent in caring for vulnerable persons who develop this illness (Dearth, Labenski, Mott & Pellegrini, 1986). In the processes, NAMI has called attention to the major issue for family study, that of the adverse impact upon the mental health of caregivers arising from the effort to provide care for schizophrenic adults across the course of adult life. While much of this attention has focused on caregiving issues for younger adult offspring, NAMI has also expressed concern regarding the problems of older parents and other family members caring for their middle-aged and older offspring. NAMI notes that the family of later life providing such caregiving focuses such problems as estate planning, wills, and trusts for disabled relatives, insurance, medicare and medicaid policy, and prevention of burden for the older patient's siblings (NAMI, 1987; Richardson, 1987).

THE OLDER PSYCHIATRIC PATIENT AND THE FAMILY

Early characterizations of schizophrenia (Bleuler, 1911/1950; Kraeplin, 1913/ 1919) portrayed this illness as a lifelong process of continuing personality deterioration. However, more recent studies, including those by Bleuler's son (M. Bleuler, 1978), suggest that earlier views regarding the course of this disorder may have been overly pessimistic. Following up a group of patients released from Vermont State Hospital in the mid-to-late 1950s, Harding and her colleagues (Harding & Brooks, 1984; Harding, Brooks, Ashikaga, Strauss, & Landerl, 1987) report that more than 90% of these patients were able to reside outside of the hospital, 43% of these patients had one or two additional admissions over the intervening period, and 20% had no further psychiatric admissions; most were functioning fairly well in the community, with three-quarters maintaining adequate social support systems. Most of these 41–79-year-old ex-patients dealt with continuing deficits by finding their niche in the community and by regulating the extent of their intimate contact to that which was comfortable, including satisfying relationships with their families.

It may also be that modern cohorts of mentally ill are better able to adjust to this disability than their counterparts from earlier eras, the result of psychopharmacologic interventions, increased awareness of the issue of stigma, increased understanding of the episodic nature of the illness, or a combination of factors. This view is supported by Clausen's (1984, 1984b) reports of two cohorts of patients discharged from the hospital with more than two decades intervening. Over this interim, with duration of in-hospital stay much reduced, persons in the more recent cohort were better able to resume their previous lives than those in the earlier cohort. Particularly in the cohort of persons hospitalized in the 1970s, as contrasted with those first hospitalized in the 1950s, patients resumed functioning at nearly premorbid levels of work and social functioning, albeit with some lasting deficits.

Midlife Changes in Symptomatology

Findings based on the study of schizophrenic and aging have shown that there is a change in the expression of positive symptoms, both among middle-aged and older adults with a first schizophrenic episode across the second half of life.

Among patients initially hospitalized in young adulthood, attainment of midlife appears to be associated with diminution of symptoms (Bridge et al., 1978; Davis, 1974; Erentheil, 1962; Kay & Roth, 1961, 1963; Lawton, 1972; Muller, 1963, 1971). This burnout of the more distressing features of the illness such as hallucinations and elaborate delusions has tremendous implications for older family caregiving. If the severity of symptoms lessens over time this may also reduce the strains encountered by family caretakers. With diminution of positive symptoms across the second half of the patient's life, there may also be changes in the patient's role within the family.

In addition to changes in the ill offspring's symptomatology and illness course, there are also changes accompanying aging that can be expected to influence subjective definitions of the caretaking experience in later life. This is true for both the ill individual and family members, with personality changes accompanying aging influencing the ways in which older caregivers and their other offspring view family caregiving. With the advent of midlife, persons stop looking forward to the future and begin to look backward to life lived to date. With the death of parents and friends, the reality of mortality becomes increasingly apparent to persons at midlife (Neugarten & Datan, 1974), leading to increased "personalization of death." While in contrast with earlier statements of the "disengagement hypothesis" proposed by Cumming and Henry (1961) there need not be actual withdrawal from continuing social ties, foreshortened sense of time may lead to increased preoccupation with the significance of the personal past, and increased reflectiveness, characterized by Neugarten (1973, 1979) as interiority, and my Munnichs (1966) as a "crisis of finitude," with the goal of attaining increased perspective on the finitude of life (Jaques, 1965, 1980; Marshall, 1975, 1981, 1986).

As patient and older parents increasingly come to share a common view of the course of life (Cohler, 1987/1988), it is likely that there is increased accommodation between the generations, reducing parental sense of burden and facilitating family adjustment to the illness. At the same time, there may be intensified concern about providing for the troubled offspring in the event of their own death and particularly about reducing possible burden on the patient's brothers and sisters. While these concerns are supported both by anecdotal evidence from our own continuing study of patients and their parents, and also reports from other studies (Hatfield, 1987a, 1987c), it is essential to begin cross-sequential study of this problem and that the psychiatric patients and their families be followed over continuing periods of time. In particular, policymakers and service providers need to know to what extent siblings and other family members are prepared to assume the burden of care from aging cohorts of parents nearing the end of life. It would be useful to know, for example, the degree of open discussion and planning which families use in order to provide for future decades.

Although we have little specific information about these and related questions among older caregivers of middle-aged and older psychiatrically ill offspring, burden studies of seriously psychiatrically ill *adults* and their *middle-aged and older parents* provide some suggestions for future study. In addition, family caregiver/ burden research on other disabilities where aging has been considered, such as *Alzheimer's disease* and caring for *mentally retarded* older offspring, can offer additional clues for understanding the nature of older family caretaking for a mentally ill relative.

VULNERABILITY, EPISODE AND FAMILY RESPONSE

Reflecting on these findings from long-term outcome studies, it is clear that schizophrenia is not necessarily the unremitting chronic disease so often portrayed. On the one hand, this is encouraging news for afflicted patients. On the other hand, this more optimistic view presents serious problems for caregiving family members. While there is some disagreement regarding the proportion of formerly hospitalized patients residing with their families and apart, such as in "board and care facilities" or transitional housing, Minkoff (1979), and Goldman (1982) have estimated that between half and three-fourths of all patients discharged from care initially return home to live with their parental family. McFarlane (1983) and Hatfield (1987a) observe that the reduction in SSI payments and other federal and state assistance plans between 1980 and 1987 have led to increased numbers of patients being forced to return home because of problems in affording alternative residence. Regardless of the length of time separated and the problems posed by hospitalization, many families accept their ill relatives back into the home (Evans, Bullard, & Solomon, 1961).

The episode nature of the disturbance, together with the magnitude of the disruption which is created in the lives of relatives living with patients, means that there may be continuing uncertainty regarding the future, and continuing anxious anticipation regarding the possibility of the outbreak of another episode. The impact of schizophrenia upon the lives of patients and their relatives, disrupting the expected sequence of life transitions, affecting the timing of expectable entrances and exits from roles associated with particular points in the course of life, together with the impact of the illness upon the life course of relatives in an ever-widening circle from the primary affected patient, take a staggering toll on the health and adjustment of caretakers. An important question is whether or not the strains of caregiving under such circumstances increase, decrease, or otherwise evolve over time as patients and their caregiving relatives grow older.

Aging Families

While there has been some study of pathways to first psychiatric hospitalization (Greenblatt, Levinson, & Williams, 1957), family response to initial encounters with the hospital (Reiss, Costell, Jones, & Berkman, 1980; Costell & Reiss, 1982), and the nature of the relationship between patient and family in the early phases of the illness (Hatfield, 1978, 1979), little is known about the reciprocal impact of patient, illness and caregiving over periods of several decades. Terkelsen (1987) maintains that there has been virtually no systematic study of this issue. Indeed, his own portrayal, based on clinical experience, of 10 phases of family struggle with psychiatric illness among offspring, is heavily weighted toward the family's response to first illness and hospitalization. Terkelsen portrays the period of time after this hospitalization as one in which the family must adjust to the reality that the patient may not return to prior levels of psychosocial adaptation:

> The patient comes home or proceeds to a new residence. Weeks go into months as the treatment continues in one form or another. The patient makes some progress, loses ground, regains his or her ability to engage in some activities but not others. Months go into years. The patient suffers a relapse and then another, appearing to worsen and to lose ground with each recurrence. In time, the family's cumulative experience with the illness leads to the conclusion that the illness is not going to simply go away, and that the whole family must make some accommodation to prolonged, possibly permanent incapacitation of the affected person. (1987, 161)

Terkelsen notes that as months stretch into years, the chronicity of the offspring's illness becomes an "assault on (the family's) ability to continue to support the patient and treatment efforts, and to bear the attendant burdens" (p. 161). The family suffers a "collapse of therapeutic optimism," compartmentalizing and isolating the patient, and directing attention away from the patient's difficulties.

A somewhat different picture is provided by the work of Tessler, Killian, and Gubman (1987), exploring nine stages in familial response to severe mental illness. Their study of 30 families showed that only 1 had given up and withdrawn from the ill member. Stages occurring later in the illness course included recognition of the illness's chronicity, followed by loss of faith in mental health professionals, followed by belief in the family's own expertise in managing the illness, and, eventually, worry about the future. Interviews with family members revealed that over many years, families come to rely less heavily on professionals and play a more active, supportive role themselves. While not tied specifically to aging issues, these results do suggest that families who choose to remain in contact and involved with their ill relative may be able to reach a balance in managing the demands of caregiving along with other life tasks.

Caretaking and the Experience of Family Burden

Reacting to the pileup of adverse events, the nature of the family caretaking burden changes both over time, and with the extent of dispositional vulnerability within the family. In their discussion of the double ABCX model of family crisis and response, McCubbin and his associates (McCubbin et al., 1982; McCubbin

& Figley, 1983; McCubbin & Patterson, 1983) emphasize that burden includes that which is both objectively and subjectively experienced. Research on family burden and mental illness has followed this conceptualization in attempting to understand the nature of strain encountered by caregiving family members (Grad & Sainsbury, 1963; Hatfield, 1978; Hoening & Hamilton, 1966; Thompson & Doll, 1982). While there is some variation across studies, *subjective burden* is typically viewed as the emotional costs of the illness to family members (e.g., feelings of embarrassment, resentment, and helplessness), while *objective burden* is defined as the disruption to everyday family life for the ill person's relatives (e.g., financial burden, loss of free time, and conflict with neighbors or law enforcement officials) (Thompson & Doll, 1982).

Beginning with Hoenig and Hamilton's (1966) pioneering study, and Hatfield's (1978) report, there has been considerable detailed study of parental response to the time following hospitalization. Much of this study has concerned specific behaviors which are objectively troublesome (objective burden), rather than the family's definition of the situation (Berger & Kellner, 1964; Blumer, 1969/1976) so important for understanding subjective aspects of burden. To date, there has been very little study of subjective experience of burden which is parallel to study of objective burden (Terkelsen, 1987).[1] Even those few studies attempting to differentiate betwen objective and subjective stress regard objective stress as a response to troublesome patient behaviors, and subjective stress as reflecting the caregiver's adjustment in response to caregiving (Grad & Sainsbury 1963, 1968; Hoenig & Hamilton, 1966; Thomspon & Doll, 1982).

Burden, Distress, and Outcome

As used in the present instance, and consistent with the Hill-Minnesota family stress research on the ABCX model (McCubbin & Figley, 1983; Mederer & Hill, 1983), the term *burden* is reserved for actual and experienced role strain and overload among relatives caring for offspring; feelings of anxiety and depression are viewed as the outcome of a process in which felt burden in response to this life change is tempered by particular coping attributes, leading to particular caregiver mental health outcomes. Investigators have not always been clear whether caregiver personal distress is a *burden* or an *outcome*. For example, Avrey and Warheit (1980) report subjective distress (anxiety and depression) experienced by more than 25% of the caregiving respondents in their study, with lower-class respondents reporting the greatest degree of affective distress. While 16% of respondents with a psychiatrically ill spouse reported anxiety or depression, percentages were higher among respondents with a mentally ill blood relative (adult offspring [23%] or parent [28%]). To date, only Noh and Turner (1987) have followed this more specific model, distinguishing between objective and experienced burden and between burden and outcome in terms of caregiver's assessing mental health.[2]

Previous study has shown the significance of the reciprocal impact of the psychiatric patient upon the family (Clausen & Yarrow, 1955a, 1955b, 1955c; Clausen, Yarrow, Deasy, & Schwartz, 1955; Hoenig & Hamilton, 1966)[3] demonstrated the extent to which psychiatric illness impacted the larger family unit. These studies suggested that more than 50% of families of schizophrenic patients are very seriously impacted by psychiatric illness, with less than 25% reporting little or no subjective impact.[4] More recently, Thompson and Doll (1982) has examined both objective and subjective burden, including the necessity for relatives (primarily middle-aged parents) to provide supervision for the patient which otherwise would not be required; neglect of brothers and sisters; feared economic consequences over long periods of time; and the patient's disruption of family routines. Half of their parental sample reported two sources of burden, another 25% reported one source of burden, and the final 25% reported no objective burden or impact. However, nearly 75% of the group reported subjective burden, primarily feelings of strain and overload in the parental role, and nearly 50% reported feelings of embarrassment in response to the patient's behavior. While there was a significant relationship between objective and subjective burden, few of the families reporting a high degree of objective burden also reported a high degree of subjective burden, suggesting some resilience when confronted with serious problems.[5]

Findings reported by our own research group (Cook & Pickett, 1985) show that among the late-middle-aged mothers and fathers of a group of recurrently ill primarily schizophrenic young adults (generally in their thirties) who resided with their parents, 94% reported worrying about the child's future, and 94% expressed concern about continuing financial dependence; 85% reported feelings of helplessness; more than 75% agreed that they yearned for the child to return to his or her "old self" again; 70% expressed concern that their offspring were too dependent upon them. Using a multi-item scale that included both subjective and objective dimensions to measure burden, analysis revealed that parents of female offspring, older offspring, and white (versus minority) families have significantly higher burden scores. Interestingly here, while *child's* age was significantly related to family burden, the *parent's* age was less important, suggesting perhaps that features related to the child and not particular features of the parent are predictive of familial burden.

In further study of the same group of parents (Cook & Pickett, 1988), the degree of parental *criticalness* was examined and related to the nature of burden for this group. Employing a crude measure of parental criticalness (interviewer rating of degree of criticism expressed toward the offspring during a face-to-face home interview), it was discovered that the two features did not always vary together or in the same direction. For example, using the means as cutoff, 23% scored low on burden but were rated as highly critical, while another 23% scored high on burden but were rated as low on criticism. This suggests that these two responses should be viewed separately, as part of a system of reactions, each varying along a continuum of intensity, perhaps with different implications for intervention.[6]

Coping with Burdens over Time

As the Minnesota group has emphasized, coping with the burdens of family crises is a consequence of longer-term life changes and the family's experience of associated burden. We have suggested that this perspective must also be considered in the context of time, particularly in understanding family response to such long-term crises as recurrent psychiatric illness among offspring. Study of coping with the impact of this burden over time has been facilitated by the intense interest in problems of coping and adjustment more generally (Lazarus & Folkman, 1984; Moos & Tsu, 1976; Pearlin & Schooler, 1978). At the same time, in virtually none of the work reported to date is there any consideration of differences in coping techniques within families of patients differing in course of disturbance or point in the life course of both patient and other family members.

In a series of reports, associates from the Center for Rehabilitation Research and Training in Mental Health at Boston University (Jung, Spaniol, & Anthony, 1983; Spaniol, Jung, Zipple, & Fitzgerald, 1987) have presented findings from a nationwide survey study of family caretakers for patients with long-standing psychiatric illness, often extending over more than a decade. A 10% sample was drawn from the membership of the National Alliance for the Mentally Ill (NAMI); within this group of families, only 29% agreed to participate, and only 22% provided sufficiently complete information to be of value for the study. Overall, nearly 67% of family members (principally parents) stated that they were managing their offspring's illness adequately or better. Those coping more effectively were parents whose offspring were recurrently ill over longer periods of time, suggesting that family members may ultimately adapt to the burden of caregiving over time. These findings also confirm earlier reports by Hatfield (1981), following 30 highly educated, high-status parents of older offspring: Effectively coping families had older offspring who had been ill over periods of many years and who exhibited lower psychosocial functioning. Consistent with the reciprocal socialization argument (Cook & Cohler, 1986; Cook & Pickett, 1988), these two studies suggest that family coping improves over time.

At the same time, these responses may be characteristic only of the minority of families willing to become involved with studies such as these. Those who agree to participate may cope more effectively and may be more willing to share their experiences. Indeed, these same attributes may have led to their being involved in a self-help group to begin with. Significantly, nearly 40% of the (assumedly) more activist, well-informed family members participating in the research reported by the Boston University group reported that they were not coping well with their offspring's psychiatric illness and that professional support was less than optimal. It is possible that these findings seriously understate the problem and that many parents of episodically troubled offspring are not coping effectively with this illness. Devoted to providing good care, even at great personal cost, and living up to their own sense of responsibility and decency, these family members may feel confused and bewildered by the unpredictable course of schizophrenia over time, as well as alienated and angered by the lack of understanding on the part of the mental health delivery system.[7]

Older Psychiatric Patients and Their Older Parents

The problems which elderly parents of an older mentally ill offspring confront include those particularly relevant to older adults. Factors contributing to elderly parents' increased feelings of strain appear to be related to particular points in the course of life and are a result of role exits and losses such as retirement, grandparenthood, and deaths of loved ones, exacerbated by the need to care for an adult offspring. For example, parents may be required to postpone retirement plans in anticipation of providing for a chronically mentally ill son or daughter who will be incapable of functioning independently. Wikler (1986) has reported that the life review process, associated with making meaning of the course of life as lived (Butler, 1963; Cohler & Galatzer-Levy, 1990), may reactivate past parental wishes for "what might have been" for both ill offspring and their parents. This longing for a different past is felt particularly strongly when the ill offspring is an only child, where parents are particularly likely to grieve failure to become grandparents. However, having the ill older offspring at home may impede the older parents' opportunity (especially that of the mother) to enjoy the "empty nest" period (Harkins, 1978; Rubin, 1978).

Retirement itself may increase role strain among the parents of psychiatrically ill older adults. Parents are no longer able to take refuge in the workplace in an effort to escape from the stress of unremitting involvement with a psychiatrically disabled offspring (Lefley, 1987a, 1987b). For the first time, recently retired fathers experience directly the 24-hour caregiving days formerly experienced by the wife and mother who has spent so many years with their ill child. Parental income now consists of Social Security and perhaps another type of pension (Stevens, 1972; Lefley, 1987c). Thus, there may be fewer financial resources to make ends meet for the entire family, adding to the levels of parental burden.

The elderly parent's social and familial support network may also be more constricted than that of younger parents (Stevens, 1972). Death of friends and spouse may leave the older person more socially isolated; the spouse's death forces the surviving aging parent, typically the mother, into the role as sole caretaker for the chronically psychiatrically ill adult offspring. Shadows of one's own death increase parental anxiety about who will care for the ill offspring after his/her death (Terkelsen, 1987). Fears about how the ill child will survive after the parent is gone are often portrayed as the most profound source of strain for the remaining older parent (Ashbaugh et al., 1983).

Older parents must count on younger relatives, particularly offspring, to assume caregiving responsibilities. However, in most instances these more resilient brothers and sisters of recurrently psychiatrically ill adult offspring have long since left the family, married, and raised their own children. Aging parents generally feel that it is unfair to burden their other children with the ill offspring's care, especially when siblings have grown up with the aversive consequences of the illness (Dearth, Labenski, Mott, & Pellegrini, 1986). In other families, well siblings' stressful life experiences with an ill brother or sister have built up walls of self-protection: they may have moved across the country, having failed to settle painful rifts in their relationships with the family (Carlisle, 1989) or have sought other ways to avoid becoming involved with their parents and their psychiatrically ill sibling (Cicirelli, 1980, 1985; Vine, 1982).

Elderly parents' declining health is also a significant concern for family members (Jacobs, Mason, & Kosten, 1986; Kasl, 1984). As the aging parents' health declines, they have less stamina, patience, and physical resources to meet the heavy demands of providing care for the ill offspring; they may not be able to depend on the mentally ill child for help in time of their own infirmity.

When, as a consequence of the role losses and exits of later life, alternative sources of confidence no longer exist, such as those derived from work and support of friends and relatives, there may be diminished belief that problems may be resolved through active mastery (Gutmann, 1987). The passive and magical mastery so often associated with later life, useful in resolving normatively expectable issues associated with life review and acceptance of mortality, provides poor solutions for older parents coping with recurrent psychiatric illness for an older adult offspring. Indeed, coming to terms with mortality is increasingly difficult when older parents face the task of providing continuing care for their troubled offspring. Lefley (1987a/1987c) argues that aging parents typically lack such resources and are more prone to greater levels of strain that result from providing for a chronically mentally ill offspring.

With increasing age, it is likely that all family members will be on some sort of public pension, making the family increasingly vulnerable to funding fluctuations and changing eligibility rules (SSI/SSDE and medicaid for the mentally ill, pensions, Social Security and medicare for the elderly family members). Roy-Byrne, Gross, and Marder (1982) see a potential for abuse of impaired older offspring by other family members who seize upon their pensions and financially exploit the patient for the benefit of the larger family. However, considering recent restrictions on eligibility requirements for SSI and SSDI (Hatfield, 1987; McFarlane, 1983), as well as significant proportions of chronically psychiatrically ill persons failing to qualify due to "loopholes" in legislation (i.e., the never-hospitalized), there are still large numbers of disabled older persons whose families must bear the entire financial burden of care.

On the other hand, there are indications that certain types of familial burden may be lessened as the ill person and his or her family enter midlife. Brunn

(1985) suggests that both increased parental concern with mortality and the very off-time nature of providing care for older offspring pose particular problems for the older parent. Cohler (1987/1988) has suggested that as offspring grow older and begin to confront the finitude of life, they increasingly share parental perspectives on self and others. Findings from studies such as Lawton's (1972) suggest that personality changes characteristic of the "crisis of finitude" take place among psychiatrically ill middle-aged men and women just as they do among psychologically well counterparts. This increased congruence of outlook may at least partially offset strains experienced by older parents caring for older offspring who are in a better position than earlier in life to understand parental concerns regarding self and future.

At the same time, a cohort effect among the ill offspring's peers may occur: same-age friends, classmates, neighbors, and cousins may also have failed in some way. These "nondisabled" adult children may have developed alcohol and drug problems, suffered divorces, lost jobs, and experienced other hardships which have forced their elderly parents to resume some type of caregiving. As a result, the ill child's role performance may not be as poor relative to same-age peers as when he or she was in the "launching" stage of adulthood with its seemingly unlimited potential. In addition, parents may also experience a cohort effect as they now find that other same-age parents are dealing with similar burdens related to providing care for their adult "problem" children.

To date, we know little about this issue, just as we know little about historical cohort differences in the experience of caring for an afflicted relative. The widespread use of antipsychotic medication and emphasis upon deinstitutionalization may lead to a group of older schizophrenic patients more competent and able to both help their parents and do household chores than among prior cohorts of older recurrently ill psychiatric patients. Educational level of parent must be considered as well: prior cohorts of older parents caring for older psychiatric patients were less well educated and less able to use community resources than the present cohort of older parents. These parents may have first encountered serious psychiatric illness among offspring at a time when psychiatry maintained that the origins of this illness were to be attributed largely to deviant family socialization processes. Self-help advocacy groups now exist to provide support, assistance, and advice, which were unknown within previous cohorts.[8]

Comparative Study of Family Caretaking Burdens in Later Life

There is some evidence that parents may ultimately accommodate to the recurrent nature of the schizophrenic offspring's illness. However, much of this evidence is based on impressionistic or clinical case observations, or on studies showing a relationship between long illnesses and lower parental burden among support group members who may be atypical family caregivers (Cohler, Borden, Groves, & Lazarus, 1988). To date, there has been little study of the impact of time upon the experience of caregiving. While some studies suggest such increased accommodation to the caregiving role over time as relatives learn to manage the illness, other studies suggest that time increases sense of burden, at least among families with a schizophrenic offspring (Hoenig & Hamilton, 1966; Noh & Turner, 1987). It is also likely that time will have a differential effect on different types of burden. For example, while financial resources may be dwindling for elderly parents, their greater understanding of the illness, stemming from increased congruence of parent and offspring outlook on the very course and meaning of life, may allow them to separate themselves emotionally from their adult child's problems, permitting them to lead increasingly productive and fulfilling lives.

A search of the literature revealed few studies addressing problems of older parents providing care for continuing episodically troubled middle-aged and older offspring. Only one report (Stevens, 1972) has provided more than anecdotal information regarding the problem of caregiving for an older relative. This study was based on a British community needs survey of 56 unemployed psychiatric patients and their elderly relatives (aged 59 to 90); in over half of the cases (67%) offspring were residing with their relatives. Stevens notes that in these cases the relative was often old and lonely, and glad of the patient's presence in the home.[9] While relatives accepted the presence of their ill family member, they also reported its disadvantages and tended to evaluate the arrangement less favorably than did the ill offspring.

Much of the parental concern expressed among parents studied by Stevens was focused on anxiety over plans for their offspring's future rather than tensions generated by living with a recurrently troubled offspring. In nearly all cases, but particularly in mother-offspring households, the parent worried about the patient's future and living circumstances after the parent's death.[10] Stevens suggests that offspring impairment might provide suitable companions for elderly parents since the impaired offspring spends much time at home, is not discontented with lack of leisure pursuits, and prefers low amounts of socialization. However, this interdependence of older parents and their impaired offspring may foster its own kind of withdrawal, reminiscent of institutionalism. Special housing arrangements are suggested as one way to avoid such withdrawal.

Caregiving Parallels for Schizophrenic and Alzheimer Patients

The scarcity of literature in this area requires comparative study in order to understand the burden and response to family caregiving across the second half of life. Significantly, two recent papers (Lefley, 1987c; Wasow, 1985) have posed a particularly interesting paradox: Older parents caring for middle-aged and older schizophrenic or retarded offspring face problems in many ways akin to the middle-aged offspring's caring for an older parent with Alzheimer's disease. In each instance (at least given present understanding of etiology), the relative's life is drastically altered as a result of a family member's illness. Caretakers are forced to deal with socially unacceptable behaviors over which the patient may have little control but which are offensive. Caregiver burden is also increased by the off-time, age-inappropriate nature of the caregiving responsibility (Cohler, Borden, Groves, & Lazarus, 1988).

In each situation, caretakers mourn for what might have been, express concern regarding the future, and must balance a complex set of role demands in order to ensure continuity of caregiving. In each instance, caretakers must deal with a health-care system that often delivers complex and ambiguous messages. Provision of certain types of care (such as home care) for afflicted adults may magnify problems of family enmeshment, making it more difficult for caretakers to differentiate their own needs from those of the afflicted family member. Problems of stigma, the social isolation of the caretaker from others who might assist in alleviating the difficulties of role strain and overload, and provision of assistance with care are all common to the two caregiving situations. Problems of violence in the enactment of frustration toward the ill family member may be observed in the case of each illness. Management of disruptive behavior and ensuing feelings of guilt, frustration, and resentment characterize each of these caregiving situations. However, middle-aged caregivers of patients with Alzheimer's disease worry somewhat less about controlling disruptive behavior than older parents looking after middle-aged and older schizophrenic offspring.

Caretakers in each instance share concern about what their death might do to the continuity of the caregiving situation. In particular, aged parents of middle-aged and older schizophrenic offspring feel unable to count on other relatives within their own age cohort and must depend upon younger relatives such as children, while caretakers of Alzheimer's patients may look to a same-age child or in-law to take over caregiving. In general, the norm of arranging for the care of impaired elderly parents is much stronger than the norm of providing care to a disabled sibling, especially when the disability is recurrent psychiatric illness. Given a greater amount of normative ambiguity, it is perhaps not surprising to find less stress among Alzheimer caretaking families than among families dealing with schizophrenia. For example, older parents caring for their older schizophrenic offspring felt less competent than family members caring for an older relative with Alzheimer's disease (Lefley, 1987a, 1987b, 1987c). Wasow (1985) notes that caretakers of patients with Alzheimer's disease mourn for the past, while caretakers of persons with schizophrenia mourn for the future and what might have been.[11]

Caregiving Parallels for Schizophrenia and Mental Retardation

Study of family caregiving for older adult mentally retarded members provides an additional perspective for understanding caregiver issues among older psychiatrically ill offspring and their older parents. While nearly all parents of developmentally disabled offspring have been coping with their child's limitations since his or her preschool years (as compared to the majority of parents whose son or daughter characteristically became psychiatrically ill during late adolescence· or early adulthood) recent studies report several problems encountered by older parents of mentally retarded adults which parents of older psychiatrically ill offspring may also face, including concern for the mentally handicapped child's future following the death of one or both parents and caregiving burdens in the parents' lives as a result of continual involvement with the disabled offspring (Farber & Rowitz, 1987; Goodman, 1978).

Mentally retarded adults and chronically psychiatrically ill offspring often have few personal resources enabling them to function independently; most developmentally disabled older adults depend heavily upon their families and/or public or private facilities to help them meet their needs. Once the developmentally disabled child reaches the age past which state and federal laws mandate schooling, there are very few programs tailored to the needs of these retarded adults (Birenbaum, 1973; Roos, McCann, & Addison, 1980). Caregiving responsibilities fall particularly heavily upon the family, for whom there are also very limited support services (Golan, 1981; Seltzer, 1985; Wikler, 1986; Wikler, Wasow, & Hatfield, 1981).

Findings from two studies (Farber & Rowtiz, 1987; Suelzle & Keenan, 1981) show that parents of older mentally retarded persons feel a particular lack of community support and social isolation. There are limited alternatives to familial care: long-term sheltered care facilities may be too expensive or have a long waiting list if available at all; workshops may provide some financial assistance but few residential services; healthy siblings may not want to take on the caregiving responsibilities; parents generally believe that it is not right to burden other children with caretaking responsibility for the care of their developmentally disabled siblings. These problems are shared by parents of adult physically ill offspring, including long waiting lists for psychiatric board and care homes, rehabilitation programs geared toward younger mentally ill patients, and the ever-present problem of providing adequate care after the parents' deaths.

Birenbaum (1971) and Farber (1968) have both reported that it becomes more difficult to cope with a mentally retarded child as the patient grows older. Romer and Berkson (1980a, 1980b, 1981) report that older mentally retarded persons have fewer friends, converse less, and are less affectionate than intellectually normal counterparts. Parents must deal on a daily basis with offspring who over the years have become increasingly dysfunctional, requiring continuing continuous care. Caregiving family members of older developmentally disabled persons who were more functionally impaired had lower activity levels and reported lower levels of life satisfaction (Mindel & Wright, 1982). This may also be true for those mentally ill adults whose symptoms increase or worsen with advancing age, making it difficult to maintain them in the family home.

CONCLUSION

Study of adults hospitalized for schizophrenia and their caregiving relatives, primarily parents, provides important information regarding the role of family processes in contemporary society, including the manner in which the family responds to crises which may extend over periods of many decades, together with factors determining variation in family use of both personal and community resources as a means of assistance in providing continuing care. Recognition that families undertake such care and discharge responsibility for this care, often over periods of many decades, calls into question claims of lessened significance of the family as a continuing source of socialization and support across the course of life. Such recognition also acknowledges the social, political, and therapeutic changes which have placed caregiving in the hands of families for certain illnesses now defined to be "in the community" treated through "home care."

While there has been some study of family response to offspring psychiatric illness, much of this study was undertaken either in an effort to prove socialization processes within the family as the "cause" of this distress or as a means of accounting for subsequent hospitalizations following discharge from care. Earlier studies of the transmission of irrationality or communication deviance within the family differ little from more recent studies of family emotional response as a precipitant of subsequent episodes of illness in their emphasis upon the family as the source of personal distress (Kanter, Lamb & Loeper, 1987). Much less often, it is realized that such distortions of expectable patterns of communication may be the consequence rather than the cause of the disturbance, the result of the patient's personal disorganization and socially unacceptable behavior.

The alternation of episodes of illness or disturbance, with periods of illness-free functioning, makes it additionally difficult for family members to respond effectively to these episodes. If the afflicted patient is an adult offspring, each episode may serve as a continuing reminder of the offspring's deficit, a disappointment to parental expectations and ambitions, and a foreshadowing of problems in providing for continuing care in the event of the parent's infirmity or death. While willing to provide care for afflicted offspring, literature reported in this chapter suggests, parents attempt to protect the patient's brothers and sisters from being emotionally or financially burdened by this caregiving.

The patient's recurrent personal distress, accompanied by inappropriate behavior, has become a nightmare for parents and other caregivers. Problems in ensuring the patient's compliance with medication whose side effects may be nearly as frightening as the illness itself has proven to be a particular burden for family members responsible for the lives of these troubled persons. Indeed, all surveys to date show marked dissatisfaction with the mental health delivery system among relatives of psychiatric patients. It is clear that mental health professionals are often not accessible and supportive of the family's caregiving efforts. Self-help advocacy groups have become an important mediating factor between cargiving families and mental health professionals, as in the case of families providing care for Alzheimer's patients and, more recently, parents of developmentally disabled persons. Family caretakers for schizophrenic patients increasingly rely upon these advocacy groups for assistance and advice.

While these organizations may be helpful for those families able to reach out to the community for support and assistance, many families react to crisis by imploding upon themselves, withdrawing from precisely those community institutions so essential for the family's continued adaptation. To date, little is known about families differing in their ability to profit from community services and differing in their response to illness by reaching out or withdrawing from formal and informal sources of support. The work of Reiss and his colleagues represents an important first step in determining aspects of family structure and process related to differences in the use of the psychiatric hospital and aftercare services (Reiss, Costell, Jones, & Berkman, 1980).

This work has important implications more generally for the study of ways in which families use services in contemporary society and hopefully will be extended to focus on the particular issues involved in help seeking by older families. Much of the study of vulnerable episodically ill psychiatric patients and their families has been confined to young adults and their parents. While there has been some work on pathways to the psychiatric hospital and adjustment in the period following first psychiatric hospitalization, including the relationship between family expectations and emotional response to the patient as a determinant of posthospital role performance, there has been little study of these issues over longer periods of time. Often, discussion of this issue trails off into generalized statements about the years of coping with episodes of illness and attendant hospitalizations.

With the aging of society, there are increasing numbers of older vulnerable family members and their older parent caregivers. The significance of caregiving for a middle-aged or older psychiatric patient is markedly different from that for a younger patient. Not only has there been a shift in the balance of positive and negative symptoms, with successive psychotic episodes often less florid across the second half of life, but also patient and parent may increasingly share a common outlook on life based on congruity in their concern with issues of interiority and finitude of life. At the same time, as parents grow older, they have less energy and ability to support troubled offspring through successive episodes. Concern about how offspring will manage without them, desire to prevent the ill offspring from becoming a burden for other family members such as brothers and sisters, and provision of continhued supervision for the activities of daily living are paramount among the concerns of these older parents.

To date, there has been little study of the older psychiatric patient and caregiving older parents. What little study has been reported has been based on anecdotal reports and extrapolation from studies of younger psychiatric patients and their families. At least two papers have noted the commonalities between provision of care in schizophrenia and Alzheimer's disease. While in the latter illness it is most often the middle-aged and older offspring who is caring for an older parent, in the former illness the older parent continues to care for the middle-aged or older offspring. However, many of the burdens and coping techniques appear common to both illnesses.

Each illness is characterized by socially disruptive and often personally threatening behavior. However, Alzheimer's disease generally occurs after a lifetime of expectable family life, while the onset of schizophrenia, often in the patient's late teens or twenties, leads to a lifetime of disrupted social relations within the family. However, each illness involves issues of stigma and behavior which is socially unacceptable. Each illness typically involves provision of care from an ever-widening radius of caregivers within the family, involving more and less distant relatives, with an impact upon the mental health of a number of family members. The parallels between the two forms of illness highlight the importance of studying the patient and the family, not following just initial episodes of disturbance but across the course of life.

Just as in the study of Alzheimer's disease, there are likely to be important differences in family caregiving response, depending on whether the caregiving relative is a spouse, sibling, or parent. If advances in community treatment result in greater numbers of schizophrenic young adults realizing normative life transitions to career, marriage, and parenthood, the relative with major caregiving responsibility may shift from the parent to the spouse. Similarly, as parents of the first cohorts of deinstitutionalized patients begin to die off, an increasing proportion of older caregivers may be siblings rather than parents. Understanding of such demographic trends may assume increasing importance in planning for successive cohorts of mentally ill now growing older in the community.

As this chapter has shown, life-course social science is able to make an important contribution not only to study of normative processes but also to the study of the course of psychiatric illness. Regardless of assumed origin, psychiatric illness is unique both in the nature of burden posed for family caregivers and coping techniques required in responding to the patient's changing impact upon the family across the adult life course. Understanding the family's response to the illness, together with the significance of particular symptoms for management by the caregiving family unit, is enhanced by adoption of a family life-course perspective. Recognition of the concept of cohort is important in studying differences over time in the way family caregivers respond to episodes of psychiatric illness. Many older parents in the present cohort of parents recall a time when the origins of schizophrenia were assumed to be related to faulty forward socialization. As a consequence, these older parents may feel greater guilt regarding their offspring's episodic illness than will be characteristic of later cohorts of parents understanding the origins of this illness in dispositionally based vulnerability.

Concepts such as reciprocal socialization—useful in explaining the frequently observed phenomena in which parents of schizophrenic offspring appear to share a disorder of interpersonal communication, sequence, and timing of anticipated entrances and exits from characteristic roles in the expectable portfolio of adult social roles and the impact of social timing upon experience of self and others—all become important in understanding the process of caregiving in families and defining problems posed for relatives attempting care of psychiatrically disabled family members. Family life-course perspectives are also important in understanding variation in use of community resources which may support family caregiving efforts and in the changing ability of the family to respond to these personal and collective crises over periods of many years. Life-course perspectives emphasize the significance of studying family caregiving in the context of society over time, fostering integration of study of family processes in responding to major psychiatric disturbance which are parallel to larger social changes such as those related to patterns of hospitalization and aftercare.

NOTES

1. While some studies have reported relatives' emotional response to the presence of a psychiatrically troubled relative (Avrey & Wahrheit, 1980; Freeman & Simmons, 1961; Thompson & Doll, 1982), this subjective sense of burden is characteristically measured by feelings of anxiety and depression, regarded in the present instance as the outcome factor, or "X," viewed in terms of Hill-Minnesota family stress model.

2. Reviewing studies to date of burden of psychiatric illness of any relative upon the family unit, Gubman, Tessler, and Willis (1987), observing that the very concept of burden assumes the same stigmatized role for the patient within the family as was once assumed for the parents, prefer the term *impact* rather than *burden*.

3. The emerging field of neuroimmunology has begun to study the manner in which role strain among caretakers may lead to impairment in health. To date, little is known regarding the complex interaction between caretaking and health. Clearly, both the nature of adversity, including the character of the afflicted patient's personally and socially threatening symptoms, as well as feelings of caring, and living up to own image of self as a caretaking person, fostering increased feelings of personal integration (Cohler & Galatzer-Levy, 1990; Kohut, 1977), may serve as a "buffering" factor in determining the extent to which caretaker strain may lead to impaired health (Terkelsen, 1987). Much more needs to be learned regarding the meaning of caregiving to family caregivers in illnesses such as recurrent schizophrenia and Alzheimer's disease.

4. While, understandably, there has been considerable concern with those families reporting significant negative impact as a consequence of offspring psychiatric illness, there has been little study of families reporting little impact of this caregiving or of the means these families use in coping with the tasks of caregiving to episodically troubled offspring.

5. Nearly half of these family members expressed feelings of resentment and frustration regarding the caretaking demands expected of them, but there is little evidence that

this feeling was translated into the "expressed (hostile) emotions" portrayed by Leff and Vaughn (1985) and believed to be enacted as a source of conflict precipitating rehospitalization.

6. Most recently, Cook (1988) has shown that both the objective burden of caregiving, and the experienced sense of interpersonal isolation as burdened caretaker, is distinctive among mothers of seriously disturbed offspring. The mental health of fathers was far less profoundly affected. Women caretakers reported both greater objective and experienced burden than men. Particularly significant in this analysis was that experienced burden was more highly associated than objective burden with overall caretaker adjustment.

7. Another possibility is that parents' ability to deal with illness actually *improves* over time: older parents of older offspring may be less burdened by psychiatric illness, both objectively and/or subjectively. It is also possible that one type of burden lessens while the other worsens. Such proposals can find foundation in the findings presented below, which indicate far from unanimously negative effects of caretaking on older parents.

8. It is interesting to note that virtually all studies of the impact of caring for a relative with Alzheimer's disease, even increased study of the disease itself, have occurred within the past few years in a cohort of both caretakers and professionals involved in Alzheimer advocacy groups. Further, Alzheimer patients don't come to the illness and caretaking situation with the degree of prior care and disappointments characteristic of schizophrenic patients.

9. The issue of social isolation is a problem both in normative studies of later life and study of mental health and aging. While Stevens assumes that having an impaired offspring living in the parental household may reduce feelings of social isolation, it must be remembered that there is little evidence to suggest that older adults are in fact socially isolated (Lowenthal, 1964; Lowenthal & Robinson, 1976). Too often, social scientists studying aging assume that reduced interpersonal contact, so important among younger adults, translates into increased sense of social isolation among older adults. While younger adults depend in large measure upon continuing ties with others as a source of support and comfort at times of infirmity, older adults may rely upon memories of the past for such solace (Cohler, 1983; Cohler & Galatzer-Levy, 1990). These memories of the past may be more significant in fostering continued adjustment among older persons than actual social ties which may be less satisfying than reminiscence, particularly when such ties demand extensive caregiving. It is still not clear whether living alone or living with an impaired elder offspring is of greater importance in fostering the adjustment among older adults.

10. Davies (1968) reports that parental death was a major factor accounting for rehospitalization of aged schizophrenic patients.

11. The historical development of information about the two illnesses is somewhat dissimilar, with models of origin stressing the family as determinant of psychotic symptoms posing a burden which is not present among caretakers of patients with Alzheimer's disease. With less family blaming and greater acceptance for a disease viewed as physical rather than mental, these families may be in a different relationship to health-care delivery systems (such as that built around gerontology, which is expanding and healthy) than families forced to deal with our nation's current mental health system, which is in disarray and underfunded (Torrey & Wolfe, 1986).

REFERENCES

Avrey, S., & Wahrheit, G. (1980). Psychological costs of living with psychologically disturbed family members. In L. Robins, P. Clayton, & J. Wing (Eds.), *The social consequences of psychiatric illness* (pp. 158-175). New York: Brunner/Mazel.

Ashbaugh, J. W., Leaf, P., Manderscheid, R., et al. (1983). Estimates of the size and selected characteristics of the adult chronically mentally ill population living in U.S. households. In J. Greenley & R. Simmons (Eds.), *Research in community and mental health*, 3, (pp. 3-24). Greenwich, CT: JAL Press.

Berger, P. L., & Kellner, H. (1964). Marriage and the construction of reality. *Diogenes, 46*, 1-10.

Birenbaum, A. (1971). The mentally retarded child in the home and the family cycle. *Journal of Health and Social Behavior, 12*, 55-65.

Bleuler, E. (1911/1950). *Dementia Praecox or the group of schizophrenias* (H. Zinkin, Trans.). New York: International Universities Press.

Bleuler, M. (1978). *The schizophrenic disorders: Long-term patient and family studies* (S. M. Clems, Trans.). New Haven, CT: Yale University Press.

Blumer, H. (1969/1976). *Symbolic interactionism: perspective and method*. Berkeley, CA: The University of California Press.

Bridge, T., Cannon, E., & Wyatt, R. (1978). Burned out schizophrenia: Evidence for age-effects on schizophrenic symptomology. *Journal of Gerontology, 33*, 835-839.

Brown, G., Birely, J., & Wing, J. (1972). Influence of family life in the course of the schizophrenic disorders: A replication. *British Journal of Psychiatry, 121*, 241-258.

Brown, G., Monck, E., Carstairs, G, & Wing, J. (1962). Influence of family life in the course of schizophrenic illness. *British Journal of Preventative and Social Medicine, 16*, 55-68.

Brunn, L. (1985, March). Elderly parent and dependent adult child. *The Journal of Contemporary Social Work*, 131-138.

Burgess, E. (1926). The family as a unity of interacting personalities. *Family, 7*, 3-9.

Butler, R. (1963). The "life review": An interpretation of reminiscence in the aged. *Psychiatry, 26*, 65-76.

Carlisle, W. (1984). *Siblings of the mentally ill*. Saratoga, CA: R & E Publishers.

Cicirelli, V. (1980). Sibling relations in adulthood. In L. W. Poon (Ed.), *Aging in the 1980s* (pp. 455-462). Washington, DC: American Psychological Association.

Cicirelli, V. (1985). The role of siblings as family caretakers. In W. Sauer & R. Coward (Eds.), *Social support networks and the care of the elderly: Theory, research, and practice* (pp. 93-107). New York: Springer Publishing Company.

Clausen, J. (1984a). Mental illness and the life course. In P. B. Baltes and O. G. Brim, Jr. (Eds.), *Life-Span Development and Behavior* (Vol. 6, pp. 204-242). New York: Academic Press.

Clausen, J. (1984b). A fifteen to twenty year follow-up of married adult psychiatric patients. In L. Erlenmeyer-Kimling, N. Miller, & B. Dohrenwend (Eds.), *Life-span Research on the Prediction of Psychopathology* (pp. 175-194). New York: Academic Press.

Clausen, J., & Yarrow, M. (1955a). Introduction: Mental illness and the family. *Journal of Social Issues, 11*, 3-5.

Clausen, J., & Yarrow, M. (1955b). Paths to the mental hospital. *Journal of Social Issues, 11*, 25-32.

Clausen, J., & Yarrow, M. (1955c). Further observations and some implications. *Journal of Social Issues, 11*, 61-65.

Clausen, J., Yarrow, M., Deasy, L., & Schwartz, C. (1955). The impact of mental illness: Research formulation. *Journal of Social Issues, 11*, 6-11.

Cohler, B. (1983). Autonomy and interdependence in the family of adulthood: A psychological perspective. *The Gerontologists, 23*, 33-39.

Cohler, B. (1987/1988). The adult daughter relationship: Perspective from life-course family study and psychoanalysis. *Journal of Geriatric Psychiatry, 21*, 51-72.

Cohler, B., Borden, W., Groves, L., & Lazarus, L. (1988). Caring for family members with Alzheimer's disease. In E. Light & B. Lebowitz (Eds.), *Alzheimer's disease, treatment, and family stress* (pp. 50-105). Washington, DC: U.S. Government Printing Office.

Cohler, B., & Ferrono, C. (1987). Schizophrenia and the adult life-course. In N. E. Miller & G. Cohen (Eds.), *Schizophrenia and aging* (pp. 189-200). New York: The Guilford Press.

Cohler, B., & Galatzer-Levy, R. (1990). Self, meaning and morale across the second-half of life. In R. Nemiroff & C. Colarusso (Eds.), *New dimensions in adult development* (pp. 214-259). New York: Basic Books.

Cook, J. (1988). Who "mothers" the chronically mentally ill. *Family Relations, 37*, 42-49.

Cook, J. A., & Cohler, B. (1986). Reciprocal socialization and the care of offspring with cancer and with schizophrenia. *Life-span Developmental Psychology, 9*, 101-129.

Cook, J. A., & Pickett, S. (1985). *Feelings of burden among parents residing with chronically mentally ill offspring.* Paper presented at the annual meeting of the National Association of Social Work, Chicago, Illinois.

Cook, J. A., & Pickett, S. (1988). Feelings of burden and disappointment among parents residing with chronically mentally ill offspring. *Journal of Applied Social Sciences, 12*, 79-107.

Costell, R., & Reiss, D. (1982). The family meets the hospital: Clinical presentation of a laboratory-based family typology. *Archives of General Psychiatry, 39*, 433-438.

Cumming, E., & Henry, W. (1961). *Growing old.* New York: Basic Books.

Davies, G. (1968). Family relationships of elderly mental hospital patients. *Australian and New Zealand Journal of Psychiatry, 2*, 264-271.

Davis, J. (1974). Use of psychotropic drugs. *Journal of Geriatric Psychiatry, 7*, 148-159.

Dearth, N., Lebanski, B., Mott, M., & Pellegrini, L. (1986). *Families helping families: Living with schizophrenia.* New York: W. W. Norton.

Erentheil, O. (1962). Behavioral changes of aging chronic psychotics. In R. Kastenbaum (Ed.), *New thoughts on old age* (pp. 99-115). New York: Springer Publishing Company.

Evans, A., Bullard, D., Jr., & Solomon, M. (1961). The family as a potential resource in the rehabilitation of the chronic schizophrenic patient. *American Journal of Psychiatry, 117*, 1075-1083.

Farber, B. (1968). *Mental retardation: Its social context and social consequences.* Boston: Houghton Mifflin.

Farber, B., & Rowitz, L. (1987). *Stress and reciprocity in kin networks: Parents of retarded offspring in later years.* Paper presented at the annual meeting of the American Sociological Association, Chicago, Illinois.

Freeman, H., & Simmons, O. (1961). Treatment experiences of mental patients and their families. *American Journal of Public Health, 51*, 1266-1273.

Golan, N. (1981). *Passing through transitions: A guide for practitioners.* New York: The Free Press.

Goldman, H. (1982). Mental illness and family burden: A public health perspective. *Hospital and Community Psychiatry, 33,* 557–560.

Goodman, D. (1978). Parenting an adult mentally retarded offspring. *Smith College Studies in Social Work, 48,* 209–234.

Grad, J., & Sainsbury, P. (1963, March 9). Mental illness and the family. *Lancet,* 544–547.

Grad, J., & Sainsbury, P. (1968). The effects that patients have on their families in a community care and a control psychiatric service—A two year follow-up. *British Journal of Psychiatry, 114,* 265–278.

Greenblatt, M., Levinson, D., & Williams, R. (1957). *The patient and the mental hospital.* New York: The Free Press/Macmillan.

Gubman, G., Tessler, R., & Willis, G. (1987). Living with the mentally ill—Factors affecting household complaints. *Schizophrenia Bulletin, 13,* 727–736.

Gutmann, D. (1987). *Reclaimed powers: Toward a psychology of men and women in later life.* New York: Basic Books.

Harding, C., & Brooks, G. (1984). Life assessment of a cohort of chronic schizophrenics discharged 20 years ago. In S. Mednick, X. Harway, & X. Finello (Eds.), *Handbook of longitudinal research* (Vol. 2, pp. 375–393). New York: Praeger.

Harding, C., Brooks, G., Ashikaga, T., Strauss, J., & Landerl, P. (1987). Aging and social functioning in once-chronic schizophrenic patients 22-62 years after first admission: The Vermont story. In N. E. Miller & G. Cohen (Eds.), *Schizophrenia and aging* (pp. 74–82). New York: The Guilford Press.

Harkins, E. (1978). Effects of e-n transition on self-report of psychological and physical well-being. *Journal of Marriage and the Family, 40,* 549–555.

Hatfield, A. (1978). Psychological costs of schizophrenia to the family. *Social Work, 23,* 355–359.

Hatfield, A. (1979). The family as partner in the treatment of mental illness. *Hospital and Community Psychiatry, 30,* 338–349.

Hatfield, A. (1981). Self-help groups for families of the mentally ill. *Social Work, 26,* 408–413.

Hatfield, A. (1987a). Systems resistance to effective family coping. In A. T. Meyerson (Ed.), *Barriers to treating the chronic mentally ill* (pp. 51–62). San Francisco: Jossey-Bass.

Hatfield, A. (1987b). Families as caregivers: A historical perspective. In A. Hatfield & H. P. Lefley (Eds.), *Families of the mentally ill: Coping and adaption* (pp. 3–29). New York: The Guilford Press.

Hatfield, A. (1987c). Social support and family coping. In A. Hatfield & H. P. Lefley (Eds.), *Families of the mentally ill: Coping and adaption* (pp. 191–207). New York: The Guilford Press.

Hoenig, J., & Hamilton, M. (1966). The schizophrenic patient in the community and his effect on the household. *British Journal of Psychiatry, 20,* 165–176.

Jacobs, S., Mason, J., & Kosten, T. (1986). Bereavement and catecholamines. *Journal of Psychosomatic Research, 30,* 489–496.

Jacques, E. (1965). Death and the mid-life crisis. *International Journal of Psychoanalysis, 46,* 502–514.

Jacques, E. (1980). The mid-life crisis. In S. Greenspan & G. Pollock (Eds.), *The course of life, III: adulthood and aging* (pp. 1–23). Washington, DC: U.S. Government Printing Office.

Jung, H., Spaniol, L., & Anthony, W. (1983). *Family coping and schizophrenia.* Unpublished manuscript, Center for Rehabilitation Research and Training in Mental Health, Boston University.

Kanter, J., Lamb, H., & Loeper, C. (1987). Expressed emotion in families: A critical review. *Hospital and Community Psychiatry, 38,* 374–380.

Kay, D., & Bergman, K. (1980). Epidemiology of mental disorders among the aged in the community. In J. Birren & R. B. Sloane (Eds.), *Handbook of mental health and aging* (pp. 34–56). Englewood Cliffs, NJ: Prentice-Hall.

Kay, D., & Roth, M. (1961). Environmental and heredity factors in schizophrenia of old age ('late paraphrenia') and their bearing on the general problem of causation in schizophrenia. *Journal of Mental Science, 107,* 649–686.

Kay, D., & Roth, M. (1963). Schizophrenia of old age. In R. Williams, C. Tibbits, & W. Donahue (Eds.), *Processing of aging: Social and psychological perspectives, vol. I* (pp. 402–448). New York: Atherton-Prentice-Hall.

Kasl, S. (1984). Stress and health. *Annual Review of Public Health, 5,* 319.

Kohut, H. (1977). *The restoration of the self.* New York: International Universities Press.

Kraeplin, E. (1913/1919). Dementia praecox and paraphrenia. In E. Kraeplin (Ed.), *Textbook of psychiatry, vol. 3: Endogenous dementias* (R. Barclay, Trans.). Edinburgh: E. S. Livingstone.

Kreisman, D., & Joy, V. (1976). The family as a reactor to the mental illness of a relative. In M. Guttentag & E. Streuning (Eds.), *Handbook of evaluation research, vol. 2* (pp. 483–516). Beverly Hills, CA: Sage Publications.

Lawton, P. (1972). Schizophrenia forty-five years later. *The Journal of Genetic Psychology, 121,* 133–145.

Lazarus, R., & Folkman, S. (1984). *Stress, appraisal, and coping.* New York: Springer Publishing Company.

Leff, J., & Vaughn, C. (1980). The interaction of life events and relatives' expressed emotion in schizophrenia and depressive neurosis, *British Journal of Psychiatry, 136,* 146–153.

Leff, J., & Vaughn, C. (1985). *Expressed emotion in families.* New York: Guilford Press.

Lefley, H. (1987a). The family's response to mental illness in a relative. In A. Hatfield (Ed.), *Families of the mentally ill: Meeting the challenges* (New Directions in Mental Health Monograph 22) (pp. 31–22). San Francisco: Jossey-Bass.

Lefley, H. (1987b). An adaptation framework: Its meaning for research and practice. In A. Hatfield & H. P. Lefley (Eds.), *Families of the mentally ill: Coping and adaptation* (pp. 307–330). New York: The Guilford Press.

Lefley, H. (1987c). Aging parents as caregivers of mentally ill adult children: An emerging social problem. *Hospital and Community Psychiatry, 10,* 1063–1070.

Lidz, T. (1973). *The origin and treatment of schizophrenic disorders.* New York: Basic Books.

Liem, J. (1974). Intrafamily communication and schizophrenic though disorder: An etiologic or responsive relationship. *The Clinical Psychologist, 29,* 28–30.

Liem, J. (1980). Family studies of schizophrenia: An update and commentary. *Schizophrenia Bulletin., 6,* 429–455.

Lowenthal, M. F. (1964). Social isolation and mental illness in old age. *American Sociological Review*, *29*, 54–70.

Lowenthal, M. F., & Robinson, B. (1976). Social networks and isolation. In R. Binstock & E. Shanas (Eds.), *Handbook of aging and the social sciences* (pp. 432–456). New York: Van-Nostrand, Reinhold.

Marshall, V. (1975). Age and awareness of finitude in developmental gerontology. *Omega*, *6*, 113–129.

Marshall, V. (1981). *Last chapters: A sociology of death and dying*. Belmont: CA: Wordsworth Publishing Company.

Marshall, V. (1986). A sociological perspective on aging and dying. In V. Marshall (Ed.), *Later life: The social psychology of aging* (pp. 125–149). Beverly Hills, CA: Sage Publications.

McCubbin, H., & Figley, C. (1983). Bridging normative and catastrophic family stress. In H. McCubbin & C. Figley (Eds.), *Stress and the family, volume I: Coping with normative transitions* (pp. 218–228). New York: Brunner/Mazel.

McCubbin, H., Nevin, R., Cauble, A. E., Larsen, A., Comeau, J., & Patterson, J. (1982). Families coping with chronic illness: The case of cerebral palsy. In H. McCubbin, A. E. Cauble, & J. Patterson (Eds.), *Family stress, coping, and social support* (pp. 169–188). Springfield, IL: Charles Thomas.

McCubbin, H., & Patterson, J. (1983). The family stress process: The double ABCX model of adjustment and adaptation. *Social stress and the family: Advances and developments in family stress theory and research. Marriage and Family Review*, *6*, 7–38.

McFarlane, W. (1983). *Family therapy in schizophrenia*. New York: Guilford Press.

Mederer, H., & Hill, R. (1983). Critical transitions over the family life span: Theory and Research. *Social stress and the family: Advances and developments in family stress theory and research. Marriage and Family Review*, *6*, 39–60.

Mindel, C., & Wright, R. (1982). Satisfaction in multigeneration households. *Journal of Gerontology*, *37*, 483–489.

Minkoff, K. (1979). A map of chronic mental patients. In J. Talbott (Ed.), *The chronic mental patient* (pp. 11–37). Washington, DC: American Psychiatric Association.

Mishler, E., & Waxler, N. (1965/1968). Family interaction process and schizophrenia: A review of current theories. In E. Mishler & N. Waxler (Eds.), *Family processes and schizophrenia* (pp. 3–62). New York: Science House.

Mishler, E., & Waxler, N. (1968). *Schizophrenia in families: An experimental study of family process and schizophrenia*. New York: Wiley.

Moos, R., & Tsu, B. (1976). A typology of family social environments. *Family Process*, *15*, 357–371.

Muller, C. (1963). The influence of age on schizophrenia. In R. Williams, C. Tibbitts, & W. Donahue (Eds.), *Processes of aging: Social and psychological aspects* (Vol. 1, pp. 504–511). New York: Atherton Press.

Muller, C. (1971). Schizophrenia in advanced senescence. *British Journal of Psychiatry*, *118*, 347–348.

Munnichs, J. (1966). *Old age and finitude: A contribution to psychogerontology*. New York: Karger.

National Alliance for the Mentally Ill. (1987). *National Alliance for the Mentally Ill: 1987 Annual Convention Program*. Arlington, VA: Authors.

Neugarten, B. (1973). Personality change in late life: A developmental perspective. In C. Eisdorfer & M. P. Lawton (Eds.), *The psychology of adult development* (pp. 311–338). Washington, DC: The American Psychological Association.

Neugarten, B. (1979). Time, age, and the life-cycle. *American Journal of Psychiatry, 136*, 887–894.

Neugarten, B., & Datan, N. (1974). The middle years. In S. Arieti (Ed.), *American handbook of psychiatry, vol. I: Foundations of psychiatry* (pp. 592–606). New York: Basic Books.

Neugarten, B., Moore, J., & Lowe, J. (1965). Age norms, age constraints, and adult socialization. *The American Journal of Sociology, 70*, 710–717.

Neugebauer, R. (1980). Formulation of hypotheses about the true prevalence of functional and organic disorders among the elderly in the United States. In B. Dohrenwend, B. Dohrenwend, M. Gould, B. Link, R. Neugebauer, & R. Wunsch-Hitzig, (Eds.), *Mental illness in the United States: Epidemiological estimates* (pp. 95–113). New York: Praeger.

Noh, S., & Turner, R. J. (1987). Living with psychiatric patients: Implications for the mental health of family members. *Social Science and Medicine, 25*, 263–271.

Pearlin, L., & Schooler, C. (1978). The structure of coping. *Journal of Health and Social Behavior, 19*, 2–21.

Reiss, D., Costell, R., Jones, C., & Berkman, H. (1980). The family meets the hospital: A laboratory forecast of the encounter. *Archives of General Psychiatry, 37*, 141–154.

Richardson, D. (1987). President's column. *National Alliance for the Mentally Ill News, 8*(2), 1.

Romer, D., & Berkson, G. (1980a). Social ecology of supervised communal facilities for mentally disabled adults. II: Predictors of affiliation. *American Journal of Mental Deficiency, 85*, 243–252.

Romer, D., & Berkson, G. (1980b). Social ecology of supervised communal facilities for mentally disabled adults. III: Predictors of social choice. *American Journal of Mental Deficiency, 85*, 243–252.

Romer, D., & Berkson, G. (1981). Social ecology of supervised communal facilities for mentally disabled adults. IV: Characteristics of social behavior. *American Journal of Mental Deficiency, 86*, 28–38.

Roos, H., McCann, B., & Addison, M. (Eds.). (1980). *Shaping the future: Community-based services and facilities for mentally retarded people.* Baltimore, MD: University Park Press.

Roth, J. (1963). *Timetables: Structuring the passage of time in hospital treatment and other careers.* Indianapolis, IN: Bobbs-Merrill.

Roy-Byrne, P., Gross, P., & Marder, S. (1982). Financial exploitation of schizophrenic patients by their families. *Hospital and Community Psychiatry, 33*, 576–579.

Rubin, L. (1978). *Women of a certain age: The mid-life search for self.* New York: Holt, Rinehart and Winston.

Seltzer, M. (1985). Informal supports for aging mentally retarded persons. *American Association on Mental Deficiency, 90*, 259–265.

Sheehan, S. (1982). *Is there no place on earth for me?* Boston: Houghton Mifflin.

Singer, M., & Wynne, L. (1963). Thought disorder and family relations of schizophrenics. IV: Results and implications. *Archives of General Psychiatry, 12*, 201–212.

Sorokin, P., & Merton, R. (1937). Social time: A methodological and functional analysis. *The American Journal of Sociology, 42*, 615–629.

Spaniol, L., Jung, H., Zipple, A., & Fitzgerald, S. (1987). Families as a resource in the rehabilitation of the severely disabled. In A. Hatfield & H. P. Lefley (Eds.), *Families of the mentally ill: Coping and adaptation* (pp. 167–190). New York: The Guilford Press.

Stevens, B. (1972). Dependence of schizophrenic patients on elderly relatives. *Psychological Medicine, 2,* 17–32.

Suelzle, M., & Keenan, V. (1981). Changes in family support networks over the life cycle of mentally retarded persons. *American Journal of Mental Deficiency, 86,* 267–270.

Terkelsen, K. (1987). The meaning of mental illness to the family. In A. Hatfield & H. P. Lefley (Eds.), *Families of the mentally ill: Coping and adaptation* (pp. 128–150). New York: The Guilford Press.

Tessler, R., Killian, L., & Gubman, G. (1987). Stages in family response to mental illness: An ideal type. *Psychosocial Rehabilitation Journal, 10,* 3–16.

Thompson, E., & Doll, W. (1982). The burden of families coping with the mentally ill: An invisible crisis. *Family Relations, 31,* 379–388.

Torrey, E. F., & Wolfe, S. M. (1986). *Care of the seriously mentally ill: A rating of state programs.* Washington, D.C.: Public Citizens Health Research Group.

Vaughn, C. (1986). Patterns of emotional response in the families of schizophrenic patients. In M. Goldstein, I. Hand, & K. Hahlweg (Eds.), *Treatment of schizophrenia: Family assessment and intervention* (pp. 97–108). New York: Springer-Verlag.

Vaughn, C., & Leff, J. (1976). The influence of family and social factors on the course of psychiatric illness. *British Journal of Psychiatry, 129,* 125–137.

Vine, P. (1982). *Families in pain: Children, siblings and parents speak out.* New York: Pantheon.

Wasow, M. (1985). Chronic schizophrenia and Alzheimer's disease: The losses for parents, spouses, and children compared. *Journal of Chronic Disease, 38,* 711–716.

Waxler, N. (1974). Parent and child effects on cognitive performance: An experimental approach to the etiological and responsive theories of schizophrenia. *Family Process, 13,* 1–23.

Weber, M. (1905-06/1955). *The Protestant ethnic and the spirit of capitalism.* (T. Parsons, Trans.). New York: Scribners. (Original work published 1905.)

Wikler, L. (1986). Periodic stresses of families of older mentally retarded children: An exploratory study. *American Journal of Mental Deficiency, 90,* 703–706.

Wikler, L., Wasow, M., & Hatfield, E. (1981). Chronic sorrow revisited: Attitudes of parents and professionals about adjustment to mental retardation. *American Journal of Orthopsychiatry, 51,* 63–70.

7

Research Focused on Intervention with Families of the Chronically Mentally Ill Elderly

Michael A. Smyer, Richard C. Birkel

This chapter has several related purposes: to provide a selective review of the literature on interventions with family members of the chronically mentally ill (CMI) and CMI elderly; to identify gaps in the current research base, along with potential barriers to pursuing research in the area; and to suggest future directions for research emphases in this domain.

In the first section of this chapter, we provide a brief overview of family-oriented research on CMI and its treatment. Next, we present our basic assumptions that provide a framework for the development, implementation, and evaluation of family interventions of the CMI elderly. In the third section, we highlight gaps in the existing literature, emphasizing both empirical and conceptual work that remains to be done. In the fourth section, we consider barriers to filling in the gaps in the knowledge base. We conclude with a discussion of future directions for intervention research with families of the CMI elderly.

Our research agenda, however, assumes a certain structure of inquiry for research and intervention. Specifically, we assume that intervention research is a process of reciprocal interaction with three basic aspects: description, explanation, and prediction or intervention (Birkel, Lerner, & Smyer, 1989; Reese & Overton, 1980; Smyer & Gatz, 1986). Some researchers (e.g., Anderson, Reiss, & Hogarty, 1986) begin with a strong theoretical framework that directs their descriptive and intervention efforts. Others begin with the significant demands of patient care and service provision; in meeting these demands, the clinician has an opportunity to begin the process of describing and explaining the CMI process. (As Bronfenbrenner, 1977, noted: If you want to understand something, try to change it!)

Our own approach to understanding families of CMI patients is to take a broad view. We believe it is useful to supplement research and theory on specific handicapping conditions (e.g., mental retardation, mental illnesss) with an awareness of important similarities and issues that cut across these conditions. Such an approach has been usefully employed by others (e.g., see Bruininks & Krantz, 1979; Moroney, 1980; Perlman, 1983). In our view, then, CMI poses unique challenges and problems for family caregivers that are best understood within a broad framework that addresses the response of families to a range of transitions and crises involving the dependency of one or more of their members.

In addition to assessing the similarities and differences between CMI in the elderly and other chronic illnesses, researchers and clinicians must make another important distinction: To what extent is CMI among the elderly similar to or different from CMI in younger populations? We will return to these themes in the concluding section of the chapter.

Throughout the chapter, we will draw from literature developed on populations facing adaptation to a variety of chronic conditions. We will also focus on literature developed from younger CMI populations. We will apply the lessons learned from these groups to CMI elderly in the absence of a comprehensive intervention literature on CMI elderly and their families.

AN OVERVIEW OF RESEARCH IN CMI AND FAMILY CARE

Because the growth of psychiatric treatment in the community and the decline of long-term hospitalization placed significant new demands on families to provide care for CMI patients (Mechanic, 1980), early research was concerned with whether family care was a viable option of psychiatric treatment. This was particularly important since social science literature of that time viewed families as largely incapable of providing such care (Parsons & Fox, 1952). However, a number of early studies demonstrated that home care of CMI patients was feasible and that a concentration of services in support of the patient and the family was effective in preventing hospitalization (Pasamanick, Scarpitti, & Dinitz, 1970). Several researchers, however, questioned the reliance on such outcome indicators as community tenure since they disregarded the social costs of retaining patients in the community (Mechanic, 1980).

In regard to social costs, British studies were among the first to demonstrate that the behavior of CMI patients in the community could have significant negative impacts on their families. For example, one early English study of 339 schizophrenic hospital patients who were returned to the community found that in the 6-month period prior to being interviewed, 14% of first admissions and 27% of previously admitted patients showed violent, threatening, or destructive behavior. Thirty-one percent of first admissions and 49% of readmissions had delusions and hallucinations. Other symptoms reported included marked social withdrawal, odd behavior, phobias, and depression. A significant proportion of the relatives of these patients reported that the patient's illness was harmful to their health, affected children adversely, created financial difficulties, and restricted leisure activity and the ability to have visitors (Brown, Bone, Dalison, & Wing, 1966). A number of other studies contributed to our knowledge of the significant burdens faced by the families of community-living CMI patients (Anderson & Lynch, 1984; Creer, 1975; Grad & Sainsbury, 1968; Herz, Endicott, & Gibbon, 1979; Hoenig & Hamilton, 1967; Rutter, 1966).

From a policy perspective, then, the next step was to determine if it was possible to have family home care for CMI patients without additional burdens being placed on caregiving families. In response, a number of controlled studies were designed to provide answers to this question, and several have suggested that it is possible to extend community tenure without significantly increasing the family burden over that experienced by hospitalized CMI patients (e.g., Anderson et al., 1986; Falloon & Pederson, 1985; Leff, Kuipers, Berkowitz et al., 1982; Reynolds & Hoult, 1984; Stein, Test, & Marx, 1979). What seem to be necessary are (1) specially trained staff, (2) the provision of structured training in problem-solving methods or strategies for families, (3) the provision of information about the illness and its course to family members, (4) readily available (24-hour) assistance with whatever problems might arise in home care, (5) the availability of hospitalization if necessary, and (6) frequent monitoring and adjustment of medication. In contrast, several studies have suggested that family home care in situations where comprehensive and responsive services are not provided is likely to result in elevated burdens for families and significant interference with family functioning (Anderson & Lynch, 1984; Creer, 1975; Grad & Sainsbury, 1968).

The direction of research, then, has been toward increasingly multivariate assessments and concern with simultaneous, multiple outcomes, including patient functioning, institutionalization, economic costs, and social costs to families and communities. It is becoming apparent that finding the proper balance of services to support family care of CMI patients will require increasingly complex field studies where significant dimensions of treatment are varied; target families represent a range of ages, economic classes, and syndromes; and multiple outcomes are assessed. Only those programs that demonstrate acceptable outcomes in several domains (e.g., patient functioning, family functioning, community costs, economic costs) across a range of family types are likely to be viewed as successful.

Anderson and her colleagues (Anderson et al., 1986, viii) recently summarized the major tasks for a successful family intervention program for relatives of CMI patients. They are applicable to relatives of CMI elderly as well:

1. Creating a treatment alliance that promotes a supportive working relationship with the patient *and* the family.
2. Providing information about the illness and its management to the patient and family members.
3. Establishing a low-key home/work/social environment that supports the patient's staying in the community.
4. Gradually integrating the patient into familial/social/vocational roles.
5. Creating a sense of continuity of care and an "institutional transference" for both the patient and the family.

Such comprehensive intervention research approaches require an understanding of the process of adaptation on the part of CMI patients and their families—a theme we return to in the next section.

BASIC ASSUMPTIONS

Several assumptions structure our approach to research on interventions with family members of the elderly CMI. These assumptions reflect our views of the nature of CMI, the family's role in responding to CMI, and the process of research. We begin with our view of CMI and the family's response.

From a research perspective, there is no consensus regarding the family's role in the development and response to a relative's CMI. Hatfield (1987a) recently reviewed several theories of the etiology of CMI, particularly schizophrenia. She noted that much of the early attention given to family members of CMI patients focused on their potential contribution as a causal factor in the illness (e.g., Bateson, Jackson, Haley, & Weakland, 1956; Fromm-Reichmann, 1948; Lidz, Fleck, & Cornelison, 1965). Other researchers have highlighted the family's role as reactors to the mental illness of their relatives (e.g., Clausen & Yarrow, 1955; Goldman, 1982; Hatfield, 1984). Research focused on expressed emotion (EE) within families is another prominent example of this point of view (e.g., Brown, Monck, Carstairs, & Wing, 1962; Leff & Vaughn, 1981; Vaughn & Leff, 1976).

Each of these research approaches to the family's role in CMI (Leff & Vaughn, 1985) has influenced clinical practice and intervention. The view of the family's role in relation to disability in one of its members is consistent across types of disability. For example, after reviewing and content analyzing 1,300 articles, books, and reports on family involvement in severe mental retardation and problems of aging relatives, Moroney (1980) concluded that families were viewed in five ways in the literature: (1) as part of the problem; (2) as a resource to the disabled person; (3) as a resource to the professional caregiver; (4) as primary caregivers in need of professional support in that role; and (5) as a unit of service with needs apart from those of the disabled member.

Naturally, views of the family's role and of the disabled relative are linked. Thus, in the case of CMI if one assumes that schizophrenia is a thought disorder "caused" by a schizophrenic mother or by faulty communication patterns within the family, then one's view of the family will focus on changing those patterns of interaction. In contrast, if one views the family not as a causal agent but as a reactor to mental illness among one of its members, then the focus of intervention and intervention research will change.

In our view, the most useful model is one that allows the broadest, most comprehensive view of family functioning and role performance. A particular family unit, at one time or another in the course of its involvement with CMI, may fill each of the roles outlined by Moroney. Thus, family interaction patterns may initially be involved in exacerbating certain genetically linked predispositions in one member and as a result be part of the "cause" of his/her florid symptomatology at one point. Later, the family may be of invaluable assistance to the therapist in providing insight into the problem and in motivating the patient toward recovery. Ultimately, with appropriate training and support, the family unit may itself provide the most meaningful and effective support during the patient's recovery. Along the way, of course, other family members may experience a range of stresses and needs unrelated to the patient but that require professional attention in order to maintain the family unit intact. This view is consistent with the work of Hogarty and his colleagues (e.g., Anderson et al., 1986).

Thus, we view the family's response to CMI as involving and often requiring a continual shifting of the family's role. As a result, we assume that families coping with a CMI elderly relative will face a series of transitional crises (Hatfield, 1987b). The characteristics of transitional crises have been highlighted by Hagestad and Smyer (1982):

- They are unscheduled.
- They are not controlled by individual choice.
- They are accompanied by little or no perceived warning.
- They result in a loss of status.
- They have no social rite of passage associated with them.

These characteristics of an unscheduled transition affect both the family's and the intervenor's capacity to plan for the transition, as well as the availability of resources to meet the demands of adapting. Within this framework, it is assumed that family strain often derives from the family's attempts to adapt to CMI. For example, strain may result from (a) blocked pathways to adaptation related to inflexibility in key family dimensions (income requirements, other dependents, lack of skills, etc.); (b) alterations and disruption of previously satisfying or essential household patterns and activities (e.g., sleep, communication, privacy, economic functioning), or interference with anticipated ones (e.g., retirement living); or (c) interpersonal conflict and tensions related to the meaning and significance of household adaptation or to interindividual differences in the ability or willingness to adapt. Some of the demands on the family stem directly from the CMI relative (e.g., Hatfield, 1984; McElroy, 1987; Terkelsen, 1987a), while others are more "normative" and a part of a general process of family change and development (e.g., Hagestad, 1986; Kingson, Hirshorn, & Cornman, 1986). In this view, then, the purpose of family intervention is designed to (1) facilitate household adaptation, (2) compensate for disruption of satisfying or essential household patterns, and (3) reduce conflict concerning the process and outcomes of adaptation itself.

Linked to our view of the family's course of responding to CMI is the assumption that family interventions are best developed within a conceptual framework that is adaptation-oriented rather than illness-oriented (Adler, Drake, & Stern, 1984; Birkel, 1987; Hatfield, 1987b; Lefley, 1987a). Again, Anderson and her colleagues (Anderson et al., 1986, vii) captured the essence of this perspective when they defined their "psychoeducational approach": "a method of care that provides attention to the family system without sacrificing the potential contributions of biological, psychological, and vocational systems."

Several authors have highlighted the adaptive tasks that families of CMI face. Terkelsen (1987b), for example, outlined ten stages that families go through in responding to the stresses and demands of a CMI relative, each stage involving a unique set of issues and tasks for family members. Before describing Terkelsen's stages, however, we want to highlight his caveats: "Since there are virtually no longitudinal investigations in this area of inquiry, the material . . . is derived from personal and clinical longitudinal experience with families" (p. 151). With this limitation in mind, consider Terkelsen's stages outlined in Table 7.1. Several elements are important in Terkelsen's work. First, he stresses that there is diversity across families in their process of coping and adaptation. No family goes through each stage in the outlined order. Instead, the process is likely to be more halting and erratic, with portions of the family working on differing aspects of adaptation at the same time. Linked to the diversity across and within families is the fluctuation of the CMI relative's functioning. Terkelsen argues that especially early in the CMI process, the patient's restoration of function can be used to minimize the importance of the issue, to maintain the family's denial of a

TABLE 7.1 Terkelsen's Phases of Family Response to Chronic Mental Illness in a Relative

Phase One:	Ignoring what is coming
	• He'll grow out of it soon enough
	• Nip it in the Bud
Phase Two:	The first shock of recognition
	• Pull yourself together
	• Get your life back on the track
Phase Three:	Stalemate
	• Things are not that bad
	• Flight to health
Phase Four:	Containing the implications of illness
	• All better now
	• Must have been the medicines
Phase Five:	Transformation to official patienthood
	• You really are a patient
	• Dangerous to self or others
Phase Six:	The search for causes
	• Who is the guilty party in the family?
	• What is the biological cause?
Phase Seven:	The search for treatment
	• Learning the system—inpatient and outpatient
	• Learning the professions
Phase Eight:	The collapse of optimism
	• The family becomes overwhelmed by caregiving
	• The patient is seen as a total invalid
Phase Nine:	Surrendering the dream
	• Mourning the loss
	• The roller coaster of recovery
Phase Ten:	Picking up the pieces
	• Compartmentalizing illness
	• Get on with the rest of life

Source: Based on Terkelsen's (1987b) discussion.

problem, or to support a particular view of etiology favored by a portion of the family (e.g., "It was his medicine; once they got the dosage right, he got much better").

Another view of the family's coping tasks comes from surveys of family members of CMI relatives. Hatfield (1979a, 1979b), for example, surveyed members of the Schizophrenic Association of Greater Washington. When asked about the types of assistance of most concern for these relatives of CMI patients, the respondents highlighted several areas (see Table 7.2).

Several elements are noteworthy about Hatfield's work. First, she is focusing on a self-selected sample of relatives of CMI—those active in a regional organization

TABLE 7.2 Assistance Desired by Caregivers

Assistance	No. Chosen[a]	% Chosen
Knowledge and understanding of patient's symptoms	51	57
Specific suggestions for coping with patient's behavior	49	55
People to talk to who have known the experience	39	44
Substitute care to relieve the family	27	30
Having patient change place of living	24	27
More understanding from friends and relatives	16	18
Relief from financial stress	16	18
Therapy for self	11	12

[a]Although three choices were requested, some mentioned fewer than three.
Source: Reprinted from Hatfield (1979b).

to mobilize support and assistance for individuals with CMI. Second, there is likely to be important variability among Hatfield's respondents in two important respects: their current status in adapting to the CMI process (e.g., where in Terkelsen's stages or other schemes of adaptation they might be); and their current family stage or life-course stage of development. Each of these elements might affect the respondent's view of the most difficult coping challenge and most readily available coping resources.

Lefley (1987b) offers another discussion of the coping tasks faced by families with CMI relatives. As outlined in Table 7.3, Lefley emphasizes three distinct types of behaviors that may affect the family's response: behaviors that "elicit anger, irritability, or exasperation" (p. 114); behaviors that "shut off human interaction" (p. 117); and behaviors that elicit "empathic pain" among family members.

Lefley's conceptualization reminds us that families must adapt and cope on a variety of levels. The types of problems that often bring families and professionals into contact are often the most pressing direct manifestations of CMI: what Lefley labeled threatening or annoying behaviors. At the same time, however, family members respond with their own expectations of "normal" interpersonal interaction. These expectations are often not met with CMI relatives. In addition, the family members' emotional reactions must be a focus of concern for family members and service providers.

Our own view of adaptation to CMI involves three primary areas: (a) interpersonal; (b) instrumental; and (c) life course. Perhaps the most difficult interpersonal task is mourning the loss of the premorbid CMI patient. Terkelsen's phrase "surrendering the dream" captures the poignancy of this process. Depending upon the age and role of the CMI relative, family members may focus on grieving for either lost functioning or lost opportunities for the development of future functioning. It is notable that this same process has been described in the literature on the elderly suffering from dementia (Berezin's 1970 notion of "partial grief"), the retarded (Olshansky's 1962 idea of "chronic sorrow"), and the physically disabled (Bray, 1987). Second, studies of discharged patients have identified a variety of patient behavior problems which require interpersonal adjustments on the part of family members. These include frequent and intense argumentativeness, withdrawal and lack of communication, bizzare and/or threatening behavior (Gubman & Tessler, 1987). These behaviors may dramatically alter the nature of the relationships that have been established between the patient and other members of the household.

What seems most important in understanding interpersonal adjustments to CMI is that the relationship of the patient to each family and household member is unique. The issues raised and their impact vary considerably, depending upon whether the relationship between the CMI patient and family member is parental (Caton, 1984; Clausen & Huffine, 1979; Rutter, 1966), sibling (Gubman & Tessler, 1987; Sheehan, 1982), or spousal (Clausen & Yarrow, 1955). Not only are emotional responses likely to differ in these instances, but the types of available adaptive responses (e.g., divorce, separation, leaving home, etc.) differ as well. For example, older siblings may have the relatively unique option of coping with a family member's CMI by leaving home in accord with prevailing norms regarding the independence of young adults (Gubman & Tessler, 1987). Other norms may limit or preclude options for relatives of CMI elderly.

TABLE 7.3 Behavioral Manifestations of Mental Illness

Threatening or annoying behaviors
- Hostile, abusive, or assaultive behaviors
- Mood swings and unpredictability
- Socially offensive or embarrassing behaviors
- Amotivation, parasitism, apparent malingering
- Self-destructive behaviors
- Behaviors disturbing to household living

Behaviors involving lack of human relatedness
- Changed relationships with family members, friends, and neighbors
- Tendency toward encapsulation
- Long-term readjustment of family lifestyle
- Potential marital and sibling conflict regarding changing family roles

Behaviors evoking empathic pain in family members
- The patient's acknowledgment of decreased self-esteem
- The patient's expression of fear or anxiety in re-entering important social contexts (e.g., school, work, family, etc.)
- The patient's acknowledgment of being a burden on the family

Source: Based on Lefley's (1987b) discussion.

Relationships beyond the household are affected as well. Research suggests that in caring for individuals with a variety of chronic disabilities, household members may become isolated as they withdraw from involvements and relationships outside the household and as the involvement of extended family and friends in the life of the household decreases (Anthony, 1970; Fengler & Goodrich, 1979; Jones, Victor, & Vetter, 1983; Kazak & Clark, 1986; Kreisman & Joy, 1974; McAlister, Butler, & Lei, 1973; Suelzle & Keenan, 1981). A national survey completed by the Social Security Administration, for example, concluded that for families taking care of disabled members, "contraction, rather than compensation, emerges as the major impact of disability on the family structure" (Franklin, 1977, p. 18). At the same time that the family is becoming increasingly cut off from its informal relations, however, it must also expand psychologically to accommodate members of the psychiatric or community mental health team. In this new working relationship, conflict may develop, and new problems of communication and linkage are likely to arise (Golodetz, Evans, Heinritz, & Gibson, 1969). Ultimately, whether the relationship between families and professionals is cooperative or adversarial has important implications for household adaptation and patient and family functioning (Appleton, 1974; Grob, Eisen, & Edinburg, 1982; Spaniol, Jung, Zipple, & FitzGerald, 1985).

In the instrumental domain, researchers in mental retardation (Birenbaum, 1971), brain injury (Lezak, 1978; Power & Sax, 1978), stroke (Overs & Healy, 1973), senile dementia (Haley, 1983; Zarit, Orr, & Zarit, 1985), schizophrenia (Falloon et al., 1982; Falloon et al., 1985), end-state renal disease and home hemodialysis (Blodgett, 1981), and family care of the frail elderly (Clark & Rakowski, 1983) have emphasized that day-to-day problem behavior associated with chronic disability is often among the most difficult for families. For example, a variety of household complaints—including awakening the family at night, failing to adhere to a regular time schedule, being uncooperative, refusing to perform household chores, and making unreasonable demands—have been identified by caregiving relatives as primary sources of strain (Creer, 1975; Grad & Sainsbury, 1968; Hatfield, 1978; Hoenig & Hamilton, 1966).

Research in this area suggests that many of these problems are common to all forms of residential settings for the CMI, including institutions, group homes, and other community residences (Gubman & Tessler, 1987). For example, Gubman and colleagues report that in an analysis of complaint data for over 1,400 CMI clients, behavioral problems of the type outlined above were best predictors of complaints for all households, regardless of type (Gubman, Tessler, & Willis, 1986, reported in Gubman & Tessler, 1987, p. 233).

Finally, each relative must assess and adapt to the likely life-course patterns of adjustment for all of the relatives of the CMI elderly patient. Any life stress has "ripple effects" throughout the family (Pruchno, Blow, & Smyer, 1984) and across the generations (Hagestad, 1986). Thus, both short-term and long-term planning must take place in anticipating changing care needs and options as the family and patient age.

The types of planning the family must undertake will vary, depending upon the course of the illness, the particular stage of the illness, and the life stage of the family. The consequences of CMI for the family are likely to be very different, for example, if there is a single episode of mental illness versus recurrent symptoms (Clausen, 1984). Also, the types of adaptation and planning required of the family are different early in the illness when shock, disbelief, and hopefulness are powerfully intertwined, compared to later when the limits of treatment are clear and a feeling of resignation may prevail (Gubman & Tessler, 1987). Finally, the types of planning facing the elderly family with CMI are likely to be dramatically different in focus and scope than those facing the very young family. Unfortunately, however, longitudinal studies of CMI elderly (e.g., Ciompi, 1987; Harding, Brooks, Ashikaga, Strauss, & Landerl, 1987; McGlashan, 1987) have provided sketchy information about the process of family adaptation across the life course.

Our theoretical view of the family's coping and adaptational tasks is summarized in Table 7.4.

In the next section we provide a brief overview of gaps of previous research efforts in CMI in order to highlight areas for future research and obstacles to carrying out that research.

GAPS IN THE LITERATURE AND BARRIERS
TO INTERVENTION RESEARCH

Our assumptions necessarily shape our assessment of areas for future research and obstacles to carrying out that work. There are several key areas for needed research. First is basic epidemiological investigation focused on the household structure of families with CMI relatives. Although there is consensus that the majority of CMI patients return to family settings for initial living arrangements, little is known of the composition of the family networks in these settings. Similarly, little is known about the household arrangements of CMI elderly. In other areas (e.g., caregiving for Alzheimer's patients or other impaired elderly), basic epidemiological investigation has carefully documented the variability of caregiving arrangements, caregiving burdens, etc. (e.g., Birkel, 1987; Zarit, 1990).

This household orientation for epidemiological study would represent a distinct departure for NIMH, since current epidemiological work (e.g., the Epidemiological Catchment Area Studies) is focused primarily on the identified patient or individual level of analysis (e.g., Klerman, 1986; Regier et al., 1984). It is our assumption, however, that the household is a basic and irreducible unit of care for the elderly CMI patient.

TABLE 7.4 Major Tasks of Family Coping and Adaptation

Interpersonal adjustment
  • Mourning the "lost" CMI relative
  • Adjusting relationships within the household
  • Maintaining relationships outside the household
  • Establishing collaborative relations with professional providers
Instrumental coping
  • Managing day-to-day challenges
  • Coordinating among formal and informal care options
  • Adjusting household schedules
  • Assigning responsibility for caregiving tasks
Life-course adaptation
  • Planning the long-term family adaptation for intergenerational continuity
  • Reassessing individual developmental trajections—for the CMI relative and
    other family members
  • Making adjustments in career and work commitments

Berkman (1983) suggested several dimensions for characterizing the social support network of impaired elderly. The criteria she outlined also apply to the caregiving household's characteristics. She highlighted the following aspects:

  • Size of the network;
  • Frequency of contact between the network members and the identified patient (in this case, the identified household member);
  • Density of interaction among the network members (i.e., how often the network members contact each other in addition to their contact with the members of the household);
  • Intimacy of the network (i.e., the level of sharing and contact that occurs);
  • Durability of the network (i.e., how lasting the network is likely to be over time);
  • Geographic dispersion of the network (i.e., how accessible it is in terms of time and distance); and
  • The reciprocity evidenced between and among members of the network.

These dimensions could be helpful in assessing the larger network within which the household of the elderly CMI patient functions.

Linked to the functional orientation implied in a descriptive epidemiology of caregiving households is an emphasis on the life-course position and prospects of the family members of CMI patients. As Elder (1979) has convincingly argued in reference to historical stresses, the age of onset for all concerned may affect the natural course of caregiving and family functioning. For example, children in middle age may bring different expectations and resources to their parent's encounter with CMI than children in young adulthood.

Hagestad (1986) has outlined the basic generational structure of families, emphasizing the difference between age and generational position. For example, the generational position of the members of the household could indicate the range of demands, responsibilities, and commitments facing the household. This distinction should be embodied in a family-oriented epidemiological investigation of CMI elderly.

A third area of needed research is in the degree of variability across conditions and across people in the course of adaptation. To what extent, for example, does chronicity of the condition affect the availability and willingness of family caregivers to provide for a CMI relative? In the aging literature, for example, Kahn (1975) suggested that the individual's history of adaptation was an important determinant of need for services and their likelihood of success: late-onset versus early-onset depression, for example, could represent differing treatment challenges, family resources, and likelihood of therapeutic success. Similarly, Birkel's research (1987) suggests that household dynamics in adapting to the care of the physically impaired, lucid elder versus the cognitively impaired elder, are quite distinct.

A fourth area that should be emphasized in future research is the link among the family characteristics, the CMI patient's characteristics, and the use of professional services. Litwak (1985), for example, suggests that a key issue for service providers to the elderly is arriving at the appropriate division of labor between formal and informal services. Similarly, an important issue for intervention research is specifying the conditions under which professional interventions will most successfully complement informal, family, or household-based caregiving and support.

To specify these interrelationships, however, requires specifying the appropriate unit of measurement (e.g., individual, family, household, community, etc.), as well as the appropriate indicator of outcome (e.g., rate of institutionalization, perceived burden, etc.). Thus far, there is no clear sense of the appropriate metrics for use in this domain.

The fifth direction that should be emphasized is increasing our understanding of the specific household and life-course adjustments that are made in adapting to CMI. As suggested earlier, current research has demonstrated that given relatively high levels of support and assistance from formal providers, families can adapt to CMI and can do so without perceiving unacceptable costs in family functioning and well-being. However, although this research tells us that adaptation outcomes are acceptable to families in terms of the level of objective and subjective stress, it tells us little about the domains in which family adaptation has occurred (e.g., work, leisure, family relations, social ties, household organization, life-course adjustments, etc.). Because some patterns of adaptation are more costly to the household, society, and different members of the household than others, knowing that adjustment states are acceptable to families (the notion of subjective burden) is not a sufficient basis on which to design interventions. In order to make informed choices in the design of intervention and policy, we must know more about the specific process of adjustment and about the trade-offs made by families.

For example, research should seek to provide information about the distinct patterns of adjustments made by families of the CMI, depending upon life-course stage (young families versus older families), age of the patient, family income, ethnicity, sex of the patient, and so on. An example of this work in the field of mental retardation is the work of Birenbaum (1971). Birenbaum found that mothers of young mentally retarded children adapted in two primary ways: (1) they emphasized expressive responses over instrumental (skill teaching) responses, and (2) they fit the child into conventional routines as a way to preserve a social appearance of "normality." Of interest, however, is Birenbaum's observation that these ways of coping *broke down* as the child passed into the normal age of independence. As a result, the mothers were forced to make major new adjustments in both their interpersonal interactions with the child and household management as the child entered into adolescence.

Similarly, research by Farber (1959) suggests that parents of mentally retarded children make life-course adjustments that may include lower incomes for husbands, fewer chances of promotion, and a general lowering of career aspirations. Thus, future research in CMI should explore life-course adjustments made by various family members in response to various presentations of the illness.

A final area of needed research is on what we call the "social ecology" of the household (Birkel, 1987). We view the home-care household as an ecological unit capable of making extensive adjustments in structure and function in order to adapt to and compensate for a member's mental illness. Household adaptation may include changes in the number of residents, the use of space, the use and patterning of time, functioning, family communication patterns, and the division of labor. How each of these household parameters is affected by CMI is an important area of research, particularly since we suspect that adjustments here are often perceived as "burdensome" to the family. Further, it is likely that household arrangements that work well in providing for individuals with one type of condition may be ineffective or inappropriate in relation to other types. As a result, the sources (correlates) of strain and tension in home-care households are likely to differ, depending upon the specifics of the patient's functioning, as are appropriate intervention activities.

The "social" aspect of this ecology refers to the fact that CMI involves fundamental changes in an individual's social identity, along with declines in role performance. Functional capabilities help define who we are and what is expected of us in relation to others. To the extent that basic cognition, orientation in time and place, and stable emotional functioning are undermined by disease or psychopathology, an individual's social presence is dramatically altered and diminished. As a result, the meaning, motivation, and dynamics of caregiving are fundamentally altered as well. The view of the patient held by household members, then, may play a critical role in determining how and how well the household is able to adapt to the patient's psychopathology. Practically, both public and private perceptions of the mentally ill may be important targets for intervention. Efforts to influence these attitudes positively may pay off in more effective interpersonal and household functioning.

SUMMARY AND CONCLUSIONS

We have suggested that the process of intervention research requires an accurate description of the household of elderly CMI patients. With the household as a unit of interest, several key dimensions become important: the structure and function of the household; the life-course positions represented in the household; the type, nature, severity, and duration of the mental illness of the affected relative; and the array of services available to supplement the family's efforts. Intervention research in the area of CMI elderly must focus on conditional analyses, explicating the conditions under which family interventions with elderly CMI patients' relatives can be effective. The goals of such interventions should encompass both improving the well-being of the elderly CMI patient and improving the functioning and adaptation of the family as a whole.

Three basic questions should guide the development, implementation, and evaluation of intervention efforts focused on families of CMI elderly:

- To what extent are CMI elderly and their families similar to other, younger CMI populations?
- To what extent are CMI elderly and their families similar to other populations responding to disability conditions (e.g., stroke; mental retardation; etc)?
- To what extent are CMI elderly and their families similar to other elderly populations?

The answers to these inquiries should help assess the generalizability of previous intervention efforts with other populations while highlighting the continued importance of interventions for this special population that blends concerns of aging and mental illness.

ACKNOWLEDGMENT

We appreciate the helpful comments of Bob Drake and Pat Piper on an earlier version.

REFERENCES

Adler, D. A., Drake, R. E., & Stern, R. (1984). Viewing chronic mental illness: A conceptual framework. *Comprehensive Psychiatry, 25*(2), 192–207.

Anderson, C. M., Reiss, D. J., & Hogarty, G. E. (1986). *Schizophrenia and the family*. New York: Guilford Press.

Anderson, E. A., & Lynch, M. M. (1984). A family impact analysis: The deinstitutionalization of the mentally ill. *Family Relations, 33,* 41–46.

Anthony, J. E. (1970). The impact of mental and physical illness on family life. *American Psychiatry, 127,* 138–146.

Appleton, W. J. (1974, June). Mistreatment of patients' families by psychiatrists. *American Journal of Psychiatry, 131,* 655–657.

Bateson, G., Jackson, D., Haley, J., & Weakland, J. (1956). Toward a theory of schizophrenia. *Behavioral Science, 1,* 251–264.

Berezin, M. A. (1970). The psychiatrist and the geriatric patient: Partial grief in family members and others who care for the elderly patient. *Journal of Geriatric Psychiatry, 4,* 53–64.

Berkman, L. F. (1983). The assessment of social networks and social support in the elderly. *Journal of the American Geriatrics Society, 31*(12), 743–749.

Birenbaum, A. (1971). The mentally retarded child in the home and family cycle. *Journal of Health and Social Behavior, 12,* 55–65.

Birkel, R. C. (1987). Toward a social ecology of the home-care household. *Psychology and Aging, 2,* 294–301.

Birkel, R. C., Lerner, R. M., & Smyer, M. A. (1989). Applied developmental psychology as an implementation of the life-span view of human development. *Journal of Applied Developmental Psychology, 10,* 425–445.

Blodgett, C. (1981). A selected review of the literature of adjustment to hemodialysis. *International Journal of Psychiatry in Medicine, 11,* 97–124.

Bray, G. P. (1987). Family adaptation to chronic illness. In B. Caplan (Ed.), *Rehabilitation psychology desk reference* (pp. 171–183). Rockville, MD: Aspen.

Bronfenbrenner, U. (1977). Toward an experimental ecology of human development. *American Psychologist, 32,* 513–531.

Brown, G. W., Bone, M., Dalison, B., & Wing, J. K. (1966). *Schizoprhenia and social care: A comparative follow-up study of 339 schizophrenic patients.* New York: Oxford University Press.

Brown, G. W., Monck, E. M., Carstairs, G. M., & Wing, J. K. (1962). Influence of family life on the course of schizophrenic illness. *British Journal of Preventive Social Medicine, 16,* 55–68.

Bruininks, R. H., & Krantz, G. C. (Eds.). (1979). *Family care of developmentally disabled members: Conference proceedings.* Minneapolis: University of Minnesota.

Caton, C. L. M. (1984). *Management of chronic schizophrenia.* New York: Oxford University Press.

Ciompi, L. (1987). Review of follow-up studies on long-term evolution and aging in schizophrenia. In N. E. Miller & G. D. Cohen (Eds.), *Schizophrenia and aging.* New York: Guilford Press.

Clark, N. M., & Rakowski, W. (1983). Family caregivers of older adults: Improving helping skills. *The Gerontologist, 23*, 637–642.

Clausen, J. A. (1984). Mental illness and the life course. In P. B. Baltes & O. G. Brim, Jr. (Eds.), *Life-span development and behavior.* New York: Academic Press.

Clausen, J. A., & Huffine, C. L. (1979). The impact of parental mental illness on children. In J. Greenley (Ed.), *Research in community and mental health* (Vol. 2). Greenwich, CT: JAI Press.

Clausen, J. A., & Yarrow, M. R. (Eds.). (1955). The impact of mental illness on the family. *Journal of Social Issues, 11*, 3–64.

Creer, C. (1975). Living with schizophrenia. *Social Work Today, 6*, 2–7.

Elder, G. H. (1979). Historical change in life patterns and personality. In P. B. Baltes & O. G. Brim, Jr. (Eds.), *Life-span development and behavior* (Vol. 2). New York: Academic Press.

Falloon, I. R. H., Boyd, J. L., McGill, C. W., Razani, J., Moss, H. B., & Gilderman, A. M. (1982). Family management in the prevention of exacerbations of schizophrenia: A controlled study. *The New England Journal of Medicine, 306*, 1437–1441.

Falloon, I. R. H., Boyd, J. L., McGill, C. W., Williamson, M., Razani, J., Moss, H. B., Gilderman, A. M., & Simpson, G. M. (1985). Family management in the prevention of morbidity of schizophrenia. *Archives of General Psychiatry, 42*, 887–896.

Falloon, I. R. H., & Pederson, J. (1985). Family management in the prevention of morbidity of schizophrenia: The adjustment of the family unit. *British Journal of Psychiatry, 147*, 156–163.

Farber, B. (1959). Effects of a severely mentally retarded child on family integration. *Monographs of the Society for Research in Child Development, 24*(2).

Fengler, A. P., & Goodrich, N. (1979). Wives of elderly disabled men: The hidden patients. *The Gerontologist, 19*, 175–183.

Franklin, P. A. (1977). Impact of disability on the family structure. *Social Security Bulletin, 40*, 12–20.

Fromm-Reichmann, F. (1948). Notes on the development of treatment of schizophrenics by psychoanalytic psychotherapy. *Psychiatry, 11*, 263–273.

Goldman, H. H. (1982). Mental illness and family burden: A public health perspective. *Hospital and Community Psychiatry, 33*, 557–560.

Golodetz, A., Evans, R., Heinritz, G., & Gibson, C. (1969). The care of chronic illness: The responsor role. *Medical Care, 7*, 385–394.

Grad, J., & Sainsbury, P. (1968). The effects that patients have on their families in a community care and a control psychiatric service—A two year follow-up. *British Journal of Psychiatry, 114*, 265–278.

Grob, M. C., Eisen, S. V., & Edinburg, G. M. (1982). Clinical social work with young adult inpatients: Perspectives of patients, parents, and clinicians. *Social Work in Health Care, 8*, 1–9.

Gubman, G. D., & Tessler, R. C. (1987). The impact of mental illness on families. *Journal of Family Issues, 8*, 226–245.

Hagestad, G. O. (1986). The family: Women and grandparents as kin-keepers. In A. Pifer & L. Bronte (Eds.), *Our aging society: Paradox and promise* (pp. 141–160). New York: W. W. Norton.

Hagestad, G. O., & Smyer, M. A. (1982). Dissolving long-term relationships: Patterns of divorcing in middle age. In S. Duck (Ed.), *Personal relationships: Dissolving personal relationships* (pp. 155-188). New York: Academic Press.

Haley, W. E. (1983). A family behavioral approach to the treatment of the cognitively impaired elderly. *The Gerontologist, 23,* 18-23.

Harding, C. M., Brooks, G. W., Ashikaga, T., Strauss, J. S., & Landerl, P. D. (1987). Aging and social functioning in once-chronic schizophrenic patients 22-62 years after first admission: The Vermont story. In N. E. Miller & G. D. Cohen (Eds.), *Schizophrenia and aging.* New York: Guilford Press.

Hatfield, A. B. (1978). Psychological costs of schizophrenia to the family. *Social Work, 23,* 355-359.

Hatfield, A. B. (1979a). The family as partner in the treatment of mental illness. *Hospital and Community Psychiatry, 30,* 338-340.

Hatfield, A. B. (1979b). Help-seeking behavior in families of schizophrenics. *American Journal of Community Psychology, 7*(5), 563-569.

Hatfield, A. B. (1982). Therapists and families: Worlds apart. *Hospital and Community Psychiatry, 33,* 513.

Hatfield, A. B. (1984). The family. In J. A. Talbott (Ed.), *The chronic mental patient: Five years later* (pp. 307-323). Orlando, FL: Grune & Stratton.

Hatfield, A. B. (1987a). Families as caregivers: A historical perspective. In A. B. Hatfield & H. P. Lefley (Eds.), *Families of the mentally ill: Coping and adaptation* (pp. 3-29). New York: Guilford Press.

Hatfield, A. B. (1987b). Coping and adaptation: A conceptual framework for understanding families. In A. B. Hatfield & H. P. Lefley (Eds.), *Families of the mentally ill: Coping and adaptation* (pp. 60-84). New York: Guilford Press.

Hatfield, A. B., & Lefley, H. P. (Eds.). (1987). *Families of the mentally ill: Coping and adaptation.* New York: Guilford Press.

Herz, M. I., Endicott, J., & Gibbon, M. (1979). Brief hospitalization: Two-year follow-up. *Archives of General Psychiatry, 36,* 701-705.

Hoenig, J., & Hamilton, M. W. (1966). The schizophrenic patient in the community and his effect on the household. *International Journal of Social Psychiatry, 12,* 165-176.

Jones, D., Victor, C., & Vetter, N. (1983). Careers of the elderly in the community. *Journal of the Royal College of General Practitioners, 33,* 707-710.

Kahn, R. L. (1975). The mental health system and the future aged. *Gerontologist, 15*(1), 24-32.

Kazak, A. E., & Clark, M. W. (1986). Stress in families of children with myelomeningocele. *Developmental Medicine and Child Neurology, 28,* 220-228.

Kingson, E. R., Hirshorn, B. A., & Cornman, J. M. (1986). *Ties that bind: The interdependence of generations.* Washington, DC: Seven Locks Press.

Klerman, G. L. (1986). The National Institute of Mental Health—Epidemiologic Catchment Area (NIMH-ECA) Program. *Social Psychiatry, 21,* 159-166.

Kreisman, D. E., & Joy, V. D. (1974). Family response to the mental illness of a relative: A review of the literature. *Schizophrenia Bulletin, 11,* 34-57.

Leff, J., Kuipers, L., Berkowitz, R. et al. (1982). A controlled trial of social intervention in the families of schizophrenic patients. *British Journal of Psychiatry, 141,* 121-134.

Leff, J. P., & Vaughn, C. E. (1981). The role of maintenance therapy and relatives' expressed emotion in relapse of schizophrenia: A two-year follow-up. *British Journal of Psychiatry, 139,* 102–104.

Leff, J. P., & Vaughn, C. (1985). *Expressed emotion in families.* New York: Guilford Press.

Lefley, H. P. (1987a). An adaptation framework: Its meaning for research and practice. In A. B. Hatfield & H. P. Lefley (Eds.), *Families of the mentally ill: Coping and adaptation* (pp. 307–329). New York: Guilford Press.

Lefley, H. P. (1987b). Behavioral manifestations of mental illness. In A. B. Hatfield & H. P. Lefley (Eds.), *Families of the mentally ill: Coping and adaptation* (pp. 107–127). New York: Guilford Press.

Lezak, M. (1978). Living with the characterologically altered brain injured patient. *Journal of Clinical Psychiatry, 39,* 592–598.

Lidz, T., Fleck, S., & Cornelison, A. R. (1965). *Schizophrenia and the family.* New York: International Universities Press.

Litwak, E. (1985). *Helping the elderly: The complementary roles of informal networks and formal systems.* New York: Guilford Press.

McAlister, R., Butler, E., & Lei, T. (1973). Patterns of interaction among families of behaviorally retarded children. *Journal of Marriage and the Family, 35,* 93–100.

McElroy, E. M. (1987). The beat of a different drummer. In A. B. Hatfield & H. P. Lefley (Eds.), *Families of the mentally ill: Coping and adaptation* (pp. 225–243). New York: Guilford Press.

McGlashan, T. H. (1987). Late onset improvement in chronic schizophrenia: Characteristics and prediction. In N. E. Miller & G. D. Cohen (Eds.), *Schizophrenia and aging.* New York: Guilford Press.

Mechanic, D. (1980). *Mental health and social policy* (2nd ed.). Englewood Cliffs, NJ: Prentice-Hall.

Moroney, R. M. (1980). *Families, social services, and social policy: The issue of shared responsibility.* Rockville, MD: U.S. Department of Health and Human Services Pub. No. (ADM) 80-846.

Olshansky, S. (1962). Chronic sorrow: A response to having a mentally defective child. *Social Casework, 43,* 191–194.

Overs, R. P., & Healy, J. R. (1973). Stroke patients: Their spouses, families, and the community. In A. B. Cobb (Ed.), *Medical and psychological aspects of disability.* Springfield, IL: C. C. Thomas.

Parsons, T., & Fox, R. (1952). Illness, therapy, and the modern urban American family. *Journal of Social Issues, 8,* 31–34.

Pasamanick, B., Scarpitti, F. R., & Dinitz, S. (1970). *Schizophrenics in the community: An experimental study in the prevention of hospitalization.* New York: Appleton Century Crofts.

Perlman, R. (Ed.). (1983). *Family home care: Critical issues for services and policies.* New York: Haworth Press.

Power, P. W., & Sax, D. S. (1978). The communication of information to the neurological patient: Some implications for family coping. *Journal of Chronic Disease, 31,* 57–65.

Pruchno, R. A., Blow, F. C., & Smyer, M. A. (1984). Life events and interdependent lives. *Human Development, 27,* 31–41.

Reese, H. W., & Overton, W. F. (1980). Models, methods, and ethics of intervention. In R. R. Turner & H. W. Reese (Eds.), *Life-span developmental psychology: Intervention.* New York: Academic Press.

Regier, D. A., Myers, J. K., Kramer, M., Robins, L. N., Blazer, D. G., Hough, R. L., Eaton, W. W., & Locke, B. Z. (1984). The NIMH Epidemiologic Catchment Area Program. *Archives of General Psychiatry, 41*(10), 934–941.

Reynolds, I., & Hoult, J. E. (1984). The relatives of the mentally ill. *Journal of Nervous and Mental Disease, 172,* 480–489.

Rutter, M. (1966). *Children of sick parents: An environmental and psychiatric study.* London: Oxford University Press.

Sheehan, S. (1982). *Is there no place on earth for me?* Boston: Houghton Mifflin.

Smyer, M. A., & Gatz, M. (1986). Intervention research approaches. *Research on Aging, 8,* 536–558.

Spaniol, L., Jung, H., Zipple, A. M., & FitzGerald, S. (1985). *Families as a central resource in the rehabilitation of the severely psychiatrically disabled: Report of a national survey.* Boston: Boston University.

Stein, L., Test, M. A., & Marx, A. (1979). Alternative to the hospital: A controlled study. *American Journal of Psychiatry, 132,* 517–522.

Suelzle, M., & Keenan, V. (1981). Changes in family support networks over the life cycle of mentally retarded persons. *American Journal of Mental Deficiency, 86,* 267–274.

Terkelsen, K. G. (1987a). The meaning of mental illness to the family. In A. B. Hatfield & H. P. Lefley (Eds.), *Families of the mentally ill: Coping and adaptation* (pp. 128–150). New York: Guilford Press.

Terkelsen, K. G. (1987b). The evolution of family responses to mental illness through time. In A. B. Hatfield & H. P. Lefley (Eds.), *Families of the mentally ill: Coping and adaptation* (pp. 151–166). New York: Guilford Press.

Vaughn, C. E., & Leff, J. P. (1976). The influence of family and social factors on the course of psychiatric illness: A comparison of schizophrenic and depressed neurotic patients. *British Journal of Psychiatry, 129,* 125–137.

Zarit, S. H. (1990). Issues and directions in family intervention research. In E. Light & B. Lebowtiz (Eds.), *Alzheimer's disease treatment and family stress: Directions for research.* New York: Hemisphere Publishing Corporation.

Zarit, S. H., Orr, N. K., & Zarit, J. M. (1985). *The hidden victims of Alzheimer's disease: Families under stress.* New York: New York University.

PART III
Research on Special Treatment Issues

8

Neuroleptic Treatment of Chronically Mentally Ill Elderly: Suggestions for Future Research

Dilip V. Jeste

Improved nutritional conditions and other medical advances have resulted in increased longevity of schizophrenic and other chronically mentally ill (CMI) patients. Unfortunately, there has not been a parallel increase in the research on changing needs for treatment of the CMI elderly. This article focuses on the treatment of the CMI elderly with neuroleptic (antipsychotic) agents, with a particular emphasis on tardive dyskinesia (TD). I will review, in brief, salient aspects of the available data, major gaps in our knowledge, and suggest strategies for trying to narrow those gaps.

BRIEF REVIEW OF LITERATURE

Neuroleptic drugs represent the most effective treatment for chronic schizophrenia. They help both to control acute psychotic symptoms and to prevent subsequent relapse, thereby facilitating rehabilitation of patients. Existing agents, however, have two main shortcomings. They do not cure schizophrenia (and do not affect aspects of the "defect state" significantly), and they have troublesome and serious side effects, especially TD.

One antipsychotic agent with a novel spectrum of activity or adverse effects that is being studied is clozapine. It was recently shown to be effective in some previously treatment-refractory patients. Its potential benefit must be balanced, however, against the relatively high risk of agranulocytosis. Nonetheless, the effectiveness of clozapine in the treatment-refractory population is encouraging because it provides evidence that some patients who have been nonresponsive to "typical" neuroleptics may be capable of drug responsiveness. It also raises questions about the assumption that all schizophrenic illnesses are treatable in the same fashion. Indeed, it suggests a need for developing and testing medications that may be useful for the management of specific subsets of patients. It will be valuable to identify and characterize treatment-relevant subgroups of schizophrenic patients. The report of the NIMH Schizophrenia-Treatment Panel (Carpenter et al., 1987) elaborates on these and other considerations relevant to the management of schizophrenia.

Tardive Dyskinesia

A serious risk of long-term use of neuroleptics is the development of TD. Tardive dyskinesia is a movement disorder characterized by choreoathetoid or repetitive movements most common in the orofacial region and extremities. The movements appear quasi-purposeful or purposeless, worsen with stress, and improve with relaxation. They can be suppressed for a short period with voluntary control. Tardive dyskinesia is a major concern with neuroleptic administration because of its frequency, its tendency to persist, and an absence of satisfactory treatment for TD (Baldessarini et al., 1980).

The prevalence of TD in chronic neuroleptic-treated patient populations in post-1975 studies has been 20% to 35% (Jeste & Wyatt, 1982). At the Long Island Jewish-Hillside Medical Center, an ongoing prospective study found the incidence of TD in relatively young outpatients being treated with low to moderate doses of neuroleptics to be 3% to 4% per year (Kane, Woerner, Lieberman, 1988).

Risk Factors

It is difficult to predict whether and when an individual patient will develop TD. Tardive dyskinesia has been discussed in the literature only in the past 30 years, and epidemiological research in this area has some serious methodological problems. For example, most of the clinical investigations looking at risk factors have been retrospective. (Only recently have prospective studies been undertaken, Kane, Woerner, et al., 1988.) The retrospective studies have been inconsistent in controlling for factors such as treatment history, concurrent medications, and duration of TD. There are likely to be complex interactions between factors such as age and duration of drug treatment. Similarly, concurrent neuroleptic treatment may mask TD, and it may be difficult to distinguish between neuroleptic-withdrawal-emergent transient dyskinesia and persistent TD in a cross-sectional investigation. There is also a dearth of practical and valid animal models of TD.

The following is a discussion of more frequently mentioned putative risk factors for TD.

Age

There is considerable evidence that older patients are at a higher risk for TD. This increased risk is not likely to be merely an artifact of differential drug treatment for older patients. A number of studies have shown that the prevalence and severity of TD rise with age, independently of dosage and duration of treatment (Baldessarini et al., 1980). The age at initiation of neuroleptic treatment can discriminate between TD and non-TD groups, with TD patients being older (Jeste, Kleinman, Potkin, Luchins, & Weinberger, 1982; Jus, Pineau, & Lachance, 1976). As compared to younger patients, elderly patients with TD have fewer remissions and slower recovery even after neuroleptics are discontinued (Kane et al., 1988).

It has been suggested that some of this increased risk may be due to a greater propensity towards senile dyskinesias in the elderly (Jeste, Krull, & Kilbourn, 1990). Some investigations reported a high prevalence of spontaneous dyskinesias (5%–10%) in older age groups, but these studies examined mostly nursing-home patients (Jeste et al., 1982). These results may have been skewed by a selection bias and the possibility that neurological disorders contributed to abnormal movements. A more valid appraisal needs unselected healthy elderly subjects.

Other possible explanations for the increased prevalence of TD in the elderly include pharmacokinetic factors and neuronal loss. There may be reduced metabolism and excretion of the drugs, as similar oral doses of neuroleptics can produce significantly higher serum neuroleptic levels in patients over 50 years than in younger patients (Jeste & Wyatt, 1987; Yesavage, Tanke, & Sheikh, 1987).

Gender

Some studies found women to have a slightly higher risk for developing TD (including severe TD), particularly in the elderly group. This is, however, not a consistent or "robust" finding.

Brain Damage

Although brain damage has been reported to contribute to higher risk of TD, it is unclear whether any specific type of brain damage predisposes to TD.

Type of Neuroleptic

All commonly used neuroleptics have been implicated in the development of TD. There are conflicting reports about specific drugs being more or less likely to cause TD. Currently it is safe to assume that all available neuroleptics given in comparable amounts carry a somewhat similar risk for TD. Some of the newer agents (e.g., clozapine) have been claimed to have a lower risk of TD, but large-scale long-term studies have not yet been done.

Dosage and Duration

There are reports of a positive association of TD with higher doses and longer duration of treatment, although the relationship is certainly not linear.

Drug Holidays

There is no satisfactory evidence that specific types of drug holidays prevent TD. On the contrary, some studies have reported a possible association between drug holidays and persistent or severe TD (Jeste, Potkin, Sinha, Feder, & Wyatt, 1979; Yassa, Nair, Iskandar, & Schwartz, 1990).

Anticholinergics

There are no hard data showing that anticholinergics increase the risk of TD. However, their use may unmask or aggravate existing TD.

Mood Disorder

Several investigators have found a high prevalence of TD in patients with mood disorders, especially depression (Casey, in press).

Extrapyramidal Symptoms

Patients with a history of other extrapyramidal symptoms (e.g., parkinsonism or dystonia) may be at a higher risk of developing TD (Crane & Sneets, 1976, Kane, Woerner, et al., 1988).

Individual Predisposition

It is often unclear why some patients develop severe TD with relatively limited exposure to neuroleptics, while other patients have no evidence of TD, even after years of large doses. Investigations of factors underlying the possible individual predisposition to TD have generally focused on biochemical abnormalities such as disturbances of dopaminergic-cholinergic balance, decreased GABAergic activity, and nonadrenergic dysfunction. We found evidence for noradrenergic overactivity in some patients with TD (Kaufmann et al., 1986), but whether this abnormality preceded or followed the development of TD was not known.

Family History

There may be genetic factors influencing development of TD. There have been no published large-scale studies of family history of TD, but this may be of potential value in determining possible risk factors.

Possible Subtypes of TD

TD may also be classified into persistent and reversible types. Response to withdrawal of neuroleptics for at least 3 months may be used as a criterion for judging reversibility of TD (Jeste et al., 1979). Patients with reversible TD are likely to respond to many nonspecific treatments, while those with persistent TD would not benefit from most of the available treatments. Approximately 35% to 45% of TD patients respond to many different types of drugs with dissimilar mechanisms of action (Jeste et al., 1988). In at least some cases, positive results may not have been due to specific actions of the drugs given but to such nonspecific factors as placebo response, spontaneous remission, and concomitant treatments such as psychotherapy or environmental modifications. These cases are probably those of reversible dyskinesia.

Casey (1976) suggested that there may be at least two subtypes of TD: one responds to cholinergic drugs, the other to antidopaminergic agents. Recent studies indicate that there may be multiple biochemical-pharmacological subtypes characterized by noradrenergic hyperactivity, GABA'ergic hypoactivity, cholinergic hypoactivity, etc. (Kaufmann et al., 1986).

Course of TD

In nearly two-thirds of patients with TD, the symptoms persist for at least 3 months after neuroleptic discontinuation. On the other hand, long-term follow-up studies now indicate that TD is not necessarily a progressive and irreversible condition (Casey, in press). Patients may have steady improvement in TD when neuroleptics are withdrawn, and improvement may be seen even years after drug discontinuation. Furthermore, TD may not worsen even when patients are kept on the same neuroleptic dose. Important unresolved issues include predictors of the course of TD both in patients maintained on neuroleptics and in those withdrawn from neuroleptics.

MAJOR GAPS IN KNOWLEDGE

It will be important to seek answers to the following questions with reference to therapeutic response to neuroleptics (Carpenter et al., 1987):

1. How long do neuroleptic drugs need to be continued in CMI patients who have been stable in terms of psychopathology for some time?
2. Does the neuroleptic response change over time after repeated episodes and courses of administration? Is the patient response related to the stage of illness? Does prior neuroleptic drug treatment affect subsequent therapeutic response?
3. What are the treatment requirements of patients with late-onset (i.e., onset after age 45) schizophrenia (Harris & Jeste, 1988)?
4. Are there gender-related differences in treatment response?
5. Why are there relatively large differences in the average dosages of neuroleptics used in the treatment of schizophrenia in different countries (Doongaji et al., 1982)?
6. How should we treat patients who show incomplete or minimal response to neuroleptic medication?
7. What is the best treatment strategy for deinstitutionalized CMI elderly patients? An ever-increasing proportion of the CMI population is deinstitutionalized and living in supported environments, in their families' homes, and even on the streets. This patient population is generally excluded from treatment research, and we therefore do not have satisfactory data on effective treatments for them.
8. What are the primary indications (other than schizophrenia) for using neuroleptics in the elderly? In clinical practice, neuroleptics are frequently prescribed in the elderly for controlling agitation (Salzman, 1987). The risk:benefit ratio of neuroleptics for such symptoms needs to be compared with that for other available treatments (e.g., benzodiazepines).

Important questions that need to be answered with respect to TD:

1. What is the risk (in terms of annual incidence) of TD in CMI elderly patients? It will be ideal to obtain risk estimates for individual variables such as diagnostic category (e.g., schizophrenia, bipolar mood disorder, etc.), gender, and age at the start of neuroleptic treatment.

2. What is the relative risk of TD with different types of neuroleptics? Are there minimum and maximum threshold durations or total amounts of neuroleptics beyond which the risk for TD is relatively low? Are there factors that protect some patients against the development of TD?

3. Can we predict the course of TD in a given patient, either in case of continuation of neuroleptics or if neuroleptics are discontinued?

4. Can one operationally define biochemical-pharmacological subtypes of TD? It would be most useful if the best treatment for TD in a patient could be determined on the basis of certain biochemical indices—e.g., low concentrations of a neurotransmitter in certain body fluids may indicate treatment with the specific neurotransmitter agonist. This is, of course, a simplistic model. Yet complex versions of the same may be applicable.

5. Is there a relationship between therapeutic response to neuroleptics and the risk of TD? A corollary would be a study of changes in therapeutic response with aging. An association between persistent TD and schizophrenic "burnout" with predominance of the so-called negative symptoms has been suggested but needs to be tested in a prospective manner.

6. Is the risk of TD reduced by measures such as avoiding polypharmacy? An association between TD and excessive smoking has been suggested, and it will be valuable to know if cessation of smoking would lower the risk of TD. The relationship of TD to alcoholism and other substance abuse also needs to be explored.

7. Do neuroleptics produce Parkinson's disease or persistent tardive parkinsonism? This question has obvious clinical and theoretical implications.

SUGGESTED RESEARCH STRATEGIES

1. There is, first and foremost, an urgent need for prospective long-term investigations of the CMI patients being treated with neuroleptics. Multidisciplinary, comprehensive, yet hypothesis-oriented evaluations of patients at the time they are started on neuroleptics, followed by repeat assessments at regular intervals, are warranted. The evaluations should include psychiatric, neurologic, other medical, neuropsychologic, and psychosocial batteries using reliable and valid instruments. Because of the large number of variables that are inevitably involved in clinical studies of this type and a likelihood of numerous dropouts, the sample sizes must be large. Videotaping of the patients under standard conditions is valuable for documentation and also for subsequent "blind" ratings by other researchers. Sophisticated statistical analyses (often multivariate) are necessary to separate out contributions of interdependent variables. Studies of this kind will provide useful information about incidence and risk factors for TD in specific types of patient populations.

2. Similar investigations of the course of TD are necessary both in the CMI patients who are maintained on neuroleptics and in those patients withdrawn from these drugs.

3. Cross-cultural comparative studies using similar designs are likely to give information about the value of different treatment strategies in different settings about the relative contributions of biological and sociocultural factors to certain phenomena—e.g., the reports that chronic schizophrenic patients in oriental countries need lower doses of neuroleptics than their Western counterparts (Doongaji et al., 1982).

4. The CMI elderly patients with clinical, neuropsychological, and brain-imaging evaluations should be followed until their death, and every effort should be made to obtain their brains for appropriate neurochemical and neuropathological studies. At the least, such investigations will help us understand better the possible "significance" of specific antemortem data.

5. It is important to try to develop better animal models of chronic mental illnesses and their treatments. While the former is likely to be more difficult, it is certainly worthwhile examining behavioral, neurochemical, and neuropathological effects of long-term (many months) administration of neuroleptics in rats and primates.

Suggestions for Well-designed Treatment Studies for TD

1. Diagnosis of TD should be based on specified criteria and confirmed by at least two investigators independently.

2. If possible, neuroleptics and anticholinergic agents should be withdrawn at least 3 months before the study. Most cases of reversible TD will then be excluded. If this procedure is not practical, neuroleptics should be maintained at a stable dose for at least 3 months before the study and throughout the treatment period.

3. Double-blind designs should include an active placebo. The groups should be similar in terms of age, psychiatric diagnosis, length of neuroleptic treatment, and location and duration of TD. Plasma concentrations of the drug should be determined when feasible.

4. Severity of the symptoms of TD, other extrapyramidal symptoms, and psychopathology should be evaluated by at least two trained raters, using standardized rating scales. Videotaping or filming is highly recommended. Patients should be assessed at the same time (of the day and the week) and the same place throughout the experiment. Long-term trials are preferable to short-term ones.

5. Data analysis should look at both the mean change in scores (absolute as well as percentage change) and the number of patients showing 50% or greater improvement.

BARRIERS TO RESEARCH AND SUGGESTIONS
FOR IMPROVEMENT

1. There are several practical difficulties in conducting long-term prospective clinical studies of neuroleptic-treated CMI patients. The most common problem is that of dropouts. Patients may drop out because of treatment resistance, side effects, physical illnesses, difficulties in transportation, migration, etc. The resulting attrition in the sample sizes not only reduces the number of patients being followed but also raises questions about the representativeness of the sample available at the end of the study. Close attention to the follow-up right from the inception of the study and use of sophisticated statistical analyses (e.g., survival analysis) are recommended.

2. The number of patients that can be studied at any single center is usually not large and may also reflect a somewhat biased sample because of the nature of the population from which the study sample is drawn. For example, a large university hospital located downtown is likely to cater to a different patient population than a small private hospital in suburbia. A nationally reputed center will attract more treatment-resistant patients from different areas. For these reasons, well-planned multicenter studies are sometimes desirable.

3. There is a lack of uniformity in the diagnostic criteria and rating scales used by different investigators. In many studies, the diagnosis of TD is not based on any explicit criteria. Although the Abnormal Involuntary Movement Scale (AIMS) (National Institute of Mental Health, 1975) and Simpson's Rockland Tardive Dyskinesia Rating Scale (Simpson, Varga, & Lee, 1978) are the most commonly employed rating scales, some investigators have used other scales with unproven validity, and some studies have not included any formal rating scales.

Furthermore, all clinical rating scales are subjective and less reliable than instrumental approaches to measuring TD (Caligiuri, Jeste, & Harris, 1989). At the same time, the validity of specific instrumental approaches must be established. Hence, a combination of clinical and instrumental assessments is optimum.

It will be helpful to have well-defined diagnostic criteria for TD in the new DSM-IV.

4. Inadequate communication across specialties is a frequent concern. Thus, research on TD conducted by psychiatrists *versus* that by neurologists is generally presented and published in different forums. One way of dealing with this problem is to encourage multidisciplinary research and to hold multidisciplinary meetings on a given topic (e.g., treatment of TD).

5. The spectacular advances in technology (such as the various brain-imaging techniques, including Magnetic Resonance Imaging, or MRI, and Positron Emission Tomography, or PET) may have led to a lowering of the emphasis on clinical

aspects of studies. This should be considered most unfortunate, because the technological "findings" are virtually uninterpretable in the absence of suitable clinical data.

6. An inherent problem in studying disorders such as schizophrenia and TD is that these are most probably heterogeneous syndromes with multifactorial etiopathology. There is, therefore, a dual risk either of generalizing results that are pertinent only to a subtype of the disorder or of a type II error (*viz.*, concluding that a specific mechanism is irrelevant to the disorder because of the absence of "positive" findings in the sample studied). Use of large and heterogeneous populations will help avoid such errors.

7. As with some other areas of research, a major problem in proper studies of TD is an inadequacy of financial resources. This makes it difficult to undertake and complete the long-term intensive studies that are needed and discourages bright young investigators from entering the field.

A concerted effort by the NIMH, VA, other federal and state government agencies, the pharmaceutical industry, and academia, as well as practicing clinicians, should result in the development of newer and better solutions to the problem of treating CMI patients without the risk of TD.

ACKNOWLEDGMENTS

I want to thank Brenda Clemons-Stribling and Susan Noblin for expert administrative assistance. This work was supported, in part, by NIMH grants #MH43693 and MH45131, and by the Veterans Affairs.

REFERENCES

Baldessarini, R. J., Cole, J. O., Davis, J. M., Gardos, G., Preskorn, S. H., Simpson, G. M., & Tarsy, D. (1980). Tardive dyskinesia, Task Force Report 18. Washington, DC: American Psychiatric Association.

Caligiuri, M. P., Jeste, D. V., & Harris, M. J. (1989). Instrumental assessment of lingual motor instability in tardive dyskinesia. *Neuropsychopharmacology, 2*, 309–312.

Carpenter, W. T., Schooler, N. R., Goldman, H., Goldstein, M. J., Hogarty, G. E., Jeste, D. V., Kane, J. M., Klerman, G. M., Liberman, R. P., Paul, S. M., Spring, B., Stahl, S. M., Tamminga, C. A., & Robinson, D. A. (1987). Relieving the pain: Research on treatment, services, and environmental factors. In *National Institute of Mental Health: Report to the National Advisory Mental Health Council on a National Plan for Research on Schizophrenia* (pp. 52–59). Washington, DC: U.S. Department of Health and Human Services.

Casey, D. E. (1976). Tardive dyskinesia: Are there subtypes? *New England Journal of Medicine, 295,* 1078.

Casey, D. E. (in press). Tardive dyskinesia. *Western Journal of Medicine.*

Crane, G. E., & Sneets, R. A. (1976). Tardive dyskinesia and drug therapy in geriatric patients. *British Journal of Psychiatry, 30,* 341–343.

Doongaji, D. R., Jeste, D. V., Jape, N. M., Sheth, A. S., Apte, J. S., Vahia, V. N., et al. (1982). Tardive dyskinesia in India: A prevalence study. *Journal of Clinical Psychopharmacology, 2,* 341–344.

Harris, M. J., & Jeste, D. V. (1988). Late onset schizophrenia: An overview. *Schizophrenia Bulletin, 14,* 39–55.

Jeste, D. V., Kleinman, J. E., Potkin, S. G., Luchins, D. J., & Weinberger, D. R. (1982). Ex uno multi: Subtyping the schizophrenia syndrome. *Biological Psychiatry, 17,* 199–222.

Jeste, D. V., Krull, A. J., & Kilbourn, K. (1990). Tardive dyskinesia: Managing a common neuroleptic side effect. *Geriatrics, 41,* 49–58.

Jeste, D. V., Lohr, J. B., Clark, K., & Wyatt, R. J. (1988). Pharmacological treatments of tardive dyskinesia in the 1980s. *Journal of Clinical Psychopharmacology, 8*(4, Supp.), 38S–48S.

Jeste, D. V., Potkin, S. G., Sinha, S., Feder, S. L., & Wyatt, R. J. (1979). Tardive dyskinesia— Reversible and persistent. *Archives of General Psychiatry, 36,* 585–590.

Jeste, D. V., & Wyatt, R. J. (1982). *Understanding and treating tardive dyskinesia.* New York: Guilford Press.

Jeste, D. V., & Wyatt, R. J. (1987). Aging and tardive dyskinesia. In N. E. Miller & G. D. Cohen (Eds.), *Schizophrenia and aging* (pp. 275–286). New York: Guilford Press.

Jus, A., Pineau, R., Lachance R., Pelchat, G., Jus, K., Pires, P., & Villeneuve, R. (1976). Epidemiology of tardive dyskinesia: Part II. *Diseases of the Nervous System, 37,* 257–261.

Kane, J. M., Honigfeld, G., Singer, J., Meltzer, H., & the Clozaril Collaborative Study Group. (1988). Clozapine for treatment-resistant schizophrenic: A double blind comparison with chlorpromazine. *Archives of General Psychiatry, 45,* 789–796.

Kane, J. M., Woerner, M., & Lieberman, J. (1988). Tardive dyskinesia: Prevalence, incidence and risk factors. *Journal of Clinical Psychopharmacology, 8,* 52S–56S.

Kaufmann, C. A., Jeste, D. V., Linnoila, M., Shelton, R., Kafka, M., & Wyatt, R. J. (1986). Noradrenergic and neuroradiologic abnormalities in tardive dyskinesia. *Biological Psychiatry, 21,* 799–812.

National Institute of Mental Health. (1975). Psychopharmacology research branch: Abnormal involuntary movement scale. *Early Clinical Drug Evaluation Unit Intercom, 4,* 3–6.

Phillipson, M., Moranville, J. T., Jeste, D. V., & Harris, M. J. (1990). Antipsychotics. In P. P. Lamy (Ed.), "Clinical Pharmacology" issue of *Clinics in Geriatric Medicine* (pp. 411–422). Philadelphia: W. B. Saunders Company.

Salzman, C. (1987). Treatment of agitation in the elderly. In H. Y. Meltzer (Ed.), *Psychopharmacology: The third generation of progress* (pp. 1167–1176). New York: Raven Press.

Simpson, G. M., Varga, E., Lee, J. H., & Zoubok, B. (1978). Tardivie dyskineseia and psychotropic drug history. *Psychopharmacology, 58,* 117–124.

Smith, J. M., & Baldessarini, R. J. (1980). Changes in prevalence, severity and recovery in tardive dyskinesia with age. *Archives of General Psychiatry, 37,* 1368–1373.

Varga, E., Sugerman, A. A., Varga, V., Zomorodi, A., Zomoradi, W., & Menken, M. (1982). Prevalence of spontaneous oral dyskinesia in the elderly. *American Journal of Psychiatry, 139,* 329–331.

Yassa, R., Nair, N. P. V., Iskandar, H., & Schwartz, G. (1990). Factors in the development of severe forms of tardive dyskinesia. *American Journal of Psychiatry, 147,* 1156–1163.

Yesavage, J. A., Tanke, E. D., & Sheikh, J. I. (1987). Tardive dyskinesia and steady-state serum levels of thiothixene. *Archives of General Psychiatry, 44,* 913–915.

9

Neuroimaging in the Elderly with Chronic Mental Illness

Andrew F. Leuchter, Mercedes M. Garcia

A major thrust in current psychiatric research is aimed at developing physiologically based diagnostic tests for the major mental illnesses. Currently, these illnesses are diagnosed by constellations of nonspecific diagnostic criteria, as in the *Diagnostic and Statistical Manual for Mental Disorders* (3rd ed., revised, 1988). For research purposes, these tests are sometimes augmented by scores on rating scales of mood, anxiety, or thought. While these scores are highly correlated with particular diagnoses, they usually represent only more quantifiable measures of nonspecific criteria.

Any quantitative physiologically based technique could add much to diagnostic accuracy, particularly in mental illnesses affecting the elderly. Many elderly people live independently and are not closely observed by others, so that the history of onset and development of their symptoms may be documented poorly. Furthermore, many of the elderly with major mental illnesses present with psychosis or confusion of sufficient magnitude to make formal interviewing or mental status testing difficult.

A potential area for the development of new diagnostic tests is in vivo imaging of the central nervous system ("neuroimaging"). The imaging technologies that have been used fall into one of two broad categories. The first category is structural imaging, which includes computed tomography (CT) and magnetic resonance imaging (MRI) scanning; these techniques are designed primarily to detect gross structural alterations of the brain. The second category of imaging technology is functional imaging, which includes emission tomography (both single photon emission computed tomography, SPECT, and positron emission tomography, PET) as well as topographic mapping of brain electrical activity (also known as quantitative electroencephalography, qEEG).

These techniques have not been extensively applied to the study of the chronically mentally ill elderly. Nevertheless, a number of studies of normal elderly subjects, young chronically mentally ill adults, and preliminary studies of chronically mentally ill elderly suggest that neuroimaging techniques could play an important role in diagnosing and understanding chronic mental illnesses among the elderly.

After a brief review of the major imaging technologies, this chapter will focus on the three categories of chronic mental disorders seen among the elderly (mood disorders, psychotic disorders, and organic mental disorders) and review the neuroimaging findings involving these disorders. The chapter will conclude with a look ahead toward new approaches to the study and diagnosis of these disorders using neuroimaging.

REVIEW OF NEUROIMAGING TECHNIQUES

Structural Imaging Techniques

X-ray computed tomography (CT scanning) constructs images of "slices" of the brain based upon measurements of brain tissue density derived from X-rays passing through the brain. Images are reconstructed through linear superimposition of filtered back-projections. This method of image reconstruction is common to all methods of computed tomography, including the functional imaging techniques discussed below.

CT scans may be performed with or without intravenously injected contrast material; contrast material may be useful for detecing disruptions of the blood-brain barrier or abnormal confluences of blood vessels as seen in tumors or vascular malformations.

For many applications, CT has been superceded by MRI. For this technique, which does not use ionizing radiation, the subject is bombarded by radio-frequency (RF) waves while resting in an intense magnetic field. Images of slices of brain tissue are constructed based on energy emission of molecules within different microchemical environments. These energy emissions are highly dependent upon proton density, magnetic susceptibility, and T1 and T2 relaxation times (i.e., time required for molecules to reorient themselves in a magnetic field following RF pulsing). Simple tissue (i.e., electron) density plays little role in MR imaging, which in part accounts for the superior contrast seen with MRI (Jernigan, 1986).

The principal molecule relied upon in clinical imaging is water, whose hydrogen molecules absorb and release RF energy differentially based on the surrounding tissue. Imaging can technically be performed based upon measuring the energy emissions of any element with an odd number of nucleons, including phosphorus.

The major advantages of CT scanning are that it can be performed relatively quickly and that the equipment is widely available. CT scanning also may be superior for the detection of acute hemorrhage. In some geographic areas, there remains a significant cost differential between CT and MRI scans, with CT as little as half the cost of an MRI. This differential is vanishing rapidly, however, as MRI equipment becomes more widely available.

MRI scans generally are superior to CT scans in image resolution, clarity, and visualization of pathology. One major advantage of MRI is its sensitivity to alterations in water content and microchemical environments within the brain. The density of gray and white matter are very similar, so that these tissues virtually are indistinguishable on CT. MRI, however, clearly distinguishes between gray and white structures, and can reveal the presence of demyelinating lesions within white matter as small as 0.5 mm or less. CT has traditionally had the advantage of intravenously infused contrast material being available. With the recent advent of gadolinium, a paramagnetic contrast medium, MRI scanning has become even more sensitive to disruptions of the blood-brain barrier.

Structural imaging has been used primarily for detection of gross structural alterations of brain tissue, such as atrophy, ventricular dilation, infarction, and hemorrhage. MRI scanning also has revealed the existence of previously undetected deep white-matter ischemic disease and periventricular hyperintensity in the elderly, the significance of which is under study.

Functional Imaging Techniques

Topographic Mapping of Brain Electrical Activity

Topographic maps of brain electrical activity display the quantitative characteristics of the brain's electrical signal production over a given period of time. For this technique, the electrical signal is recorded and processed (generally through Fourier transformation) to produce maps of a variety of characteristics, including the amplitude or power of the signal from a single location or the coherence (i.e., synchronization) of the signal between two locations in each of several frequency bands.

The evolution of a subject's electrical signal production may be mapped on a second-by-second basis; generally, however, these maps are based upon average electrical activity over a period ranging from 20 seconds to 30 minutes. The quantitative basis for these maps yields a number of advantages over conventional EEG. Since values for brain electrical activity in the maps are averaged over time, they generally are a more stable indicator than the conventional EEG of patterns of EEG signal production. Furthermore, such maps may be easily compared to previous examinations of the same subject, or to a normative database, to detect shifts in an individual's electrical signal production. The major advantage of conventional electroencephalography lies in the ability to detect paroxysmal (i.e., epileptiform) abnormalities, to which maps are insensitive because of time averaging.

Emission Tomography

Emission tomography techniques utilize one of a number of possible compounds of neurophysiologic significance, labeled with a rapidly decaying radioisotope (Jernigan, 1986). These compounds are differentially sequestered or bound in the brain based upon metabolic rates, blood flow, specific binding sites, or other parameters. The decay of the radioisotope is detected and measured for each brain region, and images are constructed in much the same manner as for CT or MRI scanning.

There are two major techniques, one utilizing single photon emitting radionuclides (SPECT), the other using positron emitting radionuclides (PET). PET uses one of many possible tracer compounds labelled with oxygen[15], fluorine[18], or other positron-emitting elements that are generally of very short half-life. PET scanning therefore requires use of a cyclotron to produce labeled compounds at or near the site of use. SPECT scanning has the advantage of relying upon photon-emitting labeled compounds with relatively long half-lives; these are easier and less costly to generate and to use. Photon-emitting compounds generally produce less energy than positron emitters, however, and the single or few detectors employed in most SPECT scanners detect a relatively small proportion of this energy. PET images generally have been of significantly higher resolution and quality than SPECT images, since more energy is produced from positron emission by the "annihilation reaction" and a higher proportion of the emitted energy is detected and used for image reconstruction through a paradigm known as "coincidence detection" (Leenders, Gibbs, Frackowiak, Lammertsma, & Jones, 1984; Raichle, 1983; Guze, Hoffman, Baxter, Mazziotta, & Phelps, in submission; Yamamoto, Thompson, Diksic, Meyer, & Feindel, 1984). The advent of improved equipment for SPECT scanning, with circumferential arrays of detectors to capture a greater proportion of emitted photon energy, is leading to production of SPECT images that rival the quality of PET.

NEUROIMAGING FINDINGS ASSOCIATED WITH NORMAL AGING

Structural Changes

Clinical experience has shown that there are a number of behavioral changes which occur in "normal" aging, such as slowed reaction time and age-associated memory impairment. Just as it is vital to distinguish these normally occurring phenomena from signs of illness, it is crucial to identify and understand the neuroimaging findings associated with normal aging.

There is abundant evidence from CT scan studies that a certain degree of brain atrophy is associated with normal aging. Mild to moderate atrophy is common, and no studies have detected an association between this degree of atrophy and cognitive deficits (Bryan, 1985; DeLeon, Ferris, & George, 1985). While there is a weak association between degree of atrophy and cognitive impairment (Earnest, Heaton, Wilkinson, & Manke, 1979), Huckman, Fox, and Topel (1975) reported moderate to severe atrophy in 15% of apparently healthy, cognitively intact individuals, making this a nonspecific finding.

A number of investigators have demonstrated that this atrophy is global, leading to increased ventricular and sulcal size (Barron, Jacob, & Kinkel, 1976; Haug, 1977; Hughes & Gado, 1981; Yamamura, Ito, Kubota, Kubota, & Matsuzawa, 1980). Miller, Alston, and Orsellis (1980) have pointed out that while this atrophy affects both gray and white matter, gray matter is lost in earlier decades while white matter is lost later in senescence.

MRI has yielded further information on structural alterations that are seen in normal aging. Two of the most common findings are multiple areas of deep white-matter hyperintensity and periventricular hyperintensity (Sarpel, Chaudry, & Hindo, 1987; Zimmerman, Fleming, Lee, Saint-Louis, & Deck, 1986). These findings may broadly be classified as "leukoencephalopathy" (Coffey et al., 1988), and have been reported to exist in 20–60% of normal elderly subjects (Brant-Zawadski et al., 1985; Fazekas, Chawiuk, Alavi, Hurtig, & Zimmerman, 1987).

The clinicopathologic significance of this leukoencephalopathy is unknown. Areas of deep white-matter hyperintensity generally are thought to represent focal demyelination, most likely related to ischemic disease that may be subclinical (Coffey et al., 1988; Kinkel, Jacobs, Polachini, Bates, & Heffner, 1985). Periventricular hyperintensity is thought to represent interstitial water reabsorption from the white matter surrounding the ventricles, although this hypothesis has not been proven (Zimmerman et al., 1986).

The functional significance of these structural alterations remains unclear. While some studies have demonstrated a correlation between leukoencephalopathy and cognitive deficits (Hachinski, Potter, & Mersky, 1987; Kluger, Gianutsos, DeLeon, & George, 1988), others have failed to demonstrate a clear association between these findings and impairment of cognitive functioning (Brandt-Zawadzki et al., 1986a; George et al., 1986b).

Functional Changes

There is abundant literature on electrophysiologic changes that occur in normal aging. In the conventional EEG, these changes consist primarily of a slight slowing of the mean frequency of the posterior dominant rhythm, as well as increased temporal slow-wave activity (Niedermeyer, 1987; Torres, Faoro, Loewenson, & Johnson, 1983).

There is surprisingly little literature on changes in topographic maps of brain electrical activity with normal aging. Studies utilizing the BEAM (Brain Electrical Activity Mapping) technique suggest that there is diminished slow-wave power seen in normal aging, as well as diminished alpha reactivity (Duffy, Albert, McAnulty, & Garvey, 1984). There is controversy surrounding these initial findings, however, with considerable evidence that in healthy older adults slow-wave power increases, while faster frequency power and mean frequency decrease (Coben, Danziger, & Storandt, 1985; Leuchter, Spar, Walter, & Weiner, 1987; Obrist, 1976).

Other physiologic parameters that have been studied with functional imaging include regional cerebral blood flow (rCBF) and regional cerebral metabolic rate of oxygen utilization (rCMRO$_2$). For decades prior to the advent of PET scanning, these parameters commonly were studied using nitrous oxide inhalation and xenon 133 clearance techniques (Butler, Dickinson, Katholi, & Halsey, 1983; Kety & Schmidt, 1948). While initial studies indicated that there were significant declines in rCBF and rCMRO$_2$ (Kety, 1956), other studies using comparable techniques concluded that there is no consistent decline in these measures with age (Datsur et al., 1963; Lying-Tunnell, Lindblad, Malmlund, & Persson, 1980).

The newer technology of PET scanning has facilitated measurement of these parameters as well as cerebral metabolic rate of glucose utilization (CMRglu) and regional CMRglu. Initial PET studies concluded that rCMRO$_2$ declines slightly with aging, but much less markedly than rCBF (Frackowiak, Lenzi, Jones, & Heather, 1980: Frackowiak, Wise, Gibbs, & Jones, 1984). Subsequent studies concluded that mean local CMRglu declines by as much as 26% between the second and eighth decades (Kuhl, Metter, Riege, & Phelps, 1982; Kuhl, Metter, & Riege, 1985). While these results point towards a consistent decline in cerebral blood flow and metabolism with age, other research casts doubt on these results. Studies by Duara and colleagues (1983, 1986) and DeLeon and co-workers (1987) that focused on CMRglu and rCMRglu suggest that cerebral metabolism is comparable in young and old adults. Even among the patients studied by Kuhl, Metter, and Riege (1985), there was significant variation in cerebral metabolic rates among elderly subjects, with some showing CMRglu comparable to young adults. The wide variation in findings among studies, and among individuals within studies, led Creasey and Rapoport (1985) to postulate that health status is the major factor accounting for disparate study results. While it is true that studies have varied widely in their exclusion criteria pertaining to general physical health, this hypothesis remains to be proved by systematic study. Another possible cause for variation in study results is failure to control rigorously for the state of the subject, to which PET scanning is highly sensitive.

Integration of structural and functional imaging studies among normal elderly subjects is still in its very early stages. Some of the initial results suggest that structural changes, most notably atrophy, can occur without a concomitant metabolic defect (DeLeon et al., 1987). The convergence of structural and functional imaging studies will be much more powerful than either alone in elucidating the significance of changes in the brain with aging.

FINDINGS ASSOCIATED WITH SPECIFIC DISORDERS
Late-onset Psychosis

There are two distinct forms of psychosis that affect the elderly: psychosis of early onset that persists into senescence (i.e., chronic schizophrenia with onset in the third decade) and psychosis of late onset with no early life history of major mental illness. The most frequent causes of late-onset psychosis are dementing illnesses and affective disorders. Primary psychotic disorders, such as schizophrenia, only uncommonly present late in life (Leuchter & Spar, 1985). Although they represent a heterogeneous group of disorders, several studies have examined the late-onset disorders together, and these studies are reviewed here.

Neuroimaging studies of late-onset psychoses are helpful in identifying possible organic etiologies for the disorders since there appears to be a significant association between structural brain alterations and late-onset psychosis. Leuchter and Spar (1985) found that of patients admitted to a psychiatric unit with late-onset psychotic symptoms, 33% had an organic mental disorder, and a substantial proportion of patients without evidence of infarction had signs of symptoms of significant atherosclerosis.

Early structural imaging findings among patients with late-onset psychosis included infarction and idiopathic basal ganglia calcification (Cummings, 1985), although the cognitive status of these patients was not carefully examined. In a small series of subjects with late-onset psychosis without obvious evidence of cognitive losses, Miller, Benson, Cummings, and Neshkes (1986) found structural brain damage, including infarction and hydrocephalus. More recently, Miller and Lesser (1988) reported on 25 patients with late-onset psychosis and found that approximately 20% had some evidence of "silent" vascular disease with significant white-matter lesions. All of Miller's patients demonstrated significant disease in the white matter underlying the frontal lobes, that appeared to correlate with impaired frontal-lobe function (unpublished data). A smaller proportion had other structural lesions, including tumors. Certainly not all or even most late-onset psychosis can be explained on the basis of gross structural changes, since 40% of Miller's subjects had no evidence of abnormalities on CT or MRI. Even among those subjects with such disease, there is no method to establish a causal link firmly (Leuchter, 1988).

Functional imaging may yield useful information regarding late-onset psychosis, but almost no results have been reported in this area. Miller and Lesser (1988) describe "abnormalities in the frontal area" seen on SPECT scanning as well as topographic mapping of brain electrical activity in a small series of patients, with research on a larger cohort in progress.

Schizophrenia

One of the most common structural alterations reported among subjects with schizophrenia at any age is that of ventricular enlargement. Several groups of investigators, including Weinberger, Cannon-Spoor, Potkin, and Wyatt (1980) and Andreasen, Olsen, Dennert, and Smith (1982) have described correlations between increased ventricular size, poorer premorbid adjustment, and "negative symptoms." Nasrallah, Kuperman, Jacoby, McCalley-Whitters, and Harma (1983) demonstrated that this cerebral atrophy, as measured by sulcal widening, is related to cognitive impairment as measured by the Mini-Mental State Examination (MMSE).

The association between atrophy, ventricular enlargement, and negative symptoms appears to be largely uninfluenced by age. In one of the few studies specifically examining the elderly, Johnstone, Crow, Frith, Husband, and Kreel, (1976) studied a group of 13 elderly chronic schizophrenics and found increases in ventricular size that were not significantly associated with increasing age. Weinberger, Torrey, Neophytides, and Wyatt (1979) corroborated the absence of an age effect in 73 chronic schizophrenics, all under 50 years of age.

The advent of the MRI has increased the capacity to detect structural detail among schizophrenic subjects. In general, MRI studies have simply corroborated the findings described with CT scanning. Although one of the first studies by Smith et al. (1984) failed to detect ventricular enlargement among schizophrenic subjects, subsequent studies have confirmed the presence of atrophy (Andreasen et al., 1986), ventricular enlargement (Kelsoe, Cadet, Pickar, & Weinberger, 1988), and other structural changes (Nasrallah et al., 1986). None of these studies focused primarily on the elderly.

Topographic mapping of brain electrical activity has not been applied to the study of elderly schizophrenic patients and among younger age groups has yielded conflicting results. Morihisa, Duffy, and Wyatt (1983) demonstrated "hypofrontality" among younger schizophrenic patients as determined by increased slow-wave activity in the frontal regions. This finding was not supported by Karson, Coppola, Morihisa, and Weinberger (1987), who found no excessive frontal slowing compared to controls when data contaminated by eye movements were rigorously eliminated. Other findings, such as the left-hemispheric dysfunction reported by Morstyn, Duffy, and McCarley (1983) and Guenther and Breitling (1985), await replication among unmedicated subjects as well as study of older chronic schizophrenic patients.

Similarly, PET scanning has not been specifically applied to the study of older schizophrenic patients. Work among younger patients has yielded a variety of interesting, albeit sometimes conflicting, results. Investigators have reported the existence of hypofrontality (Buchsbaum et al., 1982; Farkas et al., 1984; Volkow et al., 1986a; Wolkin et al., 1985; Wolkin et al., 1988), hyperfrontality (Volkow et al., 1986b), left hypofrontality induced only by treatment (Widen et al., 1983), or no significant differences in frontal blood flow or metabolism compared to controls (Kling, Metter, Riege, & Kuhl, 1986; Sheppard, Gruzelier, Manchanda, & Hirsch, 1983). A variety of focal or lateralizing abnormalities also have been noted among schizophrenic patients when compared with controls, including right-left hemispheric asymmetries (Gur et al., 1987; Wiesel, Wik, Blomqvist, Greitz, & Stone-Elander, 1987) and left hemispheric "overactivation" during verbal and spatial activation tasks (Gur, 1978; Gur et al., 1985).

Analogous to findings for structural abnormalities, increasingly severe functional abnormality has been associated with "negative symptoms," lack of reactivity to activation tasks, as well as poorer response to medications (Guenther et al., 1986; Volkow et al., 1987). Other work has suggested that "subtypes" of schizophrenics have metabolic changes in other brain regions (Kishimoto et al., 1987).

An interesting and developing line of work has focused on imaging dopamine D2 receptors in schizophrenic patients. Using (3-N-[11C]methyl) spiperone, Wong et al. (1986) and Crawley et al. (1986) have noted an increase in D2 receptors both in schizophrenics with a previous history of exposure to neuroleptics and in schizophrenics without a previous history of drug exposure. This work has focused exclusively on young schizophrenic patients.

There are several factors that probably contribute to the conflicting functional imaging results seen among schizophrenic patients. Lack of standardization in diagnostic criteria, as well as failure to control for mental activity, sensory stimulation, duration of illness, and exposure to medication, may yield differing results when studying apparently similar populations.

Mood Disorders

Structural imaging studies in the elderly with chronic affective disorders have revealed a variety of nonspecific changes. As among schizophrenic patients, ventricular enlargement appears to be the most established finding. Jacoby and Levy (1980) studied a group of older individuals (mean age 52.1) and reported that a subgroup of elderly patients with late-onset affective disorders had increased ventricular size; this group of patients did not have short-term differences in response to treatment but did have increased mortality at two-year follow-up (Jacoby, 1981). The finding of increased ventricular volume was corroborated by Coffey et al. (1988), who reported an association with refractoriness to treatment. Ventricular dilation does not appear to distinguish elderly patients with chronic depression from younger patients with affective disorder, nor does it distinguish between patients with unipolar or bipolar disease (Pearlson & Veroff, 1981; Nasrallah & Coffman, 1985), although at least one group of investigators failed to detect ventricular enlargement among younger patients with bipolar disorder (Besson, Henderson, Foreman, & Smith, 1987).

MRI scanning has revealed additional structural changes in the brains of elderly chronically depressed subjects. Coffey et al. (1988) reviewed CT and MRI scan results in 67 depressed patients preparing to undergo ECT (mean age 71.6). They reported "leukoencephalopathy" (either periventricular hyperintensity or deep white-matter hyperintensity) in 66% of this population. This finding often was associated with atrophy, lateral ventricular enlargement, and lacunar infarcts of the basal ganglia. Fifty-eight percent of these patients had a late-onset depression, and 85% had been refractory or intolerant to antidepressants. More sophisticated MRI techniques have revealed additional structural alterations associated with bipolar depressive disorder. A study of young bipolar patients revealed that while in the depressed state, they had longer T1 times in the frontal and temporal brain regions; this difference reverted to normal when the subjects were treated with lithium (Rangel-Guerra, Perez-Payan, Minkoff, & Todd, 1983).

Functional brain differences among normal controls, patients with affective disorders, and those with different types of affective disorders have been detected with functional imaging methods. These studies have been performed almost exclusively on patients below 60. Using mapping of brain electrical activity, Prichep et al. (1986) found that unipolar depressed patients could be distinguished from a group of young normal control subjects based upon composite measures of brain electrical activity, particularly increased power in the left fronto-temporal region among depressed subjects. This finding is generally consistent with the work of Shaffer, Davidson, and Saron (1983), Davidson, Schaffer, and Saron (1985), and Davidson, Chapman, and Chapman (1987) who found decreased left frontal and right posterior "activation" (i.e., increased alpha power) among depressed patients relative to controls. None of these studies focused on elderly subjects.

Using a different functional imaging method, the Xenon inhalation technique, Mathew et al. (1980) studied 13 unipolar depressed patients with a mean age of 30 and found a bilateral reduction of cerebral blood flow. Using a similar technique, Guenther et al. (1986) reported nonreactivity of rCBF to motor activation tasks.

Metabolic differences that parallel these blood flow differences also have been detected. Phelps, Mazziotta, Baxter, and Gerner (1984) studied unipolar depressed patients and reported that a bilateral decrease of glucose utilization in the striatum when compared to controls. Baxter et al. (1985) studied a larger group of patients with diagnoses of affective disorders (unipolar depressed, bipolar depressed, manic, and mixed state) as well as normal controls, all under the age of 60. They described decreased whole-brain metabolic rates among those patients with diagnoses of bipolar depression and bipolar with mixed features in comparison to the other groups. Unipolar depressed patients were best distinguished from the other groups by a ratio of metabolism in the caudate nucleus divided by the whole hemisphere that was significantly lower among these patients. These metabolic rates tended to normalize with recovery from mood disorder. Buchsbaum et al. (1986) reported decreased metabolism in the basal ganglia, as well as increased frontal to occipital metabolic ratios among unipolar depressed patients and decreased frontal to occipital ratios among bipolar depressed patients.

In one of the few reports examining an elderly patient, Kuhl (1984) examined a patient with "depressive pseudodementia," describing decreased glucose utilization of the left inferior frontal cortex in this single case.

Dementia

The dementing illnesses have frequently been examined with modern neuroimaging techniques, and not surprisingly, there are significant and fairly consistent differences between demented patients and age-matched controls. A complete review of the dementia literature is beyond the scope of this chapter. The major findings are reviewed here for the purpose of comparison to other mental illnesses among the elderly.

The study of demented patients demonstrates that the structural changes associated with dementia are nonspecific. Huckman et al. (1975) reported that some patients with cognitive impairment have no abnormal findings on CT scans, and Ford and Winter (1981) reported the similarity of scans of demented and nondemented subjects. McGeer et al. (1986) reported that degree of atrophy correlated only weakly with neuropsychiatric abnormalities among patients with dementia. Others have suggested that ventricular measurements may be more highly correlated with diagnosis and severity parameters among Alzheimer's disease patients (Soininen, Puranen, & Riekkinen, 1982), although age is still a major confounding factor in these measures (DeLeon et al., 1987).

Leukoencephalopathy as detected by MRI was first thought to be relatively specific for multi-infarct dementia (Erkinjuntti et al., 1984) but has been shown to be common in Pick's disease, Alzheimer's disease, and other forms of dementia (Johnson et al., 1987), and has been reported to be so common among normal subjects that it is of little diagnostic use (Hershey, Modic, Greenough, & Jaffe, 1987). Nevertheless, several studies have suggested that when present, the intensity of leukoencephalopathy is correlated with the severity of cognitive impairment in several different types of dementia (Besson et al., 1985; Johnson et al., 1987).

Studies of spectral analysis of the EEG have established that demented patients have increased power in low-frequency bands, decreased power in high-frequency bands, and a decrease in the mean posterior dominant rhythm (Brenner et al., 1986; Coben et al., 1985; Coben, Danziger, & Berg, 1983; Duffy, Albert, McAnulty, & Garvey, 1984; Penttila, Partanen, Soininen, & Riekkinen, 1985). It generally has been written that the EEG is insensitive to the earliest changes seen in dementia, and one study has concluded that computer analysis leads to only modest enhancements of the sensitivity of EEG (Brenner, Reynolds, & Ulrich, 1988). These studies have seldom used a comprehensive, topographic approach to data analysis, however, relying instead on one or at most a few channels of EEG data (Coben et al., 1985), sometimes pooling data from multiple channels (Brenner et al., 1986), and specifically excluding the temporal regions (Brenner et al., 1988). The topographic approach to data analysis has yielded good sensitivity in the early detection of dementia (Leuchter et al., 1987; Prichep, Gomez, John, & Ferris, 1983) and in distinguishing between different forms of dementing illness (Leuchter et al., 1987; Leuchter & Walter, 1989).

Other studies of cerebral function have utilized PET scanning and have achieved fairly consistent results. Cerebral blood flow is significantly diminished among demented patients compared to controls (Frackowiak et al., 1981). There is a generalized decrease in glucose metabolic rates among these patients (Benson, Kuhl, Phelps, Cummings, & Tsai, 1981; Farkas et al., 1982), and the metabolic deficit appears most severely to affect the temporoparietal regions bilaterally (Duara et al., 1986; Ferris & DeLeon, 1983). These findings also have been seen using SPECT scanning (Jagust & Budinger, 1988). Cutler (1988) has reported that the decrease in parietal metabolic rate may actually precede notable cognitive deficits.

DIRECTIONS FOR RESEARCH

In the area of neuroimaging research involving the chronically mentally ill, little work has focused on or even included elderly patients. The limited work that has been done does not clearly indicate that different structural or functional imaging results would be found among elderly subjects. Nevertheless, since this age group has been systematically excluded from previous studies, research is necessary to determine whether findings from younger age groups can be generalized to the elderly.

One of the highest priorities in this area must be characterization of the findings seen in "normal" aging. Many findings are commonly reported in both chronic mental illness and normal aging, and in fact no neuroimaging finding has yet been demonstrated to be both sensitive and specific for mental illness in the elderly. In the arena of structural imaging, the nonspecific findings most commonly reported among the healthy and ill are atrophy and leukoencephalopathy. In the arena of functional imaging, the most common findings are focal or generalized hypometabolism and increased slow-wave electrical activity. The literature on cerebral atrophy is a particularly good example of the difficulties confronting researchers in neuroimaging. Studies by Weinberger et al. (1979) and Johnstone et al. (1976) suggest that there is no straightforward cumulative effect of increasing age and chronic schizophrenic illness. Even among demented patients, where atrophy can be quite severe, there is not a strong relationship between the degree of atrophy and cognitive impairment (McGeer et al., 1986). Since atrophy is probably the most studied of all neuroimaging findings, it is surprising that there is still considerable confusion regarding the importance of this finding. Studies must be designed to address potentially important questions about the significance of atrophy. First, what is the impact of overall health status on degree of atrophy? This variable has seldom been addressed in studies of any of the chronic mental illnesses. Second, is there any specific pattern of atrophy that may be more indicative of pathology than normal aging? The work of Miller et al. (1980) considered the pattern of loss of gray versus white matter in normal aging, but this question has not been systematically addressed in other research. The advent of MRI will aid in visualization of cortical and subcortical gray-matter structures and should facilitate hypothesis-based research aimed at detecting specific structures subject to atrophy.

Research in functional imaging has yielded a broad range of results suggesting that the normal elderly have little or no change in cerebral blood flow and metabolism or that there are significant decreases. The only fact that these studies agree upon is that there is tremendous interindividual variation in these parameters. This variation probably is partly due to the combination of extremely sensitive neuroimaging techniques and factors in health status that have not been considered (i.e., the failure to define clearly what is meant by "normal aging").

The concept of normalcy in aging is difficult in any area of gerontologic research but is particularly problematic for neuroimaging research since advanced generation PET and MRI scanners are capable of detecting minute disruptions of brain function and structure. There is evidence to suggest that mild hypertension or hypotension, head trauma without loss of consciousness, and other physical infirmities cause subtle alterations in brain structure and function that may not be clinically apparent (e.g., detectable by neuropsychological testing). To obtain a clearer definition of the bounds of normalcy, a broad list of possible confounding factors must be considered, and to the extent possible, consistent decisions must be made regarding exclusion criteria across studies (e.g., should patients with mild hypertension be considered normal?). If such decisions are not consistent, the literature is likely to be flooded with disparate or conflicting reports of the findings in supposedly normal aging.

A review of the literature clearly indicates that better control over subject selection is necessary in future studies of neuroimaging among the chronically mentally ill elderly. Major causes for conflicting results of neuroimaging studies among young chronically mentally ill subjects are inconsistent definitions of illness, poor control over the state of the patient, and variable medication histories; these are probably the major factors accounting for diametrically opposed results among studies of schizophrenic subjects. These errors can be easily avoided in studies of the chronically mentally ill elderly by attention to potential confounding factors.

Additional comparison groups must be added for studies of elderly subjects. Among the young, subjects with affective disorders and primary psychotic disorders account for the great majority of patients with chronic illnesses of interest. Among the elderly, subjects with organic mental disorders (most notably dementia) should be used routinely as a comparison group. Dementia is one of the most common psychiatric illnesses in the elderly, and it is difficult in many cases to rule out a contribution of early Alzheimer's disease or multiple infarcts to an apparent psychotic or affective illness. This is particularly true for cases of affective disorder, which may be easily confused with dementia in the elderly. Furthermore, if the diagnostic parameters suggested by a study are likely to be of value in understanding or diagnosing an illness, they should be demonstrated to be useful in distinguishing patients with dementia from those with other mental illnesses.

A major priority in neuroimaging research must be the integration of different imaging modalities, to work toward the elimination of the dichotomy between structural and functional imaging of the brain. Virtually all of the studies discussed in this review have taken a limited perspective in the assessment of chronic mental illness, focusing on a single finding (e.g., cerebral atrophy) or a single imaging technique (e.g., PET scanning). As a result, the functional significance of atrophy or leukoencephalopathy is poorly understood, and the structural basis of focal hypometabolism remains unclear in almost all studies. For financial reasons, it is difficult to employ more than one imaging technique in any given study; in some centers, to perform both a PET and MRI scan would cost $1,500-$2,000 per subject. The great advances in neuroimaging, however, will almost certainly come through integration of structural and functional imaging, and investigators may be forced to change research designs in order to integrate techniques. First, researchers may have to limit the number of subjects studied to study more intensively individual subjects with more than one technique. Second, some researchers may have to shift from more costly imaging techniques (emission tomography) to more cost-effective technologies (topographic mapping of brain electrical activity) to achieve this integration.

There are many specific research questions that would be interesting and valuable to address early in neuroimaging research involving the elderly. Only a few of the more obvious questions are listed here. One of the first questions is Does chronic depression or schizophrenia of late onset differ from similar illness of early onset? The existence of late-onset schizophrenia was validated only in

1987 by DSM-III-R, and the physiologic characteristics of the illness have not yet been defined. Second, with the advent of ligands for specific receptor systems, it would be valuable to determine the role of changes in the density or binding characteristics of certain receptors as measured by PET scanning in chronic mental illness. For example, it would be important to determine whether cholinergic receptors are affected in depression or psychosis in the elderly and whether ligands for this system might be useful in differentiating these disorders from a dementing illness. Third, it would be important to determine if there are any neuroimaging predictors of the development of chronic mental illnesses in the elderly. Early prediction of those developing or at risk for developing a chronic mental illness would be of great clinical utility.

It is unfortunate that the elderly have been specifically excluded from most studies of neuroimaging in chronic mental illnesses since there are compelling scientific and social reasons to examine the elderly. Study of the elderly could reveal valuable information regarding the pathophysiology of chronic mental illness that is not available from studies of younger adults. The elderly are much more likely than young adults to have detectable neuropathology that may be associated with their disease. Study of the elderly may thus provide opportunities to understand the physiochemical substrates of mental illness that are not available among younger subjects.

In addition, the burgeoning population of older adults will contain large numbers of chronically mentally ill patients as longevity increases. While there are documented changes in brain structure and function with aging, the interactions between chronic mental illness and increasing age remain obscure. It is possible that the neuroimaging findings that are diagnostically useful among young adults may not be useful in the elderly. This question must be addressed if neuroimaging technologies are to be applied to the elderly patients. Research involving the elderly is therefore of interest not only to geriatric psychiatrists but also to general psychiatrists and investigators who aim to understand fully the significance of neuroimaging findings seen in chronic mental illness.

REFERENCES

Andreasen, N., Olsen, S. A., Dennert, J. W., & Smith, M. R. (1982). Ventricular enlargement in schizophrenia: Relationship to positive and negative symptoms. *American Journal of Psychiatry, 139*, 297–302.

Barron, S. A., Jacob, L., & Kinkel, W. R. (1976). Changes in the size of normal lateral ventricles during aging determined by computerized tomography. *Neurology, 26*, 1011–1013.

Baxter, L. R., Phelps, M. E., Mazziota, J. C., Schwartz, J. M., Gerner, R., Selin, C. E., & Sumida, R. M. (1985). Cerebral metabolic rates for glucose in mood disorders. *Archives of General Psychiatry, 42*, 441–447.

Benson, D. F., Kuhl, D. E., Phelps, M. E., Cummings, J. L., & Tsai, S. Y. (1981). Positron emission computed tomography in the diagnosis of dementia. *Annals of Neurology, 10*, 76.

Besson, J. A. O., Corrigan, F. M., Foreman, E. I., Eastwood, L. M., Smith, F. W., & Ashcroft, G. W. (1985). Nuclear magnetic resonance (NMR). II. Imaging in dementia. *British Journal of Psychiatry, 146*, 31–35.

Besson, J. A. O., Henderson, J. G., Foreman, E. I., & Smith, F. W. (1987). An NMR study of lithium responding manic depressive patients. *Magnetic Resonance Imaging, 5*, 273–277.

Brant-Zawadzki, M., Fein, G., Van Dyke, C., Kiernan, R., Davenport, L., & de Groot, J. (1985). MR imaging of the aging brain: patchy white matter lesions and dementia. *American Journal of Neuroradiology, 6*(5), 675–682.

Brenner, R. P., Reynolds, C. F., & Ulrich, R. F., (1988). Diagnostic efficacy of computerized spectral versus visual EEG analysis in elderly normal, demented and depressed subjects. *Electroencephalography and Clinical Neurophysiology, 69*, 110–117.

Brenner, R. P., Ulrich, R. F., Spiker, D. G., Sclabassi, R. J., Reynolds, C. F., Marin, R. S. & Boller, F. (1986). Computerized EEG spectral analysis in elderly normal, demented and depressed subjects. *Electroencephalography and Clinical Neurophysiology, 64*, 483–492.

Bryan, R. N. (1985). Imaging techniques of the aging brain. In C. M. Gaitz, & T. Samorajski (Eds.), *Aging 2000: Our health care destiny. Biomedical issues* (Vol. 1). New York: Springer-Verlag.

Buchsbaum, M. S., Ingvar, D. H., Kessler, R., Waters, R. N., Cappelletti, J., van Kammen, D. P., King, A. C., Johnson, J., Manning, R. G., Flynn, R. W., Mann, L. S., Bunney, W. E., & Sokoloff, L. (1982). Cerebral glucography with positron tomography. *Archives of General Psychiatry, 39*, 251–259.

Buchsbaum, M. S., Wu, J. C., DeLisi, L. E., Holcomb, H., Kessler, R., Johnson, J., King, A. C., Hazlett, E., Langston, K., & Post, R. M. (1986). Frontal cortex and basal ganglia metabolic rates assessed by positron emission tomography with [^{18}F]2-deoxyglucose in affective illness. *Journal of Affective Disorders, 10*, 137–152.

Butler, R. W., Dickinson, W. A., Katholi, C., & Halsey, J. H. (1983). The comparative effect of organic brain disease on cerebral blood flow and measured intelligence. *Annals of Neurology, 13*, 155–159.

Coben, L. A., Danziger, W. L., & Berg, L. (1983). Frequency analysis of the resting awake EEG in mild senile dementia of Alzheimer type. *Electroencephalography and Clinical Neurophysiology, 55*, 372–380.

Coben, L. A., Danziger, N., & Storandt, M. (1985). A longitudinal EEG study of mild senile dementia of Alzheimer type. *Electroencephalography and Clinical Neurophysiology, 61*, 101–112.

Coffey, C. E., Figiel, G. S., Djang, W. T., Cress, M., Saunders, W. B., & Weiner, R. D. (1988). Leukoencephalopathy in elderly depressed patients referred for ECT. *Biological Psychiatry, 24*, 143–161.

Crawley, J. C., Owens, D. G. C., Crow, T. J., Poulter, M., Johnstone, E. C., Smith, T., Oldland, S. R., Veall, N., Owen, F., & Zanelli, G. D. (1986). Dopamine D2 receptors in schizophrenia studied in vivo [Letter]. *Lancet, 2*, 224–225.

Creasey, H., & Rapoport, S. I. (1985). The aging human brain. *Annals of Neurology, 17,* 2–10.

Cummings, J. L. (1985). Organic delusions: Phenomenology, anatomical correlations and review. *British Journal of Psychiatry, 146,* 184–197.

Cutler, N. R. (1988). Cognitive and brain imaging measures of Alzheimer's disease. *Neurobiology of Aging, 9,* 90–92.

Dastur, D. K., Lane, M. M., Hansen, D. B., Kety, S. S., Butler, R. N., Perlin, S., & Sokoloff, L. (1963). Effect of aging on cerebral circulation and metabolism in man. In J. E. Birin, R. N. Butler, S. W. Greenhouse, L. Sokoloff, & M. R. Yarrow (Eds.), *Human aging: A biological and behavioral study* (pp. 59–76). Bethesda: U.S. Public Health, Education & Welfare, National Institute of Mental Health, DHEW publication No. 986.

Davidson, R. J., Chapman, J. P., & Chapman, L. J. (1987). Task-dependent EEG asymmetry discriminates between depressed and non-depressed subjects. *Psychophysiology, 24,* 585.

Davidson, R. J., Schaffer, C. E., & Saron, C. (1985). Effects of lateralized presentations of faces on self-reports of emotion and EEG asymmetry in depressed and non-depressed subjects. *Psychophysiology, 22,* 353–364.

DeLeon, M. J., Ferris, S. H., & George, A. E. (1985). Computerized tomography (CT) and positron emission tomography (PET) in normal and pathologic aging. In C. M. Gaitz & T. Samorajski (Eds.), *Aging 2000: Our health care destiny: Vol. I, Biomedical issues.* New York: Springer-Verlag.

DeLeon, M. J., George, A. E., Tomanelli, J., Christman, D., Kluger, A., Miller, J., Ferris, S. H., Fowler, J., Brodie, J. D., van Gelder, P., Klinger, A., & Wolf, A. P. (1987). Positron emission tomography studies of normal aging: A replication of PET III and 18-FDG using PET IV and 11-CDG. *Neurobiology of Aging, 8,* 319–323.

Diagnostic and Statistical Manual of Mental Disorders (3rd ed. revised). (1987). Washington, DC: American Psychiatric Association.

Duffy, F., Albert, M., McAnulty, G., & Garvey, A. (1984). Age-related differences in brain electrical activity of healthy subjects. *Annals of Neurology, 16,* 430–438.

Duara, R., Grady, C., Haxby, J., Sundaram, M., Cutler, N. R., Heston, L., Moore, A., Schlageter, N., Larson, S., & Rapoport, S. I. (1986). Positron emission tomography in Alzheimer's disease. *Neurology, 36,* 879–887.

Duara, V. R., Margolin, R. A., Robertson-Tchabo, A., London, E. D., Schwartz, M., Renfrew, J. W., Koziarz, B. J., Sundaram, M., Grady, C., Moore, A. M., Ingvar, D. H., Sokoloff, L., Weingartner, H., Kessler, R. M., Manning, R. G., Channing, M. A., Cutler, N. R., & Rapoport, S. I. (1983). Cerebral glucose utilization, as measured with positron emission tomography in 21 resting healthy men between the ages of 21 and 83 years. *Brain, 106,* 761–775.

Earnest, M. P., Heaton, R. K., Wilkinson, W. E., & Manke, W. F. (1979). Cortical atrophy, ventricular enlargement and intellectual impairment in the aged. *Neurology, 29,* 1138–1143.

Erkinjuntti, T., Sipponen, J. T., Iivanainen, M., Ketonen, L., Sulkava, R., & Sepponen, R. E. (1984). Cerebral MNR and CT imaging in dementia. *Journal of Computer Assisted Tomography, 8,* 614–618.

Farkas, T., Ferris, S. H., Wolf, A. P., DeLeon, M. J., Christman, D. R., Reisberg, B., Alavi, A., Abass, A., Fowler, J. S., George, A. E., & Reivich, M. (1982). ^{18}F-2-Deoxy-2-fluoro-D-glucose as a tracer in the positron emission tomographic study of senile dementia. *American Journal of Psychiatry, 139,* 352-353.

Farkas, T., Wolf, A. P., Jaeger, J., Brodie, J. D., Christman, D. R., & Fowler, J. S. (1984). Regional brain glucose metabolism in chronic schizophrenia. *American Journal of Psychiatry, 41,* 293-300.

Fazekas, F., Chawiuk, J. B., Alavi, A., Hurtig, H. I., & Zimmerman, R. A. (1987). MR signal abnormalities at 1.5 T in Alzheimer's dementia and normal aging. *American Journal of Neuroradiology, 8,* 421-426.

Ferris, S. H., & DeLeon, M. J. (1983). The PET scan in the study of Alzheimer's disease. In B. Reisberg (Ed.), *Alzheimer's disease. The standard reference* (pp. 286-291). New York: The Free Press.

Ford, C. V., & Winter, J. (1981). Computerized axial tomograms and dementia in elderly patients. *Journal of Gerontology, 36,* 164-169.

Frackowiak, R. S. J., Lenzi, G. L., Jones, T., & Heather, J. D. (1980). Quantitative measurement of regional cerebral blood flow and oxygen metabolism in man utilizing ^{15}Oxygen and positron emission tomography: Theory, procedure and normal values. *Journal of Computer Assisted Tomography, 4,* 727-736.

Frackowiak, R. S. J., Pozzilli, C., Legg, N. J., Du Boulay, G. H., Marshall, J., Lenzi, G. L., & Jones, T. (1981). Regional cerebral oxygen supply and utilization in dementia. A clinical and physiological study with oxygen-15 and positron tomography. *Brain, 104,* 753-778.

Frackowiak, R. S. J., Wise, R. J. S., Gibbs, M. J., & Jones, T. (1984). Positron emission tomographic studies in aging and cerebrovascular disease at Hammersmith Hospital. *Annals of Neurology, 15*(Suppl.), S112-S118.

George, A., DeLeon, M., Gentes, C., Miller, J., London, E., Budzilovich, G. N., Ferris, S., & Chase, N. (1986a). Leukoencephalopathy in normal and pathologic aging. 1: CT of brain lucencies. *American Journal of Neuroradiology, 7,* 561-566.

George, A., DeLeon, M., Kalnin, A., Rosner, L., Goodgold, A., & Chase, N. (1986b). Leukoencephalopathy in normal and pathologic aging. 2: MR of brain lucencies. *American Journal of Neuroradiology, 7,* 567-570.

Guenther, W., & Breitling, D. (1985). Predominant sensorimotor area left hemisphere dysfunction in schizophrenia measured by brain electrical activity mapping. *Biological Psychiatry, 20,* 515-532.

Guenther, W., Moser, E., Mueller-Spahn, F., von Oefele, K., Buell, U., & Hippius, H. (1986). Pathologic cerebral blood flow during motor function in schizophrenic and endogenous depressed patients. *Biological Psychiatry, 21,* 889-899.

Gur, R. E. (1978). Left hemisphere dysfunction and left hemisphere overactivation in schizophrenia. *Journal of Abnormal Psychology, 87,* 226-238.

Gur, R. E., Gur, R. C., Skolnick, B. E., Caroff, S., Obrist, W. D., Resnick, S., & Reivich, M. (1985). Brain function in psychiatric disorders. *Archives of General Psychiatry, 42,* 329-334.

Gur, R. E., Resnick, S. M., Gur, R. C., Abass, A., Caroff, S., Kushner, M., & Reivich, M. (1987). Regional brain function in schizophrenia. *Archives of General Psychiatry, 44,* 126-129.

Guze, B., Hoffman, J., Baxter, L. R., Mazziotta, J., & Phelps, M. E. (in submission). Functional brain imaging and Alzheimer's type dementia. A review.

Hachinski, V. C., Potter, P., & Merskey, H. (1987). Leuko-araiosis. *Archives of Neurology, 44,* 21-23.

Haug, G. (1977). Age and sex dependence of the size of normal ventricles on computed tomography. *Neuroradiology, 14,* 201-204.

Hershey, L. A., Modic, M. T., Greenough, P. G., & Jaffe, D. F. (1987). Magnetic resonance imaging in vascular dementia. *Neurology, 37,* 29-36.

Huckman, M. S., Fox, J. F., & Topel, J. (1975). The validity of criteria for the evaluation of cerebral atrophy by computer tomography. *Radiology, 116,* 85-92.

Hughes, C. P., & Gado, M. (1981). Computed tomography and aging of the brain. *Radiology, 139,* 391-396.

Jacoby, R. J. (1981). Depression in the elderly. *British Journal of Hospital Medicine, 25*(1), 40-47.

Jacoby, R. J., & Levy, R. (1980). Computed tomography in the elderly. *British Journal of Psychiatry, 136,* 270-275.

Jagust, W. J., & Budinger, T. F. (1988). A comparison of positron emission tomography and single photon emission computed tomography in the study of dementia. *Bulletin of Clinical Neurosciences, 53,* 51-57.

Jernigan, T. L. (1986). Human brain-imaging: Basic principles and applications in psychiatry. In L. L. Judd & P. M. Groves (Eds.), *Psychobiological Foundations of Clinical Psychiatry* (Vol. 4, pp. 109-116). New York: Basic Books; Philadelphia: Lippincott.

Johnson, K. A., Davis, K. R., Buonanno, F. S., Brady, T. J., Rosen, T. J., & Growdon, J. H. (1987). Comparison of magnetic resonance and roentgen ray computed tomography in dementia. *Archives of Neurology, 44,* 1075-1080.

Johnstone, E. C., Crow, T. J., Frith, C. D., Husband, J., & Kreel, L. (1976). Cerebral ventricular size and cognitive impairment in chronic schizophrenia. *Lancet, 2,* 924-926.

Karson, C. N., Coppola, R., Morihisa, J. M., & Weinberger, D. R. (1987). Computed electroencephalographic activity mapping in schizophrenia. *Archives of General Psychiatry, 44,* 514-517.

Kelsoe, J., Cadet, J., Pickar, D., & Weinberger, D. (1988). Quantitative neuroanatomy in schizophrenia. *Archives of General Psychiatry, 45,* 533-541.

Kety, S. S. (1956). Human cerebral blood flow and oxygen consumption as related to aging. *Research Publication Association for Research Nervous Mental Disorders, 35,* 31-45.

Kety, S. S., & Schmidt, C. F. (1948). The nitrous oxide method for the quantitative determination of cerebral blood flow in man: Theory, procedure and normal values. *Journal of Clinical Investigation, 42,* 951-959.

Kinkel, W. R., Jacobs, L., Polachini, I., Bates, V., & Heffner, R. R. (1985). Subcortical arteriosclerotic encephalopathy (Binswanger's disease). Computed tomographic, nuclear magnetic resonance, and clinical correlations. *Archives of Neurology, 42,* 951-959.

Kishimoto, H., Kuwahara, H., Ohno, S., Takazu, O., Hama, Y., Sato, C., Ishii, T., Nomura, Y., Fujita, H., Miyauchi, T., Matsushita, M., Upkoi, S., & Iio, M. (1987). Three subtypes of chronic schizophrenia identified using ^{11}C-Glucose positron emission tomography. *Psychiatry Research, 21,* 285-292.

Kling, A. S., Metter, E. J., Riege, W. H., & Kuhl, D. (1986). Comparison of PET measurements of local brain glucose metabolism and CAT measurement of brain atrophy in chronic schizophrenia and depression. *American Journal of Psychiatry, 143,* 175-180.

Kluger, A., Gianutsos, J., DeLeon, M. J., & George, A. E. (1988). Significance of age-related white matter lesions [Letter]. *Stroke, 19*(8), 1054–1055.

Kuhl, D. E. (1984). Imaging local brain functions with emission computed tomography. *Radiology, 150*, 625–631.

Kuhl, D. E., Metter, J., & Riege, W. H. (1985). Pattern of cerebral glucose utilization in depression, multi-infarct dementia and Alzheimer's disease. In L. Sokoloff (Ed.), *Brain imaging and brain function* (pp. 211–226). New York: Raven.

Kuhl, D. E., Metter, J., Riege, W. H., & Phelps, M. E. (1982). Effects of human aging on patterns of local cerebral glucose utilization determined by the [^{18}F] fluorodeoxyglucose method. *Journal of Cerebral Blood Flow Metabolism, 2*, 163–171.

Leenders, K. L., Gibbs, J. M., Frackowiak, R. S. J., Lammertsma, A. A., & Jones, T. (1984). Positron emission tomography of the brain: New possibilities for the investigation of human cerebral pathophysiology. *Progress in Neurobiology, 23*, 1–38.

Leuchter, A. F. (1988). Late-onset psychosis: Differential diagnosis and management. *Geriatric Medicine Today, 7*, 121–129.

Leuchter, A. F., & Spar, J. E. (1985). The late onset psychoses: Clinical and diagnostic features. *Journal of Nervous and Mental Disorders, 173*, 488–494.

Leuchter, A. F., Spar, J. E., Walter, D. O., & Weiner, H. (1987). EEG spectra and coherence in the diagnosis of Alzheimer's type and multi-infarct dementia. *Archives of General Psychiatry, 44*, 993–998.

Leuchter, A. F., & Walter, D. O. (1989). Diagnosis and assessment of dementia using functional brain imaging. *International Psychogeriatrics, 1*, 63–72.

Lying-Tunnell, U., Lindblad, B. S., Malmlund, H. O., & Persson, B. (1980). Cerebral-blood flow and metabolic rate of oxygen, glucose, lactate, pyruvate, ketone bodies and amino acid. *Acta Neurologica Scandinavica, 62*, 265–275.

Mathew, R. J., Meyer, J. S., Francis, D. J., Semchuk, K. M., Mortel, K., & Claghorn, J. L. (1980). Cerebral blood flow in depression. *American Journal of Psychiatry, 137*, 1449–1450.

McGeer, P. L., Kamo, H., Harrop, R., Li, K. B., Tuokko, H., McGeer, E. G., Adam, M. J., & Amman, W. (1986). Positron emission tomography in patients with clinically diagnosed Alzheimer's disease. *Canadian Medical Association Journal, 134*, 597–607.

Miller, A. K. H., Alston, R. L., & Orsellis, J. A. (1980). Variation with age in the volumes of grey and white matter in the cerebral hemispheres of man: Measurements with an image analyser. *Neuropathology and Applied Neurobiology, 6*, 119–132.

Miller, B. L., Benson, D. F., Cummings, J. L., & Neshkes, R. (1986). Late-life paraphrenia: An organic delusional syndrome. *Journal of Clinical Psychiatry, 47*, 204–207.

Miller, B. L., & Lesser, I. M. (1988). Late-life psychosis and modern neuroimaging. *Psychiatric Clinics of North America, 11*, 346.

Morihisa, J. M., Duffy, F. H., & Wyatt, R. J. (1983). Brain electrical activity mapping (BEAM) in schizophrenic patients. *Archives of General Psychiatry, 40*, 719–728.

Morstyn, R., Duffy, F. H., & McCarley, R. W. (1983). Altered topography of EEG spectral content in schizophrenia. *Electroencephalography and Clinical Neurophysiology, 56*, 263–271.

Nasrallah, H. A., Andreasan, N. C., Coffman, J. A., Olson, S. C., Dunn, V. D., Ehrhardt, J. C., & Chapman, S. M. (1986). A controlled magnetic imaging study of corpus callosum thickness in schizophrenia. *Biological Psychiatry, 21*, 274–282.

Nasrallah, H. A., & Coffman, J. A. (1985). Computerized tomography in psychiatry. *Psychiatric Annals, 15*, 239-249.

Nasrallah, H. A., Kuperman, G., Jacoby, C. G., McCalley-Whitters, M., & Hamra, B. (1983). Clinical correlates of sulcal widening in chronic schizophrenia. *Psychiatry Research, 10*, 237-242.

Niedermeyer, E. (1987). EEG and old age. In E. Niedermeyer & F. Lopes da Silva (Eds.), *Electroencephalography: Basic principles, clinical applications and related fields* (pp. 301-308). Baltimore: Urban & Schwarzenberg.

Obrist, W. D. (1976). Problems of aging. In G. E. Chatrian & G. C. Lairy (Eds.), *Handbook of electroencephalography and clinical neurophysiology* (Vol. 6, pp. 6A274-6A292). Amsterdam: Elsevier.

Pearlson, G. D., & Veroff, A. E. (1981). Computerized tomographic scan changes in manic-depressive illness [Letter]. *Lancet, 2*, 470.

Penttila, M., Partanen, J. V., Soininen, H., & Riekkinen, P. J. (1985). Quantitative analysis of occipital EEG in different stages of Alzheimer's disease. *Electroencephalography and Clinical Neurophysiology, 60*, 1-6.

Phelps, M. E., Mazziotta, J. C., Baxter, L., & Gerner, R. (1984). Positron emission tomographic study of affective disorders: Problems and strategies. *Annals of Neurology, 15* (suppl.), S149-S156.

Prichep, L., Gomez, M. F., John, E. R., & Ferris, S. H. (1983). Neurometric electroencephalographic characteristics of dementia. In B. Reisberg (Ed.), *Alzheimer's disease: The standard reference* (pp. 252-257). New York: Macmillan.

Prichep, L. S., Lieber, A. L., John, E. R., Alper, K., Gomez-Mont, F., Essig-Peppard, T., & Flitter, M. (1986). Quantitative EEG in depressive disorders. In C. Shagass (Ed.), *Electrical brain potentials and psychopathy*. Amsterdam: Elsevier.

Raichle, M. E. (1983). Positron emission tomography. *Annual Review of Neuroscience, 6*, 249-267.

Rangel-Guerra, R. A., Perez-Payan, H., Minkoff, L., & Todd, L. E. (1983). Nuclear magnetic resonance in bipolar affective disorder. *American Journal of Neuroradiology, 4*(3), 229-231.

Sarpel, G., Chaudry, F., & Hindo, W. (1987). Magnetic resonance imaging in periventricular hyperintensity in a Veteran's Administration hospital population. *Archives of Neurology, 44*, 725-728.

Shaffer, C. E., Davidson, R. J., & Saron, C. (1983). Frontal and parietal electroencephalogram asymmetry in depressed and nondepressed subjects. *Biological Psychiatry, 18*, 753-762.

Sheppard, G., Gruzelier, J., Manchanda, R., & Hirsch, S. R. (1983). ^{15}0 positron emission tomographic scanning in predominantly never treated acute schizophrenia patients. *Lancet, 2*, 1448-1452.

Smith, R. C., Calderon, M., Ravichandran, G. K., Largen, J., Vroulis, G., Shvartsburd, A., Gordon, J., & Schoolar, J. C. (1984). Nuclear magnetic resonance in schizophrenia: A preliminary study. *Psychiatry Research, 12*, 137-147.

Soininen, H., Puranen, R., & Riekkinen, P. J. (1982). Computer tomography findings in senile dementia and normal aging. *Journal of Neurology, Neurosurgery, and Psychiatry, 45*, 50-54.

Torres, F., Faoro, A., Loewenson, R., & Johnson, E. (1983). The electroencephalogram of elderly subjects revisited. *Electroencephalography and Clinical Neurophysiology, 56,* 391–398.

Volkow, N. D., Brodie, J., Wolf, A., Gomez-Mont, F., Cancro, R., Gelder, P., Russell, G., & Overall, J. (1986a). Brain organization in schizophrenia. *Journal of Cerebral Blood Flow and Metabolism,, 6,* 441–446.

Volkow, N. D., Brodie, J. D., Wolf, A. P., Angrist, B., Russell, J., & Cancro, R. (1986b). Brain metabolism in patients with schizophrenia before and after neuroleptic administration. *Journal of Neurology, Neurosurgery, and Psychiatry, 49,* 1199–1202.

Volkow, N. D., Wolf, A. P., Van Gelder, P., Brodie, J. D., Overall, J. E., Cancro, R., & Gomez-Mont, F. (1987). Phenomenological correlates of metabolic activity in 18 patients with chronic schizophrenia. *American Journal of Psychiatry, 144,* 151–158.

Weinberger, D. R., Cannon-Spoor, E., Potkin, S. G., & Wyatt, R. J. (1980). Poor premorbid adjustment and CT scan abnormalities in chronic schizophrenia. *American Journal of Psychiatry, 137,* 1410–1413.

Weinberger, D. R., Torrey, E. F., Neophytides, A. N., & Wyatt, R. J. (1979). Structural abnormalities in the cerebral cortex of chronic schizophrenic patients. *Archives of General Psychiatry, 36*(9), 935–939.

Widen, L., Blomqvist, G., Greitz, T., Litton, J. E., Bergstrom, M., Ehrin, E., Ericson, K., Eriksson, L., Ingvar, D. H., Johansson, L., Nilsson, L. G., Stone-Elander, S., Sedvall, G., Wiesel, F., & Wiik, G. (1983). PET studies of glucose metabolism in patients with schizophrenia. *American Journal of Neuroradiology, 4,* 550–552.

Wiesel, F. A., Wik, G., Blomqvist, I. S. G., Greitz, T., & Stone-Elander, S. (1987). Regional brain glucose metabolism in drug free schizophrenic patients and clinical correlates. *Acta Psychiatrica Scandinavica, 76,* 628–641.

Wolkin, A., Angrist, B., Wolf, A., Brodie, J. D., Wolkin, B., Jaeger, J., Cancro, R., & Rotrosen, J. (1988). Low frontal glucose utilization in chronic schizophrenia: A replication study. *American Journal of Psychiatry, 145,* 251–253.

Wolkin, A., Jaeger, J., Brodie, J. D., Wold, A. P., Fowler, J., Rotrosen, J., Gomez-Mont, F., & Cancro, R. (1985). Persistance of cerebral metabolic abnormalities in chronic schizophrenia as determined by positron emission tomography. *American Journal of Psychiatry, 142,* 564–571.

Wong, D. F., Wagner, H. N., Tune, L. E., Dannals, R. F., Pearlson, G. D., Links, J. M., Tamminga, C. A., Broussolle, E. P., Ravert, H. T., Wilson, A. A., Troung, J. K. T., Malat, J., Williams, J. A., O'Tuama, L. A., Synder, S. H., Kuhar, M. J., & Gjedde, A. (1986). Positron emission tomography reveals elevated D_2 dopamine receptors in drug-naive schizophrenics. *Science, 234,* 1558–1563.

Yamamoto, Y. L., Thompson, C. J., Diksic, M., Meyer, E., & Feindel, W. (1984). Positron emission tomography. *Neurosurgery Review, 7,* 233–251.

Yamamura, H., Ito, M., Kubota, K., Kubota, K., & Matsuzawa, T. (1980). Brain atrophy during aging: A quantitative study with computed tomography. *Journal of Gerontology, 4,* 492–498.

Zimmerman, R. D., Fleming, C. A., Lee, B. C. P., Saint-Louis, L. A., & Deck, M. D. (1986). Periventricular hyperintensity as seen by magnetic resonance: prevalence and significance. *American Journal of Neuroradiology, 146*(3), 443–450.

10

Beyond Neuroleptics: The Treatment of Agitation

Barry S. Fogel

Agitated behavior, irrespective of psychiatric diagnosis, brings mentally ill elderly people to treatment and may trigger important clinical events such as institution-alization (Ferris et al., 1985), change of institutional setting, or the use of restraints. For psychiatrists, it is a variably present feature of several different mental disorders, both chronic and acute; for geriatricians, it is one of the major symptoms, along with incontinence, immobility, and malnutrition, to which they are called upon to respond. The geriatric literature often addresses agitation as a symptom complex, without specifically employing standard psychiatric nosology (Cohen-Mansfield & Billig, 1986).

Most chronically mentally ill elderly who receive any formal treatment are served by the general health-care system and not by specialty mental health providers (Burns & Taube, 1990). Even for those chronically mentally ill elderly who were once state hospital patients, medical responsibility may shift to nonpsychiatric providers at some point after deinstitutionalization. Placement in a nursing home, for example, often entails such a shift in medical responsibility. When nonspecialist providers are called upon to deal with the chronic mentally ill, the request is often to deal with agitated, hostile, paranoid, or uncooperative *behavior* rather than systematically to diagnose and treat mental *illness*. The most common response is the prescription of a drug (Burns & Taube, 1990). Thus, the refinement of approaches to the diagnosis and drug treatment of agitation that could be practically applied in general health-care settings would facilitate better care for the large number of chronically mentally ill elderly who obtain access to care by displaying agitated behavior.

Agitation often occurs without definite evidence of psychosis; prevalence rates among demented patients are estimated at 70% to 80% for agitation and 30% to 40% for psychosis (Wragg & Jeste, 1988). Regardless, neuroleptics are the traditional mainstay of its pharmacologic treatment, whether or not delusions are present (Helms, 1985; Wragg & Jeste, 1988). The widespread use of neuroleptics in nursing homes (Beardsley, Larson, Burns, Thompson, & Kamerow, 1989; Bears, et al., 1988) and rest homes (Avorn, Dreyer, Connelly, & Soumerai, 1989), often in patients without diagnosed psychosis, probably occurs in response to agitated behavior. Despite their popularity, neuroleptics are of limited effectiveness for agitation and are probably of decisive benefit in fewer than half of the patients for whom they are prescribed (Barnes, Veith, Okimoto, Raskind, & Gumbrecht, 1982; Helmes, 1985; Wragg & Jeste, 1988). Many of their extrapyramidal side effects, however, differentially affect the elderly: tardive dyskinesia (Jeste & Wyatt, 1987), parkinsonism (Peabody, Warner, Whiteford, & Hollister, 1987), and akinesia all are more likely to occur in older patients (see chapter by Jeste, this volume). Further, falls (Tideiksaar, 1989), incontinence, and immobility, those most common problems of the frail elderly, can all be provoked by neuroleptic therapy.

There is strong support for the utility of neuroleptics in delusional depression (Kroessler, 1985), schizophrenia (Klein, Gittelman, Quitkin, & Rifkin, 1980), and in paranoid psychosis associated with Alzheimer's disease (Maletta, 1985). However, many agitated elderly people do not easily fit these diagnostic categories. It is often difficult to establish what elements of mood or thought disorder might be present in an individual with advanced dementia who cannot understand detailed mental status questions or articulate accurate responses. And there are elderly persons with only mild cognitive impairment who may become transiently agitated or explosive in response to frustrations and disappointments without being delusional or suffering from any definite mental illness.

In approaching the treatment of agitation, the following issues can be identified: (1) How can agitated patients best be categorized to aid in the selection of pharmacologic treatments and to define more homogeneous categories for research? (2) Since sequential drug trials may be necessary, in what order should they be given, and what end point should be used for terminating a drug trial? (3) When neuroleptics are employed, what is the optimal dosage? (4) What adjuncts can reduce neuroleptic dosage while preserving or improving clinical outcomes and reducing overall adverse effects? (5) What agitated patients are most likely to respond to nonneuroleptic alternatives?

This chapter will present an approach to these issues in the light of recent research and will further specify promising directions for future investigation of the treatment of agitation in the mentally ill elderly.

CLASSIFICATION OF AGITATED STATES

Agitated behavior can be approached as a syndrome sometimes seen in elderly persons, particularly those in institutional care, that can be reliably and operationally defined without regard to a conventional psychiatric diagnosis (Cohen-Mansfield, 1986; Cohen-Mansfield & Billig, 1986). Or, agitation can be seen as an accompaniment of dementia or cognitive impairment, without further subtyping, following the practice of DSM-III-R that regards organic diagnoses as taking precedence over functional diagnoses. Therefore, the presence of affective features, a past history of mental illness, or premorbid personality disturbance would not necessarily be reported in describing populations treated for agitation with various pharmacologic agents.

However, some geriatric psychiatrists have placed more emphasis on traditional psychiatric diagnoses in classifying elderly patients showing agitated behavior (Salzman, 1988a). In their review of the treatment of agitation and psychosis in the elderly, Spira et al. (1984) listed five agitation-producing syndromes: dementia, delirium, late paraphrenia, schizophrenia, and major affective disorder. In this section, arguments will be presented for expanding their list, and for differentiating subcategories within the disorders mentioned, in developing a finer and hopefully more predictive classification system for agitation. Goals include reliability, predictive validity, completeness, and acceptability to clinicians. With these goals in mind, the following observations are offered:

1. Agitation in dementia is a heterogeneous phenomenon. First, it may occur with or without delusions. Agitation driven by fixed beliefs that one is in danger usually requires specific treatment of the delusions. Nondelusional agitation may respond to a broader range of treatments and may be less likely to require neuroleptics. Second, agitation in mildly demented patients is different from agitation in severely demented patients. In mildly demented patients, agitation may be associated with a mood disorder, delusions, the aggravation of premorbid personality problems, or a direct effect of the degeneration of a specific neurotransmitter system. Agitation in severely demented patients may reflect an end-stage organic disorder relatively independent of mood, premorbid personality, or the particular sequence of development of dementing symptoms. Formed delusions (Cummings, 1985) or the full syndrome of depression or mania are rarely seen in advanced dementia.

2. Delirious agitation similarly may occur with or without delusions, or with either mild or severe impairment of cognition. Further, the etiology of the delirium is relevant to the choice of treatment for agitation. Agitation due to neuroleptic malignant syndrome would never be treated with neuroleptics; benzodiazepine withdrawal would optimally be treated with long-acting benzodiazepines.

3. Mood disorders may have atypical presentations in elderly patients. Reasons include sociocultural factors, the effects of cognitive impairment on symptom formation, and the confounding effect of comorbid physical illnesses on the assessment of symptoms. For these reasons it is not unusual to encounter agitated elderly persons meeting many diagnostic criteria for major depression or for hypomania, but with an insufficient number of criteria for diagnosis or with uncertainty whether to diagnose an organic mood disorder instead (Fogel 1990).

Mood disturbances of this kind are a relevant category for research on the treatment of agitation, as patients in this category may show dramatic responses to treatment for major mood disorders, including antidepressants, lithium, and ECT. An operational definition of this enlarged category of mood disorders is easily accomplished: It requires that a specific number of mood disorder criteria be present but that symptoms of possible organic origin be included (Cohen-Cole & Harpe, 1987). If desired, the category can be made more homogeneous by requiring the presence of a definite past history of mood disorder in the individual or a definite history of a major mood disorder in a first-degree relative.

4. Personality disorders and other characterological dispositions to impulsiveness, agitation, or violence are prominent in the differential diagnosis of agitated or disinhibited behavior in younger patients. While more florid acting-out behavior may decline with age in otherwise healthy persons with personality disorders, dispositions to violence and to demanding and disruptive behavior may be exposed in late life by the stress of physical illness, the regressive effects of dependency, or a loss of inhibition on an organic basis (Sadavoy & Fogel, in press). Since personality diagnoses are often neglected in the elderly (Fogel & Westlake, 1990), and in any case accurate histories of lifelong development and adaptation may be difficult to obtain, formal personality diagnosis probably should not be the basis for differentiating this additional group of agitated patients. Rather, a category can be defined of patients with significant maladaptive personality traits preceding the present illness, and aggravated by it. The reliability and validity of such a category might be enhanced by employing an established scale of personality disturbance, such as the Personality Assessment Schedule (PAS) (Tyrer & Alexander, 1988). The demonstration of the effectiveness of low-dose neuroleptics for borderline or schizotypal personalities (Goldberg et al., 1986; Gunderson, 1986; Soloff et al., 1986), and beta-blockers for some of the anxiety-based personality disorders (Liebowitz, Stone, & Turkat, 1986), supports the relevance of personality disturbances in a classification for research on the pharmacological therapy of agitation.

5. Primary anxiety disorders, though they usually begin in the first half of life, may persist into old age where they may produce symptomatology difficult to distinguish from the agitation that accompanies psychosis or dementia. Particularly if some cognitive impairment is present, it may be difficult for patients to articulate feelings of anxiety or panic, and they may express these feelings

nonspecifically as irritability, restlessness, or increased purposeless and/or repetitive bodily movement. Agitated patients with definite past histories of anxiety disorders earlier in life deserve a separate category, as they may turn out to be differentially responsive to anxiolytic agents such as tricyclics, MAOIs, or benzodiazepines. These agents may be less useful in treating forms of agitation due to psychosis or dementia.

Cutting across all diagnoses is a concern for distinguishing patients by the degree of cognitive impairment present, the presence or absence of delusions, and the presence earlier in life of continuous or recurrent psychiatric disorders such as schizophrenia and major depression. These distinctions are likely to be relevant both to how well particular drugs may work and how well they may be tolerated. Lumping agitated states or disruptive behavior, as is sometimes done in geriatrics, is unlikely to lead to a scientific basis for drug selection. A suggested typology for disorders causing agitation is displayed in Table 10.1.

GENERAL GUIDELINES FOR EFFICACY STUDIES

Efficacy studies for drug treatments of psychosis and agitation in the elderly should employ standard methodological precautions such as the use of control groups and reliable standardized measures (Risse & Barnes, 1986; Wragg & Jeste, 1988). However, they also should incorporate certain specific measures and considerations particularly pertinent to mental illness in old age.

First, subjects should be characterized as specifically as possible. As argued above, efforts to describe subsyndromal mood disorders or personality disorders should be made, even when a DSM-III-R diagnosis is not possible. Cognitive function should be measured in all cases. The presence or absence of delusions should be noted. When delusions are absent, the existence of less-structured paranoid cognitions should be sought and noted as well.

Second, neurological evaluation before and after treatment should pay special attention to functions often impaired by medications, including gait, muscle tone, and the EEG. Tremors and involuntary movements should be sought and noted, and a formal evaluation for tardive dyskinesia using the AIMS test should be included both before and after treatment. Even when neuroleptics are not being tested in a trial, alternate or adjunctive drug therapies may either ameliorate, aggravate, or precipitate this condition.

Third, functional capacities must be assessed before, during, and after therapy. Measures of physical ADLs, instrumental ADLs, and cognitive function are relevant. For higher-functioning patients, social ADLs also should be measured. Residence status is a face-valid measure of success of drug therapy. Effective treatment of agitation should keep people out of institutions or permit deinstitutionalization. For patients in institutions, the use of physical restraints is a similar

TABLE 10.1 Disorders Causing Agitation

Dementia

   with delusions*
   with paranoid ideation*
   with mood disorder
   with personality disorder*
   with disinhibition due to frontal lobe dysfunction

Delirium

   with delusions*
   with paranoid ideation*
   due to drug toxicity
   due to drug withdrawal

Mood Disorders

   with delusions*
   with paranoid ideation*

Personality Disorders

   borderline*
   paranoid*
   schizotypal*
   antisocial

Anxiety Disorders

   generalized
   panic

* = conditions most likely to be helped by neuroleptics.

face-valid measure. Since the prevalence of this practice ranges from 7% to 22% in hospitals and 25% to 85% in nursing homes (Evans & Strumpf, 1989), there is a reasonable chance of finding a significant change with an effective therapy.

Fourth, surveillance for adverse drug reactions and interactions must be targeted on special vulnerabilities of the elderly. The incidence of falls and incontinence, for example, should be compared between control and intervention groups. Since most patients will be on other medications for physical illnesses, the literature on reported interactions must be reviewed and studies designed to ascertain specifically the incidence of drug interactions for which study population would be especially at risk.

Finally, the satisfaction of patients and their caretakers with the treatment needs to be assessed. Since the use of psychotropic drugs in the elderly is a focus of intense feeling and controversy, caretakers' observations that a particular treatment makes a patient look more comfortable without appearing "drugged" is meaningful evidence that the treatment may be superior to its predecessor. From the clinical standpoint, such observations may mean as much as improvement on a psychopathologic rating scale.

TESTING STRATEGIES FOR SEQUENTIAL MEDICATION TRIALS

At present, initial drug therapy is successful about 70% of the time for agitated depression; initial pharmacotherapy for agitation due to other disorders is no better. Thus, it is a common experience that two or more drug regimens must be tried before symptoms improve. While a finer clinical classification of patients may enable a more specific first choice of drug, strategies will still be needed to help clinicians decide what drug to try second or third. The overall impact, including both therapeutic effects and adverse reactions, should be evaluated for *strategies of drug choice*. For example, ECT is offered early to seriously depressed patients in some localities but is seen as a last resort in others. The sequence "drugs first, then ECT" carries different risks and benefits than the sequence "ECT, then drugs." For example, there might be a higher rate of memory loss in the first group and a higher rate of suicide or falls in the second if numbers of patients were large enough.

Strategies to be tested should specify drugs, dosages, and durations; more sophisticated strategies might indicate how the *quality* of a negative or incomplete response to the first drug might influence the choice of the second.

A related problem concerns the phenomena, frequent in nursing homes, that drugs are continued even when they are not fully effective or that all drug therapy for a mental disorder is abandoned if the first drug trial is unsuccessful. Systematically tested strategies for drug selection that offer a first, second, and third choice, and specific durations for adequate trials, might offer the scientific basis for alleviating this problem.

SPECIFIC THERAPIES FOR AGITATION: RECENT OBSERVATIONS AND RESEARCH RECOMMENDATIONS

In the following brief sections, the potential efficacy of several specific therapies for agitation is discussed in relation to different classes of agitated patients. Observations are made concerning the optimal duration of treatment trials and special precautions regarding adverse effects. Each section concludes with a set of recommendations for further investigation, with emphasis on methodologic points of particular relevance. Recommendations for specific agents offer finer detailing of the general concerns presented above.

Neuroleptics: Dosing Strategies, Adjuncts, and the Mitigation of Side Effects

A central theme of recent clinical research on neuroleptics has been the determination of optimal dosage. Recent work suggest that overall function of treated schizophrenics may be better with relatively low neuroleptic dosages, even though higher dosages might more rapidly diminish some of the patient's positive symptoms (Baldessarini, Cohen, & Teicher, 1988; McEvoy, 1986).

Work on dosage has been paralleled on a smaller scale in the geriatric population. Risse, Lampe, and Cubberly (1987) demonstrated better clinical responses in agitated demented patients when smaller doses of neuroleptics were used; doses as small as five milligrams of thioridazine were employed. Gottlieb, McAllister, and Gur (1988) reported the use of very low doses (as low as .05cc) of depot fluphenazine decanoate with favorable response. Maximal response took as long as 16 weeks for some patients and often required at least 8 weeks.

In clinical settings, relatively high dosages of neuroleptics are often administered because the physician or staff cannot wait for a true antipsychotic response but are seeking immediate reduction of agitation. When high doses of neuroleptics are used for rapid tranquilization, sedative and hypokinetic effects of neuroleptics may be more relevant than antipsychotic action. While subsequent dosage reduction to a lower maintenance level is generally recommended, it is not always carried out.

Regardless of diagnosis, the only unique indication for neuroleptics is the presence of delusions or other forms of thought disorder. Since many other drugs may alleviate agitation, the core of novel strategies for employing neuroleptic adjuncts is to use the neuroleptic specifically for delusions or thought disorder and the adjunct specifically for agitation. This may permit the use of a lower dose of neuroleptic. At times, complete resolution of positive symptoms of psychosis may not be necessary for a satisfactory functional outcome.

Because older people have decreased dopaminergic function, they are particularly vulnerable to drug-induced parkinsonism, akinesia, and related phenomena. Antiparkinson drugs can be used, but the anticholinergic antiparkinson drugs have adverse effects on memory and may cause constipation, urinary retention, and tachycardia. The dopamine agonist drug amantadine may be more satisfactory: It not only lacks anticholinergic side effects on memory (Fayen, Goldman, Moulthrop, & Luchins, 1988) but may actually be helpful in *itself* for some organic agitated states (Chandler, Barnhill, & Gualtieri, 1988). Dosage strategy for this drug in the elderly has not been adequately studied. Its pharmacokinetics are nonlinear (Aoki & Sitar, 1988), and the agent may have its own toxicities, particularly confusion and orthostatic hypotension. However, a properly adjusted combination of a neuroleptic and a dopamine agonist may control psychotic symptoms better, with fewer extrapyramidal symptoms, than would a neuroleptic alone, even at optimal dosage.

In studies of schizophrenia, a full response to neuroleptic therapy may take up to 8 weeks (Klein et al., 1980). While reduction of psychomotor rate in acute mania is more rapid, resolution of manic delusions may also take several weeks. Thus the proper evaluation of a neuroleptic regimen requires studies of at least 2 months' duration.

The above-mentioned work of Gottlieb et al. (1988) on low-dose depot fluphenazine in Alzheimer's patients offers a new option for home treatment of paranoid patients with mild dementia. Not only can noncompliant patients be treated more effectively, but the consistency of dosage with depot dosage may permit even lower total neuroleptic exposure than a low-dose oral strategy.

Recommendations for Further Investigation

Studies of neuroleptics for agitation and psychosis in the elderly should address the issue of finding minimum maintenance dosages and optimizing antiparkinson medication. Motor and cognitive functions, as well as instrumental ADLs, require special attention because of the near-universal occurrence of extrapyramidal effects. Specific recommendations include (1) detailed characterization of patients, beyond diagnosis, as discussed above; (2) further exploration of very low doses of neuroleptics, either initially or after a higher-dose acute treatment period; (3) further study of low-dose depot neuroleptics; (4) study durations of at least 8 weeks; (5) systematic evaluation of dopamine agonist antiparkinson drugs for neuroleptic-induced parkinsonism—blood levels of these drugs should be considered because of the variable pharmacokinetics of these drugs in the elderly; (6) randomized controlled trials of conventional neuroleptic therapy versus low-dose therapy with adjuncts (see below).

Anticonvulsants

In recent years, anticonvulsants have entered the mainstream of psychopharmacology (McElroy, Pope, Keck, & Hudson, 1988) Carbamazepine is the equal of lithium in the treatment of bipolar disorder, and it may succeed in cases where lithium fails (Post, 1988). Valproate also is emerging as a valuable alternative or adjunct in antimanic therapy (McElroy et al., 1988). Clonazepam, a benzodiazepine anticonvulsant, has proved to have both antimanic and antipanic actions (Chouinard, 1988).

Of the three antimanic anticonvulsants, carbamazepine has been explored most extensively for other indications (Luchins, 1984). It has specifically been used to reduce agitation and violent behavior in excited psychoses (Klein, Bental, Lerer, & Belmaker, 1984), rage attacks (Mattes, 1984), dementia (Jenike, 1985; Leibovici & Tariot, 1988), and chronic severe mental disorders with nonepileptic EEG abnormalities (Neppe, 1983). Agitation in mentally retarded patients has also been helped with carbamazepine (Sovner, 1988). And in a placebo-controlled study of the pharmacotherapy of borderline personality, behavioral dyscontrol was dramatically decreased in the carbamazepine-treated group (Gardner & Cowdry, 1988).

While carbamazepine appears to ameliorate agitation in many diagnostic groups, it has toxicities of particular relevance to the elderly. Its suppressant effects on the bone marrow may be particularly troublesome in elderly persons already susceptible to anemia and leukopenia. Further, advanced age is a risk factor for hyponatremia, another carbamazepine side effect.

While carbamazepine has not been shown to be effective as sole therapy for schizophrenia, cases have been reported of thought disorder improving with the drug, especially when the thought disorder was accompanied by significant EEG abnormalities. Carbamazepine is also effective for some cases of depression, although its overall efficacy in depression is less than its efficacy in mania.

When carbamazepine is effective for mania, its therapeutic action is near-maximal at 2 weeks. Antidepressant effects are maximal at about 1 month. When carbamazepine has been used for other indications, positive effects when obtained were seen in 4 weeks or less, although clinical improvement could continue beyond that time, particularly in patients who were extremely ill prior to treatment.

The treatment of nonmanic agitation with other anticonvulsants has been less well studied. However, cases have been reported in elderly persons responding to clonazepam (Freinhar & Alvarez, 1986; Smeraski, 1988). While such reports suggest that clonazepam deserves further investigation in the elderly, its long half-life, tendency to accumulate, and the frequent occurrence of sedation and ataxia as side effects may limit its use.

Recommendations for Further Investigation

Carbamazepine deserves controlled trials for agitation in dementia, as well as for agitation due to late-life personality disturbance. Its application to the treatment of mood disorders should be systematically studied in the elderly, as the risk-benefit ratio or relative status versus lithium might be different. For schizophrenia and paraphrenia with agitation, carbamazepine should be studied as an adjunct.

In carbamazepine trials in the elderly, serum sodium deserves close monitoring, as do the usual hematologic parameters. Also, because of the possibility of additive neurotoxicity, patients receiving carbamazepine as an adjunct to other psychotropic drugs will need special attention to cognitive and motor status, and to the EEG.

Because carbamazepine is an anticonvulsant, numerous studies have attempted to associate its effectiveness with pretreatment EEG abnormalities. Excluding patients with epilepsy, results have been disappointing. However, as carbamazepine is tested systematically for new indications such as agitation in dementia, pretreatment EEG data should be obtained and tested for incremental value in predicting treatment outcome.

Of the other anticonvulsants, the antimanic anticonvulsants clonazepam and valproate offer the most promise as treatments for agitation. Clonazepam might now be tested in a controlled trial for agitation associated with dementia in view of encouraging case reports. If case reports and open studies support a similar therapeutic action of valproate, it also should be investigated in controlled trials.

Benzodiazepines

Benzodiazepines are widely employed as sedatives, hypnotics, and anxiolytics, and are known to be effective for the acute treatment of agitation, including agitation associated with mania or schizophrenia. They potentiate the effects of neuroleptics in these disorders (Cohen & Khan, 1987; Cohen, Khan, & Johnson, 1987). However, they do not have substantial antipsychotic effects. They produce tolerance and dependence, and have effects on cognition, memory, and gait to which the elderly are particularly susceptible.

Surveys of psychotropic drug use in nursing homes suggest that benzodiazepines are widely used to treat agitation and insomnia in demented people (Avorn et al., 1989; Beardsley et al., 1989; Bears et al., 1988). However, two comparative studies suggest their efficacy for agitation may be inferior to neuroleptics (Covington, 1975; Stotsky, 1984); systematic characterization of differential responders has not been carried out. The benzodiazepines are helpful in some but not all delirious states. While they are a mainstay in the treatment of delirium tremens, they may aggravate confusion or produce disinhibition in delirious states of other etiologies. Both clonazepam and lorazepam are effective for acute mania (Chouinard, 1988), while benzodiazepines, with the possible exception of alprazolam and clonazepam, do not generally help depression and may aggravate it. Adjunctive use for anxiety or agitation in neuroleptic treatment of schizophrenia has become an accepted practice (Cohen & Khan, 1987; Salzman, 1988b) which may reduce the neuroleptic dosage requirement. All of the benzodiazepines are effective for the treatment of generalized anxiety; alprazolam and clonazepam may be preferable when panic attacks are prominent. In patients with acting-out personality disorders, the benzodiazepines may have disinhibiting effects or be subject to abuse, so they are relatively contraindicated.

The effects of benzodiazepines on cognition and gait make them generally unsuitable for patients with advanced dementia. However, in patients with less severe cognitive impairment and relatively intact motor function, they may offer a less neurotoxic alternative to neuroleptics.

Patients with agitation caused or aggravated by benzodiazepine withdrawal can be treated specifically with benzodiazepines; substitution and very slow withdrawal of a long-acting agent is the treatment of choice.

In studies of benzodiazepines for various indications, therapeutic effects have often been seen immediately, and peak benefit for most indications is attained within 2 weeks after a steady-state blood level of drug is reached. Side effects of sedation, ataxia, and respiratory depression are dose-dependent and may build up gradually when long-acting agents are used.

Recommendations for Further Investigation

Studies of benzodiazepines as adjuncts to neuroleptics for the treatment of schizophrenic disorders should be extended to the elderly, with special attention to measures of physical and instrumental function, cognition, and coordination. Benzodiazepines should also be tested for residual agitation in patients with otherwise-treated mood disorders. A controlled comparison of benzodiazepines with neuroleptics for the treatment of nondelusional agitation in mild dementia should also be considered. In such a comparison, a crossover phase with characterization of differential responders should be included. Likewise, comparison of benzodiazepines to neuroleptics for nondelusional agitation might be appropriate for some delirious states if care is taken to exclude patients with intercranial pathology, chronic lung disease, and liver failure.

Beta-blockers

Beta-adrenergic blocking drugs, especially propranolol, have successfully been used for the treatment of agitation in patients with organic mental disorders associated with head injury, mental retardation, and dementia (Greendyke & Kanter, 1986; Greendyke, Kanter, & Schuster, 1986; Greendyke, Schuster, & Wooten, 1984; Petrie & Ban, 1981; Ratey, Mikkelsen, & Smith, 1986; Weiler, Mungas, & Bernick, 1988; Yudofsky, 1981; Yudofsky, Stevens, & Silver, 1984). Data has also been reported on beta-blockers as adjuncts in neuroleptic-treated schizophrenia (Sheppard, 1979; Yorkston et al., 1977). In all these studies reduction of agitation rather than resolution of thought disorder was the main effect of the beta-blockers.

The side effects of beta-blockers are well known; principal risks in frail elderly persons include hypotension, bradycardia, and aggravation of congestive heart failure or asthma. Propranolol and other beta-blockers can provoke or aggravate depression; however, they are not effective antimanic agents. Their utility in delirium depends on etiology, with evidence of benefit in post-head-injury delirium and alcohol withdrawal (Kraus, Gottlieb, Horwitz, & Anscher, 1985). They are obviously contraindicated in delirium due to heart failure or respiratory failure.

The onset of action of beta-blockers may differ among clinical populations treated. While response to propranolol in acute head injury may occur in days, Ratey's work with the mentally retarded suggests that many weeks of slow upward dosage titration may be required for optimum effect. A recent case series on propranolol for agitation in senile dementia suggested that some patients are early responders, while others require a month (Weiler et al., 1988).

Recommendations for Further Investigation

Beta-blockers deserve testing in patients with dementia or with personality disturbances who show explosiveness, agitation, or self-injury in the absence of major mood disturbance or delusions. Evaluation should allow at least 1 month of slow upward dosage titration. Since ideal dosage is not known, the maximum recommended dose of the drug (given by the manufacturer for nonpsychiatric indications) would be approached subject to limits imposed by sedation or alterations in vital signs. Side-effect monitoring should include EKGs, assessment of exercise tolerance, and evaluation for orthostatic hypotension. Because of the association of beta-blockers with depression, pre- and posttreatment depression rating scales should be included.

For patients with delusions, including those with schizophrenic disorders, beta-blockers should be evaluated as adjunctive treatment for agitation that persists despite optimal treatment of delusions with neuroleptics.

Buspirone

Buspirone is a nonbenzodiazepine anxiolytic with effects on both serotonergic and dopaminergic mechanisms (Cole, 1988; Tiller, Dakis, & Shaw, 1988). Since its introduction, it has been used with success to reduce agitated and disruptive behavior in elderly demented persons (Colenda, 1988; Tiller et al., 1988), in head-injured patients (Levine, 1988), and in mentally retarded persons (J. Ratey, personal communication), as well as to attenuate the outward behavioral manifestations of borderline personality. While buspirone may cause restlessness (Liegghio, Yeragani, & Moore, 1988), myoclonus and involuntary movements (Richie, Bridenbaugh, & Jabbari, 1988), and may precipitate the development of oral dyskinesia in patients previously treated with neuroleptics (Strauss, 1988), it has not been found to cause the frequent extrapyramidal side effects that accompany the use of neuroleptics. A 4-week open study of buspirone in 605 elderly patients showed that 80% of the patients treated with 15 mg per day showed no side effects at all. Elderly patients did not show more adverse reactions than a comparison group under 65 (Robinson, Napoliello, & Shenk, 1988).

These observations suggest that buspirone may be a valuable drug for the treatment of agitation in nondelusional patients where the basis of the agitation is dementia or personality disturbance. Buspirone might also be a useful adjunct to low-dose neuroleptics in delusional patients with thought disorders that improve with neuroleptics, when the dosage optimal for control of thought disorder with preserved mobility is inadequate to control fully their agitated behavior.

In recent reports of buspirone use, effective dosages have ranged from 15 to 60 mg per day. It is not known whether there is a "window effect," with excessively large doses producing a worse response, although Ratey has reported this phenomenon in some brain-damaged retarded patients (Ratey, 1988, personal communication). Maximum improvement with buspirone may take as long as 2 months, a time course comparable to the antidepressant response to tricyclics. An open trial of buspirone in the treatment of major depressive disorder (Schweizer, Amsterdam, Rickels, Kaplan, & Droba, 1986) showed a good response in about half of the patients with nonmelancholic major depression, at dosages of 40 to 90 mg; improvement in Hamilton Depression ratings was still continuing at the end of the fourth week of the trial.

Recommendations for Further Investigation

Buspirone should be evaluated in elderly persons with agitation who do not have delusions or who have delusions that have been optimally treated with a neuroleptic. In the latter case, the neuroleptic should be maintained at a stable dosage during the buspirone trial. Buspirone does not appear suitable for the primary treatment of delusional disorders, and its role in mood disorders is limited as it appears less effective than standard tricyclics for major depression (Schweizer et al., 1986).

When buspirone is given to the elderly, the dosage should begin at a low dose of no more than 10 mg per day and be increased gradually until the maximum tolerated dose or 60 mg per day is reached. Maximal dosage should then be maintained for at least 6 weeks.

Because of the possibility that buspirone may produce or aggravate motor side effects, special attention to gait, motor function, and involuntary movements should be included in the evaluation, and patients with current or *prior* treatment with neuroleptics should be distinguished as a subgroup in the evaluation of side effects.

Lithium

Lithium is an effective treatment for bipolar disorder in the old, as well as in the young (Liptzin, 1984). It can augment the therapeutic action of antidepressants in delusional (Lafferman, Solomon, & Ruskin, 1988; Lieff & Herrmann, 1988; Pai, White, & Dean, 1986) and nondelusional depression (Heninger, Charney, & Sternberg, 1983; Kushnir, 1986). When agitation is associated with mood disorder, lithium can reduce agitation by alleviating the mood disturbance. (As discussed elsewhere in this chapter, the diagnosis of mood disorder may be difficult in the presence of cognitive impairment, particularly if the latter is severe. Further, the diagnosis of bipolar disorder may be hampered by inaccuracy or incompleteness of the available history regarding possible past attacks of mania or hypomania or by atypical presentation in the manic phase. Thus, the apparent benefits from lithium in conditions other than bipolar disorder may sometimes be based on an underdiagnosis of bipolar disorder.)

Lithium has also been shown to be helpful in a number of conditions other than mood disorders that are associated with aggressiveness, explosiveness, or rage (Sheard, Marini, Bridges, & Wagner, 1976). Populations studied have included aggressive prison inmates (Tupin et al., 1972) and individuals with borderline personality (Shader, Jackson, & Dodes, 1974). These observations suggest that episodic agitation in older patients due in part to disorders of personality might be lithium-responsive. Lithium has been tried, but with a small sample and inconclusive results, for specific treatment of agitation in demented elderly patients (William & Goldstein, 1979). Some experts have suggested that both dosages and blood levels in this population should be substantially lower than those usually used for manic illness (Salzman, 1988a).

Lithium use in old age is limited by a greater susceptibility of older people to lithium neurotoxicity, whether the drug is used alone or in combination with neuroleptics (Himmelhoch, Neil, May, Fuchs, & Licata, 1980; Miller, Menninger, & Whitecup, 1986). Patients with Alzheimer's disease may be particularly susceptible to extrapyramidal side effects of lithium (Kelwala, Pomara, Stanley, Sitaram, & Gershon, 1984). Essential tremor, a common but potentially disabling neurologic problem that increases in prevalence with age, is aggravated by lithium (VanPutten, 1978). Further, many drugs commonly prescribed for elderly persons interact adversely with lithium; calcium-channel blockers have recently been included in the list (Price & Shalley, 1987).

Lithium neurotoxicity in the elderly may occur at lithium levels within the usual adult therapeutic range. Neurotoxicity at these levels may entail gross delirium and dramatic EEG abnormalities (Smith & Kocen, 1988). Thus, the appropriate dosage, target blood level, and list of contraindications to lithium therapy may well be different in the elderly than in the young. The selection of dosage and target blood level may have a profound influence on the negative as well as the positive outcomes of lithium trials.

When lithium is used to treat mania, 2 weeks or more may be needed for full therapeutic effect. Reports of lithium for antidepressant augmentation suggest that a shorter duration of action is possible (Kushnir, 1986; Heninger et al., 1983), but that 3 weeks may be required in some cases (Lafferman et al., 1988). However, in conditions not due to mood disorder, longer trials may be needed. In one study of episodic aggressiveness not due to mood disorder, increasing benefit over three months was noted (Sheard et al., 1976).

Recommendations for Further Investigation

Lithium deserves further systematic study in agitated elderly patients with possible mood disorders (see the above section on classification regarding this issue) and intermittent agitation due to personality disturbance or mild dementia. Among demented patients, it would probably be better tolerated on those with milder cognitive impairment and fewer extrapyramidal signs, as well as by those on fewer medical drugs with known interactions with lithium. Patients with subsyndromal mood symptoms in addition to dementia or with premorbid explosiveness and irritability might be especially promising for study.

In controlled studies of lithium, trials at low dosage (blood levels between .2 and .5 mEq/Liter) should be attempted before trials at full dosage (blood levels between 0.5 and 1.0). Levels above 1.0 should generally be avoided for nonmanic elderly patients because of the greater susceptibility of elderly patients to toxic side effects and their greater vulnerability to dehydration that may rapidly raise lithium levels to a severely toxic range. The trial of lithium at each level should be at least 2 weeks in mood disorder cases, and 1 month in other conditions.

In monitoring study patients, special attention should be given to memory function, tremors, rigidity, and involuntary movements. An EEG should be obtained before and during lithium treatment. This might aid in the detection of pretreatment EEG patterns that predict a high risk of neurotoxicity or of poor clinical response.

Trazodone

Trazodone, a bicyclic antidepressant with predominant effects on serotonergic transmission, has been used successfully to treat disruptive behavior in dementia (Greenwald, Marin, & Silverman, 1986; Simpson & Foster, 1986; Tingle, 1986). The reported effects appear to go beyond mere sedation, although trazodone is highly sedative (Feighner, Merideth, & Hendrickson, 1981). The drug has not specifically been tested for adjunctive treatment of agitation in psychotic disorders, nor has it been tested for agitated delirium. As trazodone may precipitate mania (Knobler, 1986), it would be relatively contraindicated for manic agitation.

Postural hypotension is a frequent side effect (Robinson, 1984), suggesting that trazodone may, like tricyclic antidepressants, increase the risk of falls. Also, trazodone may affect bladder function and precipitate incontinence.

Recommendations for Further Investigations

Trazodone deserves systematic study for agitation accompanying dementia, especially when syndromal or subsyndromal depression is present. Further, it might be considered as an adjunct for the treatment of agitation in delusional patients, where delusions have been treated with optimal doses of neuroleptics and agitation still persists.

In trials of trazodone for these indications, a minimum of 4–6 weeks should be permitted for assessment, as would be done with any other antidepressant: there is insufficient evidence to suggest that more rapid responses can be relied upon. In monitoring for side effects, special attention should be paid to alertness in view of the sedative effects of trazodone, as well as to falls, incontinence, and orthostatic hypotension.

Electroconvulsive Therapy (ECT)

Electroconvulsive therapy is an effective treatment for major depression and probably the treatment of choice for delusional depression (Kroessler, 1985). It is also an effective treatment for acute schizophrenia (Brandon et al., 1985) and for mania (Small, Kellams, & Milstein, 1986; Small, Klapper, & Kellams, 1988), although it is rarely used for these indications because alternative treatments usually are employed. There are few absolute contraindications to ECT, and it has been given safely and effectively for treatment of mood disorders in patients with Alzheimer's Disease (Dubovsky, 1986), Parkinson's disease (Young, Alexopoulos, & Shamoian, 1985), and stroke (Coffey et al., 1987; Murray, Shea, & Conn, 1986).

Because of its broad range of efficacy, ECT may be useful in a number of agitated psychotic conditions not responsive to neuroleptics or to combinations of neuroleptics with other drugs. ECT is particularly attractive in patients unable to tolerate the extrapyramidal effects of neuroleptics since the treatment does not aggravate parkinsonian symptoms.

However effective ECT may be in inducing remissions of acute mental illness, it does not prevent relapses. Maintenance ECT, involving regularly scheduled booster treatments, is anecdotally helpful in preventing relapses of mood disorders, but it has not been evaluated in controlled clinical trials.

Evaluating the literature on response to ECT, there is marked variability in the number of treatments necessary to attain a remission of symptoms, and this variability may be even greater in elderly patients (Fogel, 1988a). While 4 to 12 treatments are typical for the treatment of major depression, some elderly patients require substantially more, and patients with schizophrenia have frequently been reported to require more than 12 treatments. Numerous issues of technique, including the optimal stimulus, seizure duration, and unilateral versus bilateral stimulus, are also incompletely resolved and require further study (Fogel, 1988a).

Recommendations for Further Investigation

Controlled trials of ECT are desirable in the following populations of psychotic and/or agitated elderly mentally ill:

1. Patients with severe depression who remit incompletely with drug therapy or have side effects from optimal drug therapy that significantly compromise their function or quality of life.

2. Patients with other psychoses, including schizophrenic, paraphrenic, and schizoaffective psychosis, who are either unresponsive to or intolerant of neuroleptics, even with appropriate adjuncts.

3. Patients with dementia and intractable agitation, a partial syndrome of major depression or mania, and a prior history of definite mood disorder in themselves or in a first-degree relative.

The patients in these categories who respond well to ECT acutely but who relapse rapidly despite maintenance with standard pharmacotherapy should be considered for a controlled trial of maintenance ECT.

Because of the concerns that ECT is a more drastic treatment than medication and that it may aggravate cognitive impairment, studies of ECT should employ systematic, sensitive and repeated measures of cognitive function before and after treatment and at follow-up, and should make use of medication-only control groups. Further, functional assessment, particularly of physical and instrumental ADL, should be used to establish whether detected side effects are significant to everyday life. In this regard, it is possible that the orthostatic hypotension induced by tricyclic antidepressant drugs may be more functionally disabling than a mild defect in autobiographical memory induced by ECT (Fogel, 1988b).

In ECT studies, conventional end points for ECT are defined in terms of an arbitrary number of treatments (e.g., 12) or with respect to the attainment of remission, a plateau in response or side effects requiring discontinuation of treatment. If the use of ECT in the elderly is to be expanded to broader indications, the end-point issue becomes increasingly subtle because the number of treatments that typically relieves major depression may be too many for a moderately demented patient and too few for a paraphrenic. These issues would best be resolved by a careful study of responders and nonresponders to ECT and by the development of appropriate biologic markers of treatment adequacy (Fogel, 1988a). In any case, the present state of knowledge argues for a flexible end point for ECT, so that a patient who was continuing to show improvement but was not fully remitted and did not have severe side effects would not have treatments discontinued after an arbitrary number.

CONCLUSION

For all of their drawbacks, neuroleptics are frequently prescribed for the elderly mentally ill for lack of anything better. Physicians tolerate incomplete remissions, extrapyramidal side effects, and an often negative functional impact of neuroleptic drugs because the alternative of uncontrolled agitation is unacceptable both clinically and socially. The development of more specific and effective, and less toxic, treatments for agitated and psychotic states in the elderly deserves a high priority in future research. While a biologically based classification of agitated states might ultimately be more useful than one based on phenomenology alone, finer clinical classification of agitated patients and systematic trials of alternative and adjunctive therapies in relatively homogeneous groups make sense now. The application of functional measures and carefully planned surveillance for side effects and drug interactions are necessary modifications of usual psychopharmacologic procedures when drug trials are to be carried out in frail and physically ill elderly patients. Special attention must be paid to differences in desirable drug dosage and optimal duration of treatment trials when drugs are used for novel indications. Ultimately, evaluating sequences of prescribing behavior, and not just individual drugs, may be necessary to develop the knowledge base for disseminating more sophisticated psychopharmacology to settings where the services of specialty mental health providers are rarely available.

REFERENCES

Aoki, F. Y., & Sitar, D. S. (1988). Clinical pharmacokinetics of amantadine hydrochloride. *Clinical Pharmacokinetics, 14*, 35–51.

Avorn, J., Dreyer, P., Connelly, K., & Soumerai, S. B. (1989). Use of psychoactive medication and the quality of care in rest homes: Findings and policy implications of a statewide study. *New England Journal of Medicine, 320*, 227–232.

Baldessarini, R. J., Cohen, B. M., & Teicher, M. H. (1988). Significance of neuroleptic dose and plasma level in the pharmacological treatment of psychoses. *Archives of General Psychiatry, 45*, 79–91.

Barnes, R., Veith, R., Okimoto, J., Raskind, M., & Gumbrecht, G. (1982). Efficacy of antipsychotic medications in behaviorally disturbed dementia patients. *American Journal of Psychiatry, 139*, 1170–1174.

Bears, M., Avorn, J., Soumerai, ScD., Everitt, D. E., Sherman, D. S., & Salem, S. (1988). Psychoactive medication use in intermediate-care facility residents. *Journal of the American Medical Association, 260*, 3016–3020.

Beardsley, R. S., Larson, D. B., Burns, B. J., Thompson, J. W., & Kamerow, D. B. (1989). Prescribing of psychotropics in elderly nursing home patients. *Journal of the American Geriatrics Society, 37*, 327–330.

Brandon, S., Crowley, P., McDonald, C., Neville, P., Palmer, R., & Wellstood-Eason, S. (1985). Leiucester ECT trial: Results in schizophrenia. *British Journal of Psychiatry, 146*, 177–183.

Burns, B., & Taube, C. (1990). Mental health services in general medical care and in nursing homes. In B. S. Fogel, A. Furino, & G. L. Gottlieb (Eds.), *Mental health policy for older Americans: Protecting minds at risk* (pp. 63–84). Washington, DC: American Psychiatric Press.

Chandler, M. C., Barnhill, J. L., & Gualtieri, C. T. (1988). Amantadine for the agitated head-injury patient. *Brain Injury, 2*, 309–311.

Chouinard, G. (1988). Clonazepam in the treatment of psychiatric disorders. In S. L. McElroy & H. G. Pope (Eds.), *Use of anticonvulsants in psychiatry* (pp. 43-58). Clifton, NJ: Oxford Health Care.

Coffey, C. E., Hinkle, P. E., Weiner, R. D., Nemeroff, C. B., Krishnan, K. R., Varia, I., & Sullivan, D. C. (1987). Electroconvulsive therapy of depression in patients with white matter hyperintensity. *Biological Psychiatry, 22,* 629-636.

Cohen-Cole, S. A., & Harpe, C. (1987). Diagnostic assessment of depression in the medically ill. In A. Stoudemire & B. S. Fogel (Eds.), *Principles of medical psychiatry* (pp. 23-36). Orlando, FL: Grune & Stratton.

Cohen, S., & Khan, A. (1987). Adjunctive benzodiazepines in acute schizophrenia. *Neuropsychobiology, 18,* 9-12.

Cohen, S., Khan, A., & Johnson, S. (1987). Pharmacological management of manic psychosis in an unlocked setting. *Journal of Clinical Psychopharmacology, 7,* 261-264.

Cohen-Mansfield, J. (1986). Agitated behaviors in the elderly. II: Preliminary results in the cognitively deteriorated. *Journal of the American Geriatrics Society, 34,* 722-727.

Cohen-Mansfield, J., & Billig, N. (1986). Agitated behaviors in the elderly. I: A conceptual review. *Journal of the American Geriatrics Society, 34,* 711-721.

Cole, J. O. (1988). The drug treatment of anxiety and depression. *Medical Clinics of North America, 72,* 815-822.

Colenda, C. C. (1988). Buspirone in treatment of agitated demented patient. *Lancet,* May 21, 1169.

Covington, J. S. (1975). Alleviating agitation, apprehension, and related symptoms in geriatric patients: A double-blind comparison of a phenothiazine and a benzodiazepine. *Southern Medical Journal, 68,* 719-724.

Cummings, J. L. (1985). Organic delusions: Phenomenology, anatomic correlations, and review. *British Journal of Psychiatry, 146,* 184-197.

Dubovsky, S. L. (1986). Using electroconvulsive therapy for patients with neurological disease. *Hospital and Community Psychiatry, 37,* 819-824.

Evans, L. K., & Strumpf, N. E. (1989). Tying down the elderly: A review of the literature on physical restraint. *Journal of the American Geriatrics Society, 37,* 65-74.

Fayen, M., Goldman, M. B., Moulthrop, M. A., & Luchins, D. J. (1988). Differential memory function with dopaminergic versus anticholinergic treatment of drug-induced extrapyramidal symptoms. *American Journal of Psychiatry, 145,* 483-486.

Feighner, J. P., Merideth, C. H., & Hendrickson, G. (1981). Maintenance antidepressant therapy: A double blind comparison of trazadone and imipramine. *Journal of Clinical Psychopharmacology, 1*(Suppl.), 45S-48S.

Ferris, S. H., et al. (1985). Institutionalization of Alzheimer's patients: Reducing precipitating factors through family counseling. *Archives of the Foundation of Thanatology, 12,* 7.

Fogel, B. S. (1988a). Electroconvulsive therapy in the elderly: A clinical research agenda. *International Journal of Geriatric Psychiatry, 3,* 181-190.

Fogel, B. S. (1988b). Combining anticonvulsants with conventional psychopharmacologic agents. In S. L. McElroy & H. G. Pope (Eds.), *Use of anticonvulsants in psychiatry* (pp. 77-93). Clifton, NJ: Oxford Health Care.

Fogel, B. S. (1990). Major depression versus organic mood disorder: A questionable distinction. *Journal of Clinical Psychiatry, 51,* 53-56.

Fogel, B. S., & Westlake, R. (1990). Personality disorder diagnoses and age in inpatients with major depression. *Journal of Clinical Psychiatry*, *51*, 232–235.

Freinhar, J. P., & Alvarez, W. A. (1986). Clonazepam treatment of organic brain syndromes in three elderly patients. *Journal of Clinical Psychiatry*, *47*, 525–526.

Gardner, D. L., & Cowdry, R. W. (1988). Anticonvulsants and personality disorders. In S. L. McElroy & H. G. Pope (Eds.), *Use of anticonvulsants in psychiatry* (pp. 127–139). Clifton, NJ: Oxford Health Care.

Goldberg, S. C., Schulz, S. C., Schulz, P. M., Resnick, R., Hamer, R. M., & Friedel, R. O. (1986). Borderline and schizotypal personality disorders treated with low-dose thiothixene vs. placebo. *Archives of General Psychiatry*, *43*, 680–686.

Gottlieb, G. L., McAllister, T. W., & Gur, R. C. (1988). Depot neuroleptics in the treatment of behavioral disorders in patients with Alzheimer's disease. *Journal of the American Geriatrics Society*, *36*, 619–621.

Greendyke, R. M., & Kanter, D. R. (1986). Therapeutic effects of pindolol on behavioral disturbances associated with organic brain disease: A double-blind study. *Journal of Clinical Psychiatry*, *47*, 423–426.

Greendyke, R. M., Kanter, D. R., & Schuster, D. B. (1986). Propranolol treatment of assaultive patients with organic brain disease: A double-blind crossover placebo-controlled study. *Journal of Nervous and Mental Disease*, *174*, 290–294.

Greendyke, R. M., Schuster, D. B., & Wooten, J. A. (1984). Propranolol in the treatment of assaultive patients with organic brain disease. *Journal of Clinical Pharmacology*, *4*, 282.

Greenwald, B. S., Marin, D. B., & Silverman, S. M. (1986). Serotonergic treatment of screaming and banging in dementia [Letter]. *Lancet*, *2*, 1464–1465.

Gunderson, J. G. (1986). Pharmacotherapy for patients with borderline personality disorder. *Archives of General Psychiatry*, *43*, 698–699.

Helms, P. M. (1985). Efficacy of antipsychotics in the treatment of the behavioral complications of dementia: A review of the literature. *Journal of the American Geriatrics Society*, *33*, 206–209.

Heninger, G. R., Charney, D. S., & Sternberg, D. E. (1983). Lithium carbonate augmentation of antidepressant treatment: An effective prescription for treatment-refractory depression. *Archives of General Psychiatry*, *40*, 1335–1342.

Himmelhoch, J. M., Neil, J. F., May, S. J., Fuchs, C. Z., & Licata, S. M. (1980). Age, dementia, dyskinesia and lithium response. *American Journal of Psychiatry*, *137*, 941–945.

Jenike, M. A. (1985). *Handbook of geriatric psychopharmacology*. Littleton, MA: PSG Publishing.

Jeste, D. V., & Wyatt, R. J. (1987). Aging and tardive dyskinesia. In N. E. Miller & G. D. Cohen (Eds.), *Schizophrenia and aging* (pp. 275–286). New York: Guilford Press.

Kelwala, S., Pomara, N., Stanley, M., Sitaram, N., & Gershon, S. (1984). Lithium-induced accentuation of extrapyramidal symptoms in individuals with Alzheimer's disease. *Journal of Clinical Psychopharmacology*, *45*, 342–344.

Klein, E., Bental, E., Lerer, B., & Belmaker, R. H. (1984). Carbamazepine and haloperidol versus placebo and haloperidol in excited psychoses. *Archives of General Psychiatry*, *41*, 165–70.

Klein, D. F., Gittelman, R., Quitkin, F., & Rifkin, A. (1980). *Diagnosis and drug treatment of psychiatric disorders: Adults and children* (2nd ed.). Baltimore, MD: Williams & Wilkins.

Knobler, H. (1986). Trazadone-induced mania. *British Journal of Psychiatry*, *149*, 787–789.

Kraus, M. L., Gottlieb, L. D., Horwitz, R. I., & Anscher, M. (1985). Randomized clinical trial of atenolol in patients with alcohol withdrawal. *New England Journal of Medicine, 313,* 905–909.

Kroessler, D. (1985). Relative efficacy rates for therapies of delusional depression. *Convulsive Therapy, 1,* 173–182.

Kushnir, S. L. (1986). Lithium-antidepressant combinations in treatment of depressed, physically ill geriatric patients. *American Journal of Psychiatry, 143,* 378–379.

Lafferman, J., Solomon, K., & Ruskin, P. (1988). Lithium augmentation for treatment-resistant depression in the elderly. *Journal of Geriatric Psychiatry and Neurology, 1,* 49–52.

Leibovici, A., & Tariot, P. N. (1988). Carbamazepine treatment of agitation associated with dementia. *Journal of Geriatric Psychiatry and Neurology, 1,* 110–112.

Levine, A. M. (1988). Buspirone and agitation in head injury. *Brain Injury, 2,* 165–167.

Liebowitz, M. R., Stone, M. H., & Turkat, I. D. (1986). Treatment of personality disorders. In A. I. Frances, & R. E. Hales (Eds.), *American Psychiatric Association annual review* (Vol. 5, pp. 390–393). Washington, DC: American Psychiatric Press.

Lieff, S., & Herrmann (1988). Combined drug therapy for an elderly depressed patient. *American Journal of Psychiatry, 145,* 1034–1035.

Liegghio, N. E., Yeragani, V. K., & Moore, N. C. (1988). Buspirone-induced jitteriness in patients with panic disorder and one patient with generalized anxiety disorder. *Journal of Clinical Psychiatry, 49,* 165–166.

Liptzin, B. (1984). Treatment of mania. In C. Salzman (Ed.), *Clinical geriatric psychopharmacology.* New York: McGraw-Hill.

Luchins, D. J. (1984). Carbamazepine in psychiatric syndromes: Clinical and neuropharmacological properties. *Psychopharmacology Bulletin, 20,* 569–71.

Maletta, G. J. (1985). Medication to modify at home behavior of Alzheimer's patients. *Geriatrics, 40*(12), 31–42.

Mattes, J. A. (1984). Carbamazepine for uncontrolled rage outbursts. *Lancet, 2,* 1164–5.

McElroy, S. L., Pope, H. G., Keck, P. E., & Hudson, J. I. (1988). Valproate in primary psychiatric disorders: Literature review and clinical experience in a private psychiatric hospital. In S. L. McElroy, & H. G. Pope (Eds.), *Use of anticonvulsants in psychiatry* (pp. 25–41). Clifton, NJ: Oxford Health Care.

McEvoy, J. P. (1986). The neuroleptic threshold as a marker of minimum effective neuroleptic dose. *Comprehensive Psychiatry, 27*(4), 327–335.

Miller, F., Menninger, J., & Whitecup, S. M. (1986). Lithium-neuroleptic neurotoxicity in the elder bipolar patient. *Journal of Clinical Psychopharmacology, 6,* 176–177.

Murray, G. B., Shea, V., & Conn, D. K. (1986). Electroconvulsive therapy for poststroke depression. *Journal of Clinical Psychiatry, 47,* 258–260.

Neppe, V. M. (1983). Carbamazepine as adjunctive treatment in non-epileptic chronic inpatients with EEG temporal lobe abnormalities. *Journal of Clinical Psychiatry, 44,* 326–31.

Pai, M., White, A. C., & Deane, A. G. (1986). Lithium augmentation in the treatment of delusional depression. *British Journal of Psychiatry, 148,* 736–738.

Peabody, C. A., Warner D., Whiteford, H. A., & Hollister, L. E. (1987). Neuroleptics and the elderly. *Journal of the American Geriatrics Society, 35,* 233–238.

Petrie, W. M., & Ban, T. A. (1981). Propranolol in organic agitation [Letter]. *Lancet, 1,* 324.

Post, R. M. (1988). Effectiveness of carbamazepine in the treatment of bipolar affective disorder. In S. L. McElroy, & H. G. Pope (Eds.), *Use of anticonvulsants in psychiatry* (pp. 1-23). Clifton, NJ: Oxford Health Care.

Price, W. A., & Shalley, J. E. (1987). Lithium-verapamil toxicity in the elderly. *Journal of the American Geriatrics Society, 35*, 177-178.

Ratey, J. J., Mikkelsen, E. J., & Smith, G. B. (1986). Beta-blockers in the severely and profoundly mentally retarded. *Journal of Clinical Psychopharmacology, 6*, 103-107.

Risse, S. C., & Barnes, R. (1986). Pharmacologic treatment of agitation associated with dementia. *Journal of the American Geriatrics Society, 34*, 368-376.

Risse, S. C., Lampe, T. H., & Cubberley, L. (1987). Very low-dose neuroleptic treatment in two patients with agitation associated with Alzheimer's disease. *Journal of Clinical Psychiatry, 48*, 207-208.

Ritchie, D. E., Bridenbaugh, R. H., & Jabbari, B. (1988). Acute generalized myoclonus following buspirone administration. *Journal of Clinical Psychiatry, 49*, 242-243.

Robinson, D. S. (1984). Adverse reactions, toxicities, and drug interactions of newer antidepressants: anticholinergic, sedative, and other side effects. *Psychopharmacology Bulletin, 20*, 280-290.

Robinson, D., Napoliello, M. J., & Shenk, J. (1988). The safety and usefulness of buspirone as an anxiolytic drug in the elderly versus young patients. *Clinical Therapeutics, 6*, 740-746.

Sadavoy, J., & Fogel, B. (In press). Personality disorders in old age. In J. E. Birren, R. B. Sloan, & G. Cohen (Eds.), *Handbook of mental health & aging* (2nd ed.). Orlando, FL: Academic Press.

Salzman, C. (1988a). Treatment of agitation, anxiety, and depression in dementia. *Psychopharmacology Bulletin, 24*, 39-42.

Salzman, C. (1988b). Use of benzodiazepines to control disruptive behavior in inpatients. *Journal of Clinical Psychiatry, 49(Suppl.)*, 13-15.

Schweizer, E. E., Amsterdam, J., Rickels, K., Kaplan, M., & Droba, M. (1986). Open trial of buspirone in the treatment of major depressive disorder. *Psychopharmacology Bulletin, 22*, 183-185.

Shader, R. I., Jackson, A. H., & Dodes, L. M. (1974). The antiaggressive effects of lithium in man. *Psychopharmacologia, 40*, 17-24.

Sheard, M. H., Marini, J. L., Bridges, C. I., & Wagner, E. (1976). The effect of lithium in impulsive aggressive behavior in man. *American Journal of Psychiatry, 133*, 1409-1413.

Sheppard, G. P. (1979). High-dose propranolol in schizophrenia. *British Journal of Psychiatry, 134*, 470-476.

Simpson, B. M., & Foster, B. (1986). Improvement in organically disturbed behavior with Trazadone treatment. *Journal of Clinical Psychiatry, 47*, 191-193.

Small, J. G., Kellams, J. J., & Milstein, V. (1986). Complications with electroconvulsive therapy in the treatment of manic episodes. In S. Malitz, & H. A. Sackeim (Eds.), *Annuals of the New York Academy of Sciences: Vol. 462. Electroconvulsive therapy: Clinical and basic research issues.* New York Academy of Sciences.

Small, J. G., Klapper, M. H., & Kellams, J. (1988). Electroconvulsive treatment compared with lithium in the management of manic states. *Archives of General Psychiatry, 45*, 727-732.

Smeraski, P. J. (1988). Clonazepam treatment of multi-infarct dementia. *Journal of Geriatric Psychiatry and Neurology, 1*, 47-48.

Smith, S. J., & Kocen, R. S. (1988). A Creutzfeldt-Jakob like syndrome due to lithium toxicity. *Journal of Neurology, Neurosurgery, and Psychiatry, 51,* 120–123.

Soloff, P. H., George, A., Nathan, R. S., Schulz, P. M., Ulrich, R. F., & Perel, D. M. (1986). Progress in pharmacotherapy of borderline disorders. *Archives of General Psychiatry, 43,* 691–697.

Sovner, R. (1988). Anticonvulsant drug therapy of neuropsychiatric disorders in mentally retarded persons. In S. L. McElroy & H. G. Pope (Eds.), *Use of anticonvulsants in psychiatry.* Clifton, NJ: Oxford Health Care.

Spira, N., Dysken, M. W., Lazarus, L. W., Davis, J. M., & Salzman, E. (1984). Treatment of agitation and psychosis. In E. Salzman (Ed.), *Clinical geriatric psychopharmacology.* New York: McGraw-Hill.

Stotksy, B. (1984). Multicenter study comparing thioridazine with diazepam and placebo in elderly, non-psychotic patients with emotional and behavioral disorders. *Clinical Therapeutics, 6,* 546–559.

Strauss, A. (1988). Oral dyskinesia associated with busiprone use in elderly women. *Journal of Clinical Psychiatry, 49,* 322–323.

Tideiksaar, R. (1989). *Falling in old age: Its prevention and treatment* (pp. 21–48). New York: Springer Publishing Company.

Tiller, J. W., Dakis, J. A., & Shaw, J. M. (1988). Short-term buspirone treatment in disinhibition with dementia. *Lancet,* August 27, 510.

Tingle, D. (1986). Trazodone in dementia [Letter]. *Journal of Clinical Psychiatry, 47,* 482.

Tupin, J. P., Smith, D. B., Clanon, T. L., et al. (1973). The long-term use of lithium in aggressive prisoners. *Comprehensive Psychiatry, 14,* 311–317.

Tryer, P., & Alexander, J. (1988). Personality assessment schedule. In P. Tryer (Ed.), *Personality disorders: Diagnosis, management, and course* (pp. 43–62). London: Wright.

VanPutten, T. (1978). Lithium-induced disabling tremor. *Psychosomatics, 19,* 27–31.

VanPutten, T., Marder, S. R., Mintz, J., & Poland, R. E. (1988). Haloperidol plasma levels and clinical response: A therapeutic relationship. *Psychopharmacology Bulletin, 24,* 112–115.

Weiler, P. G., Mungas, D., & Bernick, C. (1988). Propranolol for the control of disruptive behavior in senile dementia. *Journal of Geriatric Psychiatry & Neurology, 1,* 226–230.

William, K. H., & Goldstein, G. (1979). Cognitive and affective responses to lithium in patients with organic brain syndrome. *American Journal of Psychiatry, 136,* 800–803.

Wragg, R. E., & Jeste, D. V. (1988). Neuroleptics and alternative treatments: Management of behavioral symptoms and psychosis in Alzheimer's disease and related conditions. *Psychiatric Clinics of North America, 11,* 195–213.

Yorkston, N. J., Sakis, S. A., Pitcher, D. R., Gruzelier, J. H., Hollander, D., & Sergeant, H. G. S. (1977). Propranolol as an adjunct to the treatment of schizophrenia. *Lancet, 2,* 575–578.

Young, R. C., Alexopoulos, G. S., & Shamoian, C. A. (1985). Dissociation of motor response from mood and cognition in a parkinsonian patient treated with ECT. *Biological Psychiatry, 20,* 566–569.

Yudofsky, S. (1981). Propranolol in the treatment of rage and violent behavior in patients with chronic brain syndrome. *American Journal of Psychiatry, 138,* 218–230.

Yudofsky, S., Stevens, L., & Silver, J. (1984). Propranolol in the treatment of rage and violent behavior associated with Korsakoff's psychosis. *American Journal of Psychiatry, 141,* 114–115.

PART IV

Research on Service Delivery to the CMI Elderly

11

The Chronic
Mentally Ill Elderly:
Service Research Issues

Carl I. Cohen

Service strategies for the chronic mentally ill (CMI) can be roughly divided into four principal areas (Bellak & Mueser, 1986; Liberman & Phipps, 1987; Test & Stein, 1978):

1. Treatment alternatives to long-term hospitalization. This consists of programs such as brief inpatient treatment, partial hospitalization, continuing treatment, subacute units, mobile units, etc. Included under this rubric are programs that teach patients social and vocational skills to survive in the community and special pharmacological strategies used to treat this population.
2. Residential alternatives to long-term hospitalization. This includes alternatives such as halfway houses, family (foster) care, SRO projects, board and care homes, and other congregate care living facilities.
3. Community support programs. These include work with case managers, natural networks, and gatekeepers.
4. Psychoeducational programs. These are programs that teach families how to cope with their mentally ill relatives.

In recent years there have been some attempts to evaluate these programs systematically. With few exceptions, these programs have focused primarily on younger persons, and when elderly persons have been included, they are rarely dissected out for special examination. For example, in Braun and associates' (1981) review article of 20 community studies, the mean age of the samples ranged between 22 and 49. Similarly, Stroul's (1986) survey of community support services for persons with "long-term mental illness" indicated that the mean age of participants was generally under 45, and most were in their thirty's. In Stroul's report, the only programs targeted toward the older CMI were the community worker projects (e.g., Human Service Center in Rhinelander, Wisconsin, and Compeer in Rochester, New York), which rely on lay citizens to provide support and care.

Although there have been a few studies describing community mental health services for the elderly, particularly outreach services (Brown & Lieff, 1982; Raschko, 1988; Reifler et al., 1982; Rocca, Storer, Robbins, Tlasek, & Rabins, 1990; Sherr, Eskridge, & Lewis, 1976), when reported, the percentage of clients with chronic mental illness has been below 25%. During 1986–1987, the NIMH Community Support Program (CSP) funded 16 service programs targeted specifically for the aging mentally ill. These programs have employed a variety of service strategies, including (a) extensive outreach services with assessments conducted in homes and other community sites; (b) the development of more coordinated and highly linked services for the CMI elderly; (c) the modification of existing mental health programs to accommodate the special needs of the aging; (d) efforts to enhance clients' social support networks; (e) the creation of self-help programs; (f) the training of peer counselors, caregivers, and other persons who work with the CMI elderly such as board and care managers, meals-on-wheels staff, etc. (*Community Support Network News*, 1987). All these programs have an evaluation component, and their reports should be forthcoming.

In spite of the paucity of services and service research for the elderly CMI, judging from the foci of the CSP projects, it would seem that the four broad areas delineated above are also the most likely candidates for intervention with the aging mentally ill. Programs for the CMI elderly, however, have to adapt their programs to the special biopsychosocial characteristics of older persons. Thus, programs must pay more attention to physical health, neuropsychological functioning, disability, various personal and social losses, special psychotherapeutic approaches, and the like.

One of the basic tenets of this chapter is that it is highly desirable to conduct health and social needs research on the targeted population before the actual services are introduced. As a practical matter, this cannot always be done. Nevertheless, it is usually best to begin with the ideal and then make the necessary alterations demanded by the real world. Therefore, initially, I will delineate those methodological issues that should be considered when undertaking research of the CMI elderly. Then I shall present those issues relevant to service provision and evaluation. I have drawn heavily from my work with the homeless elderly in which we were able to adhere to the sequence of population research followed by service program and evaluation (Cohen & Sokolovsky, 1989; Cohen, Teresi, & Holmes, 1988a, 1988b; Cohen, Teresi, Holmes, & Roth, 1988).

ELEMENTS TO CONSIDER IN CONDUCTING COMMUNITY RESEARCH OF THE CHRONIC MENTALLY ILL ELDERLY

Several areas have been commonly identified as necessary prerequisites for community mental health research (Bachrach 1984-N, 1987).

The Study Population Must Be Delimited

The source populations for the sample must be determined. For example, if an investigator wishes to study the CMI elderly living in the community, it is necessary to decide whether to conduct a survey of elderly persons in the general population and then identify those persons within this population who have chronic mental illness. Alternatively, the investigator can employ a stratified random sampling technique with subsamples derived from various sites serving the elderly mentally ill such as adult homes, HRFs, mobile units, mental health clinics, etc. The first approach is broader in scope, and with respect to service delivery, it can be extremely useful in ascertaining which persons evade the mental health system. However, depending on the size of overall population to be studied, this approach is often expensive and time-consuming. At the initial stages of research, the second approach may be more sensible in providing preliminary data and guidelines for refining service delivery.

Similarly, we wished to learn more about the elderly homeless mentally ill. It was necessary to decide between two potential source populations: older homeless individuals with chronic mental illness or older chronic mentally ill who are homeless. Because we were studying a particular subsample of elderly homeless—those older men living on New York City's skid row ("the Bowery")—it was possible to do a random sampling of the entire population (which we estimated to be approximately 2,700). Such an approach also had important clinical implications as we were especially interested in determining to what extent homeless older men were being serviced by the existing Bowery agencies.

The Study Population Must Be Well Defined

In investigating the CMI elderly living in the community, it is necessary to define at least four terms: *chronic, mentally ill, elderly,* and *community.* (The issue of psychopathology and disability will be discussed below.) The term *elderly* requires a decision. Should it be the Social Security cutoff of age 65? Should it be at age 75, when many of the serious disabilities of old age seem to increase dramatically? In our Bowery research, we selected age 50 as "old." This is because previous research had indicated that most skid row men were physically and physiologically like community men who were 10–15 years older (Bogue, 1963).

Likewise, in mental health, the word *community* generally means not residing in a mental hospital. However, should *community* include nursing homes or board and care homes? Indeed, such community placements have been termed transinstitutionalization (Talbott, 1987).

In our research of the older homeless, one of our first tasks was to define *homeless*. Should we study only men living on the street, or should we include men living in the flophouses? We opted to include street and flophouse men. This was because it had been well documented that the biographies, health profiles, drinking habits, and lifestyles of street and nonstreet men were quite similar (Wallace, 1965). Indeed, many of the flophouse men had spent considerable time on the street, and many of the street men would periodically live in the flophouses, especially during inclement weather.

It Is Necessary to Define Psychopathology

As noted above, the investigator must decide the parameters of *chronic* and *mentally ill*. In general, four variables are available: diagnosis, disability, symptoms, duration of illness or time spent in institutions or other supervised settings (Goldman, Gattozzi, & Taube, 1981; Minkoff, 1978; Talbott, 1987). Selecting different variables or combinations of variables can omit important subgroups. For example, evidence suggests that many schizophrenics improve considerably in old age (Harding, Zubin, & Strauss, 1987). Using stringent disability criteria might neglect this important subgroup of the mentally ill.

In our work with the elderly homeless, the use of standard diagnostic criteria was made especially difficult because of the ubiquitous abuse of alcohol, the debilitating effects of the men's lifestyles on their mental and physical health, and the potential for developing a "social breakdown syndrome," a condition of social withdrawal or aggressivity in response to overwhelming stress that cuts across diagnoses (Gruenberg, 1967). Such widespread problems have led some workers to suggest that all homeless must be considered mentally ill (Bachrach, 1987). Because of these difficulties, we used primarily symptom scores rather than diagnoses, although we established some tentative diagnostic cutoff scores and employed community comparison groups to determine relative psychopathology.

Overlapping with Other Populations

Because community-dwelling CMI elderly may overlap with other populations, it may be more difficult to define and identify them. For example, they may overlap with "the homeless," "the physically frail," and "the organic mentally ill."

Heterogeneity within the Study Population

In studying the CMI elderly there are several sources of "within group" variation. These include diagnosis, premorbid functioning, age of onset, symptomatology, institutional history, and disability. Initially it would be best to establish broad criteria and then eliminate those variables with low prevalence. However, here again, cost and time factors may make such a broad approach impractical.

Other Sampling Problems

Critics of mass epidemiological surveys such as the Epidemiological Catchment Area study have pointed out that many mentally ill elderly were overlooked because sampling techniques did not focus on where the more impaired elderly might reside—e.g., senior housing, SRO hotels (Rabins, this volume). Thus, future community studies of the CMI elderly will require adjustments in sampling techniques to obtain adequate representations. Likewise, studies of the homeless have pointed to the fact that some sections of the city may be more prone to attract the mentally ill. For example, in New York City, those homeless living in Central Park are thought to exhibit more psychopathology and less substance abuse than the homeless living on the Upper West Side (Bachrach, 1987). In our homeless study, we selected the Bowery because of its heavy concentration of elderly homeless versus other areas.

Another important issue concerns participation and refusals. It can be assumed that a substantial number of the chronic mentally ill are no longer engaged by or are quite hostile to the mental health system. How does one enlist such persons in studies? In our Bowery study, we offered men ten dollars for participating in a 2-3 hour interview. We also used the men to help recruit others. We also worked closely with desk clerks, hotel managers, and agency staff. Various creative strategies boosted our acceptance rate to approximately two-thirds of those men approached.

Problems with Tracking This Population

There is a great need to conduct longitudinal studies on the chronic mentally ill elderly. Such data are necessary for basic research as well as to measure outcome of service programs. Community studies, however, will be made more difficult because respondents move frequently or prove to be uncooperative. Such problems have plagued studies of the younger chronically ill. Whether their older counterparts prove to be similarly elusive remains to be determined.

In the Bowery study, we found that the median time men had been living in their flophouses was 3 years, thus affording some degree of stability if we wished to conduct follow-up studies of the flophouse men. On the other hand, tracking street men depended on knowledge of their social support system. It's been possible to locate particular men by the meal programs, lounge programs, missions, taverns, parks, or restaurants that they frequent. When persons are missing from their usual haunts, not uncommonly one of their "associates" or an agency staff member has helped us locate them. Nonetheless, such procedures are quite time-consuming, thereby making longitudinal studies of homeless persons an extremely laborious undertaking.

Problems with Validity and Reliability

A major concern for researchers is to have instruments available that are appropriate to the population under study. In recent years a variety of assessment tools have been developed for use with older persons (Kane & Kane, 1981). In particular, those instruments that have attempted to keep questions simple, reduce the number of choices, and present items in the here and now are especially well suited for older samples. Of course, virtually none of these instruments have been used with the CMI elderly. At the very minimum, instruments to be used should be validated for the particular educational and social class of the population to be tested. As others in this volume (see Gurland, Shulz) have noted, we will need measures that are sensitive to broader dimensions such as quality of life in addition to measures of diagnosis and psychopathology. Instruments appropriate to measuring family caregiver burdens need to be developed. This may be accomplished by revising instruments currently being used for Alzheimer families or for parents of younger schizophrenics (Platt, 1985; Zarit, Todd, & Zarit, 1986).

Validity confronts the question of how well an instrument measures what you want to measure. A thorny issue, especially among the elderly, is the problem of the underreporting of symptoms or the use of categorizations that may differ from those for younger persons. When an investigator works with indigent or marginal populations, these problems are further compounded by class and cultural differences. Our work (Cohen & Sokolovsky, 1989) with homeless older men can illustrate some of the issues that must be addressed:

1. The need to avoid limited-choice and predetermined response items. In our research it was important to use instruments that were sufficiently flexible to avoid pigeonholing social relationships into categories such as "friends" or "intimates." Homeless men had their own taxonomy of relationships subdivided into acquaintances, associates, and friends. Sometimes acquaintances or associates were intimates, and often friends were sources of material assistance rather than emotional succor. By using social network analysis techniques in which respondents were asked to name all their contacts, what they do with them, and how they feel about them, we were able to explore all the subtle nuances of interaction.

2. The need to avoid excessive reliance on external norms, or conversely, an excessive reliance on self-reports. Heavy reliance on external norms may make

researchers more prone to view a marginal population as deviant or pathological. For example, using standards of the general population, the social world of older homeless men would seem relatively small and constricted. Indeed, the literature has commonly characterized these men as "undersocialized," "retreatist," or "disaffiliated." Utilizing network measures, however, we were able to demonstrate that these men were clearly not isolates, nor were they incapable of intimacy and complex social formations. Moreover, they were able to enlist the support of their compeers in helping to fulfill their daily needs. On the other hand, it is important to be wary of self-reports and not to neglect comparison groups. For example, in order to demonstrate their autonomy, some homeless men would at first fiercely deny that they had friends and or that they did anything with other men. Yet, on careful probing using network analysis techniques and field observation, we often found that they had extensive support systems. Furthermore, having comparison groups available enabled us to place the study population in a broader perspective. Hence, we were able to show that although homeless older men were not complete isolates, they were relatively isolated versus their age peers in the community.

SERVICE INTERVENTION PROGRAMS

What should a program for the CMI elderly look like? Because there are few well-studied programs, we must extrapolate from studies of the CMI in general or from anecdotal reports of senior programs. Although each program for the CMI elderly will have to be tailored to the characteristics of the population to be served, there is a three-stage intervention hierarchy that virtually all programs have identified as necessary to engage clients (Cohen & Sokolovsky, 1989). The first stage is "contact." For highly resistant persons, this stage may take months or years. It may require outreach visits or work with local agencies, neighbors, or community gatekeepers. The second stage involves the provision of "basic necessities." Work must be done to help the client with entitlements, food, physical health, and shelter. The last stage involves "specialist help" such as psychiatric services, alcohol counseling, social and vocational counseling, etc. Within this hierarchy, each program needs to determine the best methods for accomplishing each task, which types of clients are most receptive, and which clients are apt to be failures.

Bachrach (1980) and Talbott (1987) have enumerated 13 features that typically characterize model programs for the CMI. Presumably, these would be applicable to programs serving older persons.

1. Chronic patients targeted. Successful programs assign top priority to those who are most severely impaired (i.e., to those who are persistently ill) rather than

seeing them as undesirable or as second-rate teaching cases. Conversely, they avoid the pitfalls of many mental health programs that have focused on the "healthy but unhappy."

2. Linkage with other resources. Because of the diverse treatment needs of those who are chronically ill, model programs rely heavily on linking patients with a variety of special services in the community.

3. Functional integrity. Either by themselves or in combination with other resources, model programs attempt to address the totality of needs of the chronic population. This encompasses many of the items that had been provided previously by institutions such as health care, nutrition, shelter, monetary entitlements, socialization, rehabilitation, and psychiatric treatment. Evidence suggests that the variety of services received in community by recently discharged patients is a more important determinant of community tenure than the extent of individual therapy and case management (Solomon, Davis, & Gordon, 1984).

4. Individually tailored treatment. Model programs make a point of providing patients with personally tailored treatment regimens.

5. Cultural relevance and specificity. Successful programs are adapted to local realities of the communities in which they are situated.

6. Specially trained staff. Personnel who are trained for the special survival problems of the noninstitutionalized chronic patient is another essential ingredient.

7. Hospital liaison. Because of the growing realization that some patients will require periods of hospital care, successful programs have linkages to inpatient settings.

8. Lifetime perspective. Treating each episode of illness or treatment as only one part of a patient's entire lifetime risk for illness and need for availability of treatment.

9. Active engagement. Providing all services in an assertive manner; for example, by active outreach and engagement of reluctant patients.

10. Accountability. Feeling accountable for care delivered to this population and actually being held accountable.

11. Multimodality. Providing both psychosocial and psychopharmacologic interventions together.

12. Survival skill training. Focusing on the training of patients in survival skills (i.e., the skills of daily living).

13. Internal evaluation. This may not be the usual formal evaluation, which is often a slow process, but rather a more informal internal assessment process that allows for feedback from staff and management.

Finally, continuity of care is a key element of any program targeted for the CMI (Bellak & Mueser, 1986). Bellak & Mueser (1986) emphasize that a good program must assume the role of a "treatment coordinator," guiding patients to appropriate resources as they are required and preserving contact during stable periods, as well as during crises. Bachrach (1981) identified seven dimensions associated with continuity of care: (1) a longitudinal dimension that ensures that patient services vary according to their needs over time; (2) an individual dimension, which means that the treatment program is tailored to a specific patient and his or her family; (3) comprehensiveness, a multidisciplinary approach which addresses the full range of a patient's needs; (4) flexibility of care, so that a rapid response can be made to unforeseen life circumstances or changes in the patient's condition; (5) accessibility of care, ensuring that backup services such as inpatient hospitalization are readily available; (6) a constant relationship between patient and staff; (7) communication channels between patient and staff remaining open to promote rapport and to facilitate more appropriate rendering of services.

To cite an example from our work with the elderly homeless, we have attempted to develop a service program that is culturally specific as well as capable of providing the broad range of services that this population requires. Based on our earlier research, Project Rescue was created to address the identified needs of the Bowery population. The overall aim of Project Rescue was the following:

1. To operate a Respite Center for Bowery seniors as a place where they can find refuge, acceptance, social interaction, and welcome.
2. To meet the nutritional needs of Bowery seniors by providing balanced meals.
3. To improve the health of Bowery seniors by linking them with professional health care.
4. To provide psychiatric and alcohol counseling services to the Bowery seniors.
5. To assure shelter and housing for Bowery seniors by providing advocacy, referral, and placement services to those who are homeless or in danger of becoming homeless.
6. To help stabilize the finances of Bowery seniors by assisting in securing and maintaining government benefits for which they qualify.
7. To avoid isolation and abandonment of Bowery seniors through outreach to people on the streets and the homebound.
8. To provide opportunities for work and vocational rehabilitation.
9. To serve as a training, educational, and resource center for other agencies servicing homeless persons.

To meet these objectives, the following services were developed:

1. *Respite*: A specific area at the Bowery Residents' Committee (BRC) on Chrystie Street, one block from the Bowery, was set aside for the use of the seniors. It is opened 9:00 A.M.–5:00 P.M. (2:00 P.M. Saturdays), 6 days per week. It

includes a large cafeteria and activities area as well as a smaller area for TV viewing and peace and quiet. There are also shower facilities. Seniors are free to come and go as they please during the day. The area is reserved for their use, and this became the base of operations for Project Rescue.

2. *Nutrition*: With the support of the New York City Department for the Aging and donated foodstuffs, the BRC provides breakfast, lunch, and a snack for 115 seniors 6 days a week, Monday through Saturday. The meals are nutritionally balanced and hot.

3. *Physical health*: The BRC has on-site a medical clinic operated in conjunction with The Robert Wood Johnson Health Care for the Homeless Project. A health team is available 3 days per week. The seniors, however, do not take advantage of this service without encouragement and follow-up, and Project Rescue provides this. Individual work with seniors helps them overcome their fears of receiving medical attention and helps them follow medical instructions with regard to medication and follow-up visits. Without this type of assistance, seniors remain isolated from health services.

4. *Psychiatric and alcohol services*: The BRC has a part-time psychiatrist available for seniors. Here again, those mentally ill elderly need encouragement and support before seeing the psychiatrist. There is also a Community Support System program linked to the BRC that can assist the mentally ill seniors with case-management issues such as obtaining entitlements, specialized housing, long-term psychiatric care, and the like. The BRC has a very large alcohol rehabilitation program with many counselors, group meetings, and an AA program. Seniors are encouraged to participate in these programs.

5. *Housing*: Project Rescue staff assist homeless seniors and seniors facing eviction to secure or maintain shelter and housing. The BRC works with Mobilization for Youth Legal Services so seniors have access to the legal help they need. Project Domicile, an effort of Partnership for the Homeless with which the BRC works, makes available city-owned apartments to the homeless. Project staff work with seniors to avoid the loss of present housing and to find alternative housing. The BRC has also secured several apartments that can temporarily house homeless seniors so that they can attain medical, psychiatric, and social stability, as well as find suitable permanent housing.

6. *Finances and vocational assistance*: Most Bowery seniors are eligible for government benefits to live on. However, not all receive the benefits to which they are entitled, and others are cut off due to unwarranted bureaucratic actions. Project Rescue staff assist seniors to obtain and retain government entitlements by helping them in the paperwork and advocacy generally needed in the application and appeals processes. Counselors assist those able-bodied individuals for jobs or vocational training. Various prevocational activities are available at the BRC such as volunteer work, etc.

7. *Training/resource center*: The workers from Project Rescue make available to other agencies their expertise in dealing with homeless seniors. They provide

training programs ahd lectures, are available for telephone consultation, and accept referrals from other agencies.

SERVICE RESEARCH

Every program should make an effort to assess its effectiveness. Such assessments include determining (a) Whether the objectives of the program are being implemented; for example, is there a match between a project's philosophy and its outcome? Initially, this may include such basic information as the actual number and demographics of the persons participating in the overall program and its various components. (b) Whether there are any quantifiable or qualitative changes in the client's clinical status, functioning, or satisfaction. (c) Whether staff are satisfied with the program. In general, the specific questions to ask will be determined by the project administrators and service staff.

Strayhorn (1987) has proposed four levels of internal program analysis:

1. Experimental program versus no control group. Such an approach makes no attempt to distinguish the specific therapeutic aspects of a program from nonspecific aspects (e.g., staff warmth, staff enthusiasm) that may be common to most programs. This type of evaluation is most appropriate when there are no alternative therapeutic programs and the treatment is clearly necessary for the participants' well-being. If alternative programs are available, such an approach helps accumulate sufficient evidence for the experimental program before it is tested against alternative programs. Given the paucity of programs available for CMI elderly, this analysis approach may be most appropriate at this time.

2. Experimental program versus a minimal but useful control group. Here again, there is no attempt to identify the specific and nonspecific aspects of the experimental program. A control group exists, but it provides only a limited amount of intervention. Thus, participants in an experimental program might be contrasted with a control group of persons receiving brochures or tapes about mental health.

3. Experimental program versus another program. In this instance, the experimental program is contrasted with another existing program. Thus, participants in a program targeted specifically for the CMI elderly would be contrasted with CMI elderly attending a general outpatient clinic. Here again, no effort is made to distinguish specific and nonspecific elements of the programs.

4. "Dismantling." This method approaches the gold standard of a true control group. Here the experimental and control groups are identical except for one element. Thus, any difference would be due to that one specific element. This is the final level of analysis; it requires the ability to be able to specify the various elements of a program. Clearly, such targeted assessments should be the ultimate goal of evaluation.

A program's failure to achieve its objectives can likewise be subjected to systematic evaluation. For example, Pratt and Kethley (1980) identified various potential barriers to the development of mental health services for the elderly such as lack of agency commitment, scarcity of funds, conflicting agency priorities, inadequate staff, lack of qualified personnel, overly bureaucratized agencies, and resistance from elderly clients. Each of these items can be examined to determine their relative influence on outcome.

Bachrach (1980) further suggests that beyond the internal assessment, programs should be evaluated for their generalizability, reproducibility, and relevance. Many model programs may be specific to a particular community or cultural context. Often model programs have received special funding that is not compatible with the reality of community budgets. It is also important to take account of a possible "Hawthorne effect," brought on by exceptionally devoted persons participating in an experimental program. Liberman and Phipps (1987) have proposed that rather than reproducing an entire model program, organizations can adopt one or several aspects ("modules") of the model program, thereby reducing costs and enhancing acceptability. They urge model projects to develop such modules that can be more easily transported to other programs. Finally, the impact or broader relevancy of the program must be considered. That is, not only is it important that the program fulfills traditional evaluations, but a program should be assessed for its impact on the entire population of the CMI in a given community.

SUMMARY

This chapter was written with the notion of providing the reader (a potential proposal writer) with a kind of cookbook outline of items to be considered in community research and model service development. A three-tier process is proposed in which the first stage involves a systematic investigation of the population to be served. The second stage, the institution of a service program, is based on the preceding investigation. The last stage, an evaluation of the service program, can entail research within the particular program as well as its effects on the overall population. Services research can in turn be used to modify the existing program. Hence, there is a complex process of research begetting service begetting new research, and each tier acting on and modifying the other.

ACKNOWLEDGMENTS

Dr. Cohen's work was supported by the NIMH grants R01-MH37562, H84-MH42443, and 1-K07-MH00523. The author thanks Eric Roth and Carole Lefkowitz for their assistance.

REFERENCES

Bachrach, L. L. (1980). Overview: Model programs for chronic mental patients. *American Journal of Psychiatry, 137,* 1023-1031.

Bachrach, L. L. (1981). Continuity of care for chronic mental patients. A conceptual analysis. *American Journal of Psychiatry, 138,* 1449-1456.

Bachrach, L. L. (1984a). The concept of young adult chronic psychiatric patients: Questions from a research perspective. *Hospital and Community Psychiatry, 35,* 573-580.

Bachrach, L. L. (1984b). Research on services for the homeless mentally ill. *Hospital and Community Psychiatry, 35,* 910-913.

Bachrach, L. L. (1984c). Interpreting research on the homeless mentally ill: some caveats. *Hospital and Community Psychiatry, 35,* 914-917.

Bachrach, L. L. (1984d). The homeless mentally ill and mental health services: An analytic review of the literature. In H. R. Lamb (Ed.), *The Homeless Mentally Ill* (pp. 11-54). Washington, DC: American Psychiatric Press.

Bachrach, L. L. (1987). The homeless mentally ill. In W. W. Menninger & G. T. Hannah (Eds.), *The Chronic Mental Patient* (Vol. 2, pp. 65-92). Washington, DC: American Psychiatric Press.

Bellak, A. S., & Mueser, K. T. (1986). A comprehensive treatment program for schizophrenia and chronic mental illness. *Community Mental Health Journal, 22,* 175-189.

Bogue, D. J. (1963). *Skid row in American cities.* Chicago: University of Chicago Press.

Braun, P., Kochansky, G., Shapiro, R., Greenberg, S., Gudeman, J. E., Johnson, S., & Shore, M. F. (1981). Overview: Deinstitutionalization of psychiatric patients, a critical review of outcome studies. *American Journal of Psychiatry, 138,* 736-749.

Brown, R., & Lieff, J. D. (1982). A program for treating isolated elderly patients living in a housing project. *Hospital and Community Psychiatry, 33,* 147-150.

Cohen, C., & Sokolovsky, J. (1989). *Old men of the Bowery: Survival strategies of homeless men.* New York: Guilford Press.

Cohen, C., Teresi, J., & Holmes, D. (1988a). The physical well-being of old homeless men. *Journal of Gerontology, 43,* S121-128.

Cohen, C., Teresi, J., & Holmes, D. (1988b). The mental health of old homeless men. *Journal of American Geriatrics Society, 36,* 492-501.

Cohen, C., Teresi, J., Holmes, D., & Roth, E. (1988). Survival strategies of older homeless men. *The Gerontologist, 28,* 58-65.

Community Support Network News, 3(3), Boston University Center for Psychiatric Rehabilitation, January 1987.

Goldman, H. H., Gattozzi, A. A., & Taube, C. A. (1981). Defining and counting the chronically mentally ill. *Hospital and Community Psychiatry, 32,* 21-27.

Gruenberg, E. M. (1967). The social breakdown syndrome: Some origins. *American Journal of Psychiatry, 123,* 1481-1489.

Harding, C. M., Zubin, J., & Strauss, J. S. (1987). Chronicity in schizophrenia: Fact, partial fact, or artifact. *Hospital and Community Psychiatry, 38,* 477-486.

Kane, R. A., & Kane, R. L. (1981). *Assessing the elderly.* Lexington, MA: Lexington Books.

Liberman, R. P., & Phipps, C. C. (1987). Innovative treatment and rehabilitation techniques for the chronic mentally ill. In W. W. Menninger & G. Hannah (Eds.), *The chronic mental patient* (Vol. 2, pp. 93-130). Washington, DC: American Psychiatric Press.

Minkoff, K. (1978). A map of the chronic mental patient. In J. A. Talbott (Ed.), *The chronic mental patient* (pp. 11–38). Washington, DC: American Psychiatric Press.

Platt, S. (1985). Measuring the burden of psychiatric illness on the family: An evaluation of some rating scales. *Psychological Medicine, 15*, 383–393.

Pratt, C. C., & Kethley, A. J. (1980). Anticipated and actual barriers to developing community mental health programs for the elderly. *Community Mental Health Journal, 16*, 205–216.

Raschko, R. (1988). Assertive at home case management for impaired elderly persons. *Hospital and Community Psychiatry, 39*, 1201–1202.

Reifler, B. V., Kethley, A., O'Neill, P., Hanley, R., Lewis, S., & Stenchever, D. (1982). Five-year experience of a community outreach program for the elderly. *American Journal of Psychiatry, 139*, 220–223.

Rocca, R. P., Storer, D. J., Robbins, R. M., Tlasek, M. E., & Rabins, P. V. (1990). Psychogeriatric assessment and treatment in urban public housing. *Housing and Community Psychiatry, 41*, 916–920.

Sherr, V. T., Eskridge, O. C., & Lewis, S. (1976). A mobile mental-hospital-based team for geropsychiatric service in the community. *Journal of the American Geriatrics Society, 24*, 362–365.

Solomon, P., Davis, J., & Gordon, B. (1984). Discharged state hospital patients' characteristics and use of aftercare: Effect on community tenure. *American Journal of Psychiatry, 141*, 1566–1570.

Stroul, B. A. (1986). *Models of community support services: Approaches to helping persons with long-term mental illness.* Boston, MA: Boston University Center for Psychiatric Rehabilitation.

Strayhorn, J. M. (1987). Control groups for psychosocial intervention outcome studies. *American Journal of Psychiatry, 144*, 275–282.

Talbott, J. A. (1987). The chronic mentally ill: What do we now know, and why aren't we implementing what we know? In W. W. Menninger & G. Hannah (Eds.), *The chronic mental patient* (Vol. 2, pp. 1–29). Washington, DC: American Psychiatric Press.

Test, M. A., & Stein, L. I. (1978). Community treatment of the chronic patient: Research overview. *Schizophrenia Bulletin, 4*, 350–364.

Wallace, S. (1965). *Skid row as a way of life.* Totowa, NJ: Bedminster Press.

Zarit, S. H., Todd, P. A., & Zarit, J. M. (1986). Subjective burden of husbands and wives as caregivers: A longitudinal study. *The Gerontologist, 26*, 260–266.

12

Mental Health Services Research on the Hospitalized and Institutionalized CMI Elderly

Barbara J. Burns

This country is continuing to deinstitutionalize the chronically mentally ill, including the elderly, albeit at a much slower rate than 20 years ago. The emphasis on returning patients to the community is heightened by concern about the increasing costs of long-term care. For the mentally ill elderly, living in the community usually means a nursing home. However, recent legislation to change Medicaid requirements for nursing facilities could have the effect of further reductions in nursing home care for this population (Freiman et al., 1991). Will the CMI elderly be once again pushed out of the hospital and into the streets?

Treatment alternatives available to the public patient are strongly determined by the reimbursement system. The long-term psychiatric patient can benefit only briefly from Medicare with its 180-day lifetime hospitalization benefit, its 90-day post-hospital discharge benefit for a nursing home stay and its annual outpatient mental health benefit (recently this dollar cap was lifted, but there is a 50% co-payment). Medicaid becomes the source of reimbursement for persons who need long-term care and meet the poverty standard of a state—and many do after an extended psychiatric illness. Medicaid, however, does not pay for care in state psychiatric facilities or community institutions for mental disease (IMD) for persons between 22 and 64 years of age (Doty, Liu, & Weiner, 1985). These regulations, which avoid shifting the costs of psychiatric care previously paid by states to the federal government, were intended in part to prevent nursing homes from becoming facilities that treat the mentally ill. Although the preceding regulations do not technically restrict care for the elderly, the perception of the nursing home industry that mental illness is not covered does this on a de facto basis. Further, nursing homes are not allowed to have more than 50% of their patients with a primary diagnosis of mental disorder or to be seen as places that treat mental illness. States restrict care in other various ways (DRGs and other limits on inpatient stays and visit limitations for outpatient care). This tends to leave the public CMI patient with the options of a state hospital or a nursing home bed, whichever is available.

Even with the above limitations, half of the Medicaid budget goes to nursing homes, and half of the reimbursement to nursing homes is from Medicaid (Doty, Liu, & Weiner, 1985). These facilities are full of psychiatric patients, about 70%, including those with organic brain syndrome (OBS), based on the recent 1985–1986 National Nursing Home Survey. This cannot be acknowledged on a home-by-home basis without a threat of change in status to an IMD and loss of Medicaid funds, even though OBS is no longer considered as part of the 50% with mental disorder.

The competition between state and federal policies to avoid paying for care for the long-term mental patient has resulted in a standoff. State hospitals have not been able truly to close down—$5.3 billion is still being spent annually on them (Manderscheid & Barrett, 1987) while about five times that amount is being spent by Medicaid on nursing homes (Doty, Liu, & Weiner, 1985). States have tried to capitalize on a 50% contribution (instead of 100%) under Medicaid for nursing home care for mental patients; in doing this they have moved patients into nursing homes without mental health treatment while they have continued to operate state hospitals at a high cost. This has prevented funds from becoming available for the development of true community alternatives.

At a policy level, the most critical need is to sort out the federal and state responsibility for the CMI as it impacts directly on service system and clinical care issues. At this time states do not have any true incentive to provide care for nursing home patients with mental illness, and the new legislation that may require states to pay for treatment of mental patients in nursing homes may end up threatening nursing home care, however limited, for these patients. What has been hidden previously (the current number with mental illness) will become obvious with the requirement that all patients with mental illness have a treatment plan.

Can services research do anything to respond to this very difficult dilemma? Some ideas about this will be outlined subsequently, but first some data on the extent of the problem and the nature of the care provided in hospital and institutional settings are presented. The unfortunate picture for the CMI elderly that will emerge is one of an inverse relationship between an investment of public (federal and state) dollars and the quality of care provided.

EXTENT OF THE PROBLEM

In order to obtain an estimate of the number of CMI elderly in these facilities, it is necessary to define the population. A challenge is posed as this is a new task (see Gurland, this volume). The usual criteria for CMI—diagnosis, duration, and disability—are either not fully available or not necessarily applicable to a chronically ill elderly population. For diagnosis, all mental conditions except organic brain syndrome and mental retardation are included. The assumption is that for institutionalized persons 65 and older with current mental illness that these conditions are likely to have existed prior to age 65. This is not easily documented as information on duration of illness is difficult to obtain. The traditional disability criteria (related to work and social functioning) do not apply to the elderly mentally ill in the same way they do to younger groups. A disability measure related to dependency is needed—which goes beyond the usual activities of daily living functions (eating, bathing, dressing, toileting, mobility), not always a problem for the elderly CMI. Assessing instrumental activities of daily living (IADL) to determine clinical management needs could be useful. Criteria might include a combination of IADL items and additional behaviors that require nursing care such as aggressive behavior, suicidality, and psychotropic medication changes.

Using diagnosis as the sole criteria for chronic mental illness (since duration and disability estimates are not available) may inflate the estimates presented. Failing to include the mentally ill elderly in general hospital scatter beds may balance this off to some extent—although since most patients are short stay they would not be identified as part of the institutionalized population. An initial estimate of CMI elderly residents in hospitals and nursing homes might look like the data in Table 12.1. These data are from the census of mental health facilities conducted periodically by the NIMH and the National Nursing Home Survey conducted by the National Center for Health Statistics.

As displayed above it is immediately apparent that the great majority of the institutionalized CMI elderly reside in nursing homes—almost 90%. State and county hospitals with 8% of the CMI elderly are not a close second; however, relative to the other classes of hospitals, state and county hospitals represent an

TABLE 12.1 Census of Persons 65+ in Hospitals and Nursing Homes (OBS and Mental Retardation Excluded)

Facility type	Number	Percent
State and county hospitals (1983)	17,415	8.1
Private psychiatric hospitals (1983)	1,400	0.7
VA medical centers (1983)	2,707	1.3
General hospital psychiatry units	2,625	1.2
Nursing homes (1985)	190,700	88.8
Total:	214,847	100.1

Sources: NIMH Facility Surveys and National Nursing Home Survey by NCHS.

important source of care. While the total group represents less than 1% of the U.S. elderly population (based on the 1980 census of 29.4 million over 65), extensive resources are being invested in care that may not be appropriate to the illness—nursing homes cost around $20,000 per person a year and state hospitals about $50,000.

Specific diagnostic information is not available from the hospital census, so admissions diagnoses are used. Diagnoses for elderly admissions to these facilities are lumped into substance abuse, affective disorders, and psychoses. State and county hospitals admit about equal proportions of all three conditions, while private psychiatric hospitals and general hospitals are much more likely to admit affective disorders. The highest percentage of admissions to VA hospitals is for substance abuse, along with a substantial group with affective disorders. The hospital type most likely to admit elderly persons with schizophrenia or other psychotic disorders is the state hospital (Manderscheid & Barrett, 1987).

As current diagnoses rather than admission diagnoses are available for nursing home residents, a comparison with the hospital data is problematic. Also, a larger number of diagnostic categories were used for nursing homes, and many persons had multiple conditions—an average of three. To unduplicate the 190,700 persons with any mental disorder diagnosis (excluding OBS-dementia) they were put into a 100% distribution by dividing diagnostic groups into total diagnoses made. This may not be the best approach to unduplicate diagnoses (e.g., a hierarchical approach could be used), but it does provide a sense of the diversity of conditions reported. These data were obtained from a nurse who knew the patient and provided this information in conjunction with medical record information. (Hing, 1987) (see Table 12.2).

This diagnostic distribution points to higher rates of anxiety and affective disorders than would be predicted from general population studies like the Epidemiology Catchment Area studies (Myers et al., 1984). An overall rate of psychoses in around 12% of nursing home patients represents a significant

TABLE 12.2 Mental Disorder in Elderly Nursing Home Patients
National Nursing Home Survey, 1985

Condition	Number (N = 190,700)	Percent (unduplicated)
Alcohol abuse dependence	27,700	4.8
Drug abuse/dependence	9,850	1.7
Affective	163,600	28.3
Schizophrenia	43,400	7.5
Other psychoses	28,900	5.0
Anxiety	172,600	29.8
Personality/character	132,900	23.0

clinical management concern. Overall patients with these conditions constitute 15% of elderly residents, which clearly does not approach the Medicaid 50% limit. However, this proportion is likely to vary by nursing home.

TREATMENT PROVIDED

Shifting to a brief discussion of treatment of the hospitalized or institutionalized elderly CMI, we find major differences among hospital types. Although it has not been possible to exclude the elderly with OBS from the treatment information, the comparisons across settings are not likely to vary much, except for state hospitals, which have a larger group of OBS patients. State hospital care for other diagnostic groups might look somewhat better with the OBS group removed, assuming that minimal active treatment is given to them. Major findings include

1. General hospitals and private psychiatric hospitals provide individual therapy and drug treatment to the majority of their elderly patients while only half of elderly patients in state or VA hospitals receive either type of treatment. A lower rate of treatment with psychotropic drugs in the VA hospitals may be appropriate, given the high rate of alcoholism.
2. Low rates of rehabilitation services (around 30%), like self-care and social skills training, were found for elderly patients across hospital types, possibly indicating a general tendency not to offer such services to older patients (Milazzo-Sayre, Benson, Rosenstein, & Manderscheid, 1987).

For nursing home patients with mental illness (all ages), only 5% saw any type of mental health professional. Psychotropic drugs tended to be prescribed at somewhat lower rates to the older mental patients (Burns et al., 1988). Of

TABLE 12.3 Psychotropic Medications for Nursing Home Residents
by Age, National Nursing Home Survey Pretest, 1984

Drug class	Mental disorder (except OBS)	No mental disorder
Sedatives/Hypnotics		
−65	10.0	10.0
65+	11.0	7.5
Antianxiety		
−65	2.5	5.0
65+	5.4	6.4
Antidepressants		
−65	15.9	5.0
65+	9.5	3.7
Antipsychotics		
−65	67.5	20.5
65+	32.4	5.3

concern is the large proportion of drug prescriptions for persons with no mental disorder (see Table 12.3).

In summary, these limited data on the treatment of elderly patients in hospitals and nursing homes point to minimal clinical care of patients in state hospitals and nursing homes. While these public or publically supported facilities may see their purpose as providing maintenance instead of active treatment and criticism can be directed at the study methods (e.g., lack of precision about diagnosis), there is an overall picture that cannot be ignored.

RESEARCH DIRECTIONS

Research needs to be conducted that can address issues of policy, organization of services, and clinical practice. It is important that mental health service research be relevant to policy while also incorporating service systems and clinical considerations. In the absence of useful data, policy decisions may be made that will be detrimental to the welfare of the elderly mentally ill. Thus, research needs to be directed toward potentially more favorable policies. Current policies seem to be based on unrealistic fears about overuse of mental health services. While in the literature there is substantial evidence that the elderly CMI are hesitant and even resistant to use any mental health services, and use services at a low rate (Burns et al., 1988). Policies are needed that won't scare the legislators and will improve the quality of life of the elderly CMI in institutions. There is some precedent in the federal government for a balance between cost efficiency and quality care, as evidenced by a recent Health Care Financing Administration (HCFA) supported study being conducted the by Rand Corporation to examine whether the quality of inpatient care changed following implementation of DRGs.

As policy is largely occupied with reimbursement issues, potential changes in the three sources of reimbursement for the public patient are reviewed. First, Medicare is not likely to change much, given its long-term focus on acute care. Second, returning to states the responsibility for mental health treatment would most likely further exacerbate the current disparities in mental health care across states. Thus, as a third option there is a *pressing* need to make a strong case with Medicaid to recognize the needs of the CMI elderly. The proposed research agenda is limited to nursing homes because the most patients and dollars are there.

Research to inform Medicaid policy should focus on three broad areas:

1. Determining eligibility for nursing homes placements;
2. Assessing treatment needs for nursing home patients; and
3. Developing community services that can substitute for nursing home or other institutional care.

For the first foci, services researchers need to develop better estimates of the need for care in institutions. These estimates need to be based on criteria which are in addition to diagnosis. As nursing homes require that patients need nursing care, CMI patients who need ADL assistance meet the requirement for nursing home care and do not represent an eligibility issue unless they require "active mental health treatment." Persons without ADL problems are no more than a fourth of nursing home residents with mental illness (Burns et al., 1988). Among this group, many questions need to be addressed, such as how many are inappropriately placed and could be moved to a less restrictive setting? To obtain such an estimate, a measure is needed to capture other nursing care needs related to the management of behavioral problems (e.g., a dependency measure, referred to earlier). This effort could help reduce a perception that many elderly patients are inappropriately placed in nursing homes, while it may also identify a small group who could be served better elsewhere.

The second topic, assessing the need for active treatment, is more costly and difficult to address and will take on new meaning under Public Law 100–203, the fiscal year 1988 Omnibus Budget Reconciliation Act as the regulations are finalized. It is also more threatening to the policymakers as it may open the "Pandora's box" of costly long-term therapy. Nevertheless, there are a number of questions for which we currently do not have answers. They include

1. Who needs active treatment?
2. What types of treatment are needed for what duration and cost?

3. Who will accept treatment?
4. Who will benefit from treatment?

These questions might be examined with a limited set of treatment options (i.e., case management, brief psychotherapy, drugs, ECT, and social skills training) and would require obtaining consensus by clinicians either through assessment of actual cases or case vignettes. This also requires efficacy studies which consider stage of illness and improve quality of life.

A third focus, substitution of institutional for community care, represents a more long-term research agenda. Recent research on the treatment of schizophrenia shows that length of stay in the hospital is not necessarily associated with outcome and that alternatives to hospitalization, like a family intervention at home, may be as effective as hospital treatment (Hargreaves and Shumway, 1989). Unfortunately, the only elderly study on preventing nursing home placements, the HCFA Channeling Demonstration, did not report positive findings (i.e., that case management in the community did not prevent nursing home placements), but mental illness was not addressed specifically (Christianson, 1986).

Currently HCFA plans to conduct a major Alzheimer's demonstration that will use Medicaid waivers to provide home-based services, family counseling, day hospital, respite care, to prevent placing these patients in institutions. Given the magnitude of the problem, the opportunity to make a difference in the lives of the CMI elderly, a similar type of research-based demonstration for the CMI elderly should be undertaken. (This demonstration might also include supervised or staffed apartments, as many CMI do not have families and need more supervision than can reasonably occur when living alone.) In the absence of special demonstrations, natural experiments at the Spokane CMHC (Washington) and Abbey CMHC (Iowa) which include aggressive case identification, case management and home-based interventions could be evaluated to see whether outcomes like nursing home and hospital admissions, suicide rates, quality of life and costs are improved over comparable communities without such programs (see chapters by Raschko and Buckwalter, this volume).

In order to convince policymakers about the value of such interventions, outcomes have to be convincing. The provision of additional services to populations in need is not a priority for policymakers concerned with cost containment. Outcomes need to be assessed at multiple levels. At a clinical level, measures of changes in illness (or at least in relapse rates) and changes in symptoms, functioning, and quality of life of patients are needed, as well as measures of burden on the family. At a systems level, it is important to assess whether mental health interventions have an influence on variables like staff turnover (particularly a problem in caretaking of chronic patients) or on the demands on staff. From a policy perspective, it is essential to know whether community interventions affect the rate of admissions or length of stay in hospitals or nursing homes and to know the relationship between the cost of comprehensive community care and institutional care. Other public health measures like morbidity, mortality, and suicide rates are also relevant to policy-makers. Finally, the interrelationships between clinical variables and those with implications for saving money are important to assess (cost effectiveness) within studies and it is useful to understand why some cases succeed and others fail in response to specific interventions.

REFERENCES

Burns, B. J., Larson, D. L., Goldstrom, I. D., Johnson, W. E., Taube, C. A., Miller, N. E., & Mathis, E. S. (1988). Mental disorders among nursing home patients. *International Journal of Geriatric Psychiatry, 3*, 27–35.

Christianson, J. B. (1986). Channeling effect on informal care. Report of DHHS Contract No. HHS-100-80-0157.

Doty, P., Liu, K., & Weiner, J. (1985). An overview of long-term care. *Health Care Financing Review, 6*(3), 69–78.

Freiman, M. P., Arons, B., Goldman, H. H., & Burns, B. J. (1991). Nursing home reform and the mentally ill. *Health Affairs, 9*, 47–60.

Hargreaves, W. A., & Shumway, M. (1989). Effectiveness of mental health services: A review of controlled studies. In C. A. Taube, D. Mechanic, & A. Homan (Eds.), *The future of mental health services research.* Washington, DC: U.S. Government Printing Office.

Hing, E. (1987). National Center for Health Statistics: Use of nursing homes by the elderly, preliminary data from the 1985 National Nursing Home Survey. Advance data from vital and Health Statistics. No. 135, DHHS Pub. No. (PHS) 87-1250. Public Health Service, Hyattsville, MD.

Manderscheid, R. W., & Barrett, S. A. (Eds.). (1987). *Mental Health United States, 1987* (DHHS Publication No. ADM 87-1518). Washington, DC: U.S. Government Printing Office.

Milazzo-Sayre, L. J., Benson, P. R., Rosenstein, M. J., & Manderscheid, R. W. (1987). *Use of inpatient services by the elderly age 65 and over, United States, 1980, Statistical Note No. 181* (DHHS Publication No. ADM 87-1516). Washington, DC: U.S. Government Printing Office.

Myers, J. K., Weissman, M. M., Tischler, G. L., Holzer, C. E., Leaf, P. J., Orvaschel, H., Anthony, J. C., Boyd, J. H., Burke, J. D., Kramer, M., & Stolzman, R. (1984). Six month prevalence of psychiatric disorders in three communities. *Archives of General Psychiatry, 41*(10), 959–967.

13

The Chronically Mentally Ill Elderly in Rural Environments

Kathleen C. Buckwalter

Little is known about the chronically mentally ill elderly (CMIE) in rural areas, in part because of the lack of services designed to identify and treat community-dwelling rural elderly with long-term mental illness. Further, when researchers, clinicians, and policymakers think of the CMIE population, they most often envision settings such as single-room-occupancy dwellings, nursing homes, and state mental hospitals. And yet, as the data presented elsewhere in this volume suggest, the CMIE are not in these areas alone. It therefore behooves us to examine other settings, such as rural environments, and to describe characteristics of the CMIE in these areas to determine in what ways they may be similar to and different from the CMIE in other environments. Such comparisons can yield valuable information to guide the development of setting—specific services, interventions, and research agendas for the CMIE.

This chapter begins with a discussion of the mental health needs of the elderly in rural areas and provides an overview of a rural outreach program designed to meet those needs. A sample of CMIE identified by this outreach model is described, and sociodemographic and comorbidity issues are highlighted, using case studies. Comparative data from a recent statewide survey of young (18–55) and old (55 plus) chronically mentally ill persons in Iowa ($N = 9,151$) are also presented. Finally, implications for services research, discharge planning in acute hospital settings, access to services, and research issues in terms of interactive paradigms between mental and physical illness in this population are examined.

NEED FOR RURAL ELDERLY OUTREACH PROGRAMS

The panel on rural mental health of the President's Commission on Mental Health contended that the rural elderly population is vastly underserved by the mental health system (President's Commission on Mental Health, 1978). The panel emphasized (p. 1164) that rural areas have unique mental health service needs:

> Rural communities tend to be characterized by higher than average rates of psychiatric disorders, particularly depression, by severe intergenerational conflicts, by an exodus of individuals who might serve as effective role models for coping, by an acceptance of fatalistic attitudes and minimal subscription to the idea that change is possible.

Despite the clear need for services, the rural elderly account for only between 4–6% of community mental health center (CMHC) patients nationally and less than 2% of the caseload of private psychiatrists. Review of the National Institute of Mental Health (NIMH) Inventory of CMHCs reveals a $-.20$ correlation between the ratio of rural elderly clients to total clients and that the CMHCs in rural areas serve proportionately fewer elderly than CMHCs in more urban areas (National Institute of Mental Health, 1977).

Scheidt and Windley (1982) found that only 1% of small-town elderly used mental health services, whereas between 12–23% were "at risk" for mental disorders. Other epidemiological studies have similarly estimated that up to 25% of the elderly have significant mental health problems (Rosen, Coppage, Troglin, & Rosen, 1981). The chronically mentally ill elderly have a need for community treatment that is not adequately addressed in rural settings, as illustrated by the following statistics from the state of Iowa. Since fiscal year 1982, admissions to the geriatric medical units at the four state mental institutes have dropped nearly 83%. However, this decline is not indicative of decreased utilization but rather a dramatic increase in the lengths of stay for treatment that precludes new admissions. Iowans admitted to the mental health institutes are growing older and experiencing more debilitating mental and physiological problems that increase the difficulty of providing services in the rural community. Unfortunately, it also does not appear that those elderly remaining in the community and in need of mental health care are being served by community-based providers. Although the NIMH *State Mental Health Program Indicators—1983* indicated that slightly more than 7,000 elderly Iowans were provided outpatient services, this represents only 1.9% of the state's elderly population. Clearly, there is a need to reach a greater percentage of the rural elderly in order to identify and attract those persons in need of mental health services, including the CMIE.

Effective mental health services delivery in rural America requires innovative approaches, which includes coordination and cooperation among mental health, medical, and social service providers. A more appropriate rural mental health delivery system must maximize limited resources, address community needs, provide continuity of care, and use professional, paraprofessional and lay personnel appropriately (Palmer & Cuningham, 1983).

The limited medical and social resources in rural areas increase the likelihood that correctable illnesses and sensory deficiencies will remain undetected and untreated. Because there are few mental health services available in rural America and rural Americans are reluctant to accept such services even where they are available, care alternatives are frequently restricted to crisis intervention or long-term institutionalization. More often than not, the mentally ill elderly remain uncared-for at home.

These problems can only proliferate as the number of rural elderly increases and those individuals experience life changes known to precipitate mental health problems. Geographic and cost factors associated with the accessibility of services, plus cultural norms and the stigma of mental illness, make delivery of mental health services in rural settings problematic.

Problems in the delivery of services to the rural elderly are currently exacerbated by the farm economic crisis. In recent testimony before the Joint Economic Committee of Congress, Heffernan (1985) identified depression as the primary stress reaction of rural families and communities to the farm crisis. Based on a sociological study, Heffernan recommended the development and funding of *mental health outreach programs* as an important approach to counteracting stresses associated with the farm crisis.

Outreach programs have been suggested as one effective approach to delivering services to the rural elderly because those most at risk do not present themselves to mental health and social service agencies (Toseland, Decker, & Bliesner, 1979). Such programs would teach professionals and nonprofessionals, in health and social service agencies and in the general public, how to identify elderly who may need mental health services and how to refer these people to a special outreach team for assistance. An outreach team consisting of a psychiatrist, social worker, and nurse can overcome some of the limitations of rural mental health services by providing coordinated assessment, treatment, and aftercare of the rural elderly in their own homes (Lazarus & Weinberg, 1979). Outreach can provide diagnosis and treatment for homebound rural elderly who have physical limitations, major psychiatric illnesses of both an acute and chronic nature (e.g., dementia, schizophrenia, paranoia, affective disorders), are socially isolated, or are experiencing a combination of problems.

Outreach approaches have proved helpful in treating urban elderly patients who might not otherwise enter mental health programs until a crisis necessitates hospitalization (Wasson et al., 1984). In general, evaluations of these urban outreach efforts suggest that they provide rapid and effective disruptions due to premature institutionalization of elderly patients (Kahn & Tobin, 1981; Raskind, Alvarez, Pietrzyk, Westerlund, & Herlin, 1976; Reifler et al., 1982).

However, the effectiveness of these programs in providing a viable alternative to hospitalization and long-term institutionalization for the rural elderly has not been adequately tested. This is especially true for application of the outreach model to identification and treatment of the chronically mentally ill rural elderly. Service providers must understand and be sensitive to the value system and social ecology of the area. Otherwise, mental health workers may find themselves addressing assumed rather than real needs. Borrowing successful urban techniques such as outreach programs and imposing them without modification in rural settings may not be appropriate or effective.

The Elderly Outreach Project (EOP) described next was designed to identify rural elderly individuals who are in need of mental health care, to deliver needed services, and to initiate and coordinate referrals to appropriate medical and social services agencies. It addresses the problem of inadequate mental health services and inappropriate hospitalization by taking services to the people most in need of them—the rural elderly. It also addresses another service delivery problem common in rural areas, the sparse concentration of mental health professionals available to identify and treat the rural elderly.

PROJECT OVERVIEW

Iowa has had dramatic increases in the number of elderly persons in its rural areas over the past decade. Their mental health service needs have been a priority of the state mental health authority for the past 2 years. However, several barriers have impeded the effective delivery of services: inadequate number of staff knowledgeable in psychogeriatrics, limited service delivery models for elderly in rural areas, and lack of coordination among human services, mental health, medical and aging service providers. In an effort to overcome these barriers and to clearly identify the mental health needs of the rural elderly, the Abbe Center for Community Mental Health (ACCMH), in cooperation with the Heritage Agency on Aging, developed a model outreach program to identify and deliver outpatient mental health services to the rural elderly with serious and persistent mental disorders. Data from Linn County's Long Range Planning Task Force estimated that 20% of the elderly in rural Linn and Jones Counties were in need of mental health services but were not receiving them.

In this rural elderly outreach program (EOP), persons in need of mental health, medical, and social services are identified through a combination of five approaches: (1) psychosocial screening at local sites, such as congregate meals; (2) referrals through the county case management team and its associated agencies; (3) training of nontraditional referral sources, known as gatekeepers, such as rural mail carriers, to locate and refer high-risk elderly (Raschko, 1985); (4) mental health outreach specialists who serve as liaison between the EOP and elderly services agencies; and (5) contact with discharge planning departments of mental health and health care institutions. The outreach model is illustrated in Figure 13.1.

Following referral, a multidisciplinary outreach team conducts comprehensive in-home mental health evaluations and implements and coordinates an appropriate treatment plan, including referrals to medical and social service agencies. Services are provided to mentally impaired elderly through either existing service delivery mechanisms or home-based care provided by the EOP team.

A multifaceted evaluation of the program is ongoing. Program efficacy is being analyzed in terms of (1) ability to identify rural elderly who are in need of services; (2) effectiveness of the mental health services in alleviating symptomatology and improving functioning; and (3) cost-effectiveness of the program. This

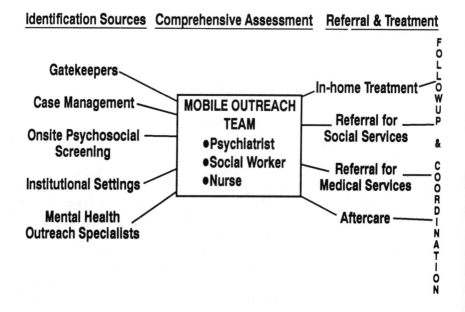

FIGURE 13.1 Rural outreach model.

TABLE 13.1 Sociodemographic Data

Sex: Male = 7 (26%)	Average age = 70.3 years
Female = 17 (63%)	Average age = 72.8 years
Missing data = 3 (11%)	Average age of sample = 72.1 years

Marital Status:	Single =	3	(11.1%)
	Married =	9	(33.33%)
	Widowed =	10	(37.04%)
	Divorced =	3	(11.11%)
	Missing data =	2	(7.41%)

Living Arrangements: Alone = 14 (51.86%)
With family or friends = 11 (40.74%)
Supervised (sheltered) living = 0
Other = 2 (7.41%)

Location of significant other:
Same dwelling = 9 (33.33%)
Same county = 13 (48.15%)
Same state = 2 (7.41%)

independent evaluation is conducted by the Center for Health Services Research (CHSR) at the University of Iowa.

Although the EOP operates essentially on an acute care, crisis-intervention model, many CMIE have been identified and referred to the project since its inception 18 months ago. To understand better the CMIE in rural areas, a random sample of 100 clients from the EOP project was selected from all the first year (October 1986–October 1987) records ($N = 247$). Of these 100 elderly clients, 27 (27%) met the criteria for "chronic mental illness." Dimensions of the term are discussed in detail by Gurland elsewhere in this volume. However, for purposes of this analysis, clients who had been diagnosed as mentally ill more than 5 years ago and had experienced persistent mental health problems requiring either outpatient, inpatient, or psychopharmacological treatment over time were included. Sociodemographic data from this sample are presented in Table 13.1.

Patients with dementia were excluded from this analysis unless the dementia developed subsequent to another psychiatric disorder. The diagnoses of CMIE clients in this sample are listed in Table 13.2.

Finally, concurrent medical diagnosis in the CMIE were examined, suggesting very high levels of comorbidity (37.04%). These coexisting medical problems are set forth in Table 13.3.

TABLE 13.2 Diagnosis

Depression = 11 (40.74%)
Dementia, developed in addition to dysthymic disorder = 1 (3.70%)
Dementia, developed in addition to histrionic personality disorder = 1 (3.70%)
Alcoholism = 1 (3.70%)
Paranoid schizophrenia = 2 (7.41%)
Anxiety disorder = 1 (3.70%)
Multiple problems: depression and personality disorder = 2 (7.41%)
Multiple problems: dementia, depression, paranoia = 1 (3.70%)
Unknown or deferred = 5 (18.52%)
Missing data = 2 (7.41%)

CASE STUDIES

D.Y. is a 68-year-old widow who lives alone in a dilapidated apartment building. According to her records, she first became ill in 1959 when she was diagnosed as having a "nervous breakdown." Since that time she has undergone numerous hospitalizations, outpatient treatments, and psychopharmacological interventions. Her last reported hospitalization prior to this referral was in 1975. At that time her diagnosis was "schizophrenia with delusions of persecution."

Presenting Problem: D.Y.'s landlord became concerned when she kicked a hole in her doorway "to get rid of the gases coming out of the wall." When assessed by the EOP team, D.Y. was found to have malignant hypertension which was out of control (BP = 220/135), in addition to her delusions. Despite her dangerously high blood pressure, D.Y. refused to take her prescribed antihypertensive medications because she felt they were "poison." It appeared that she was similarly noncompliant with her antipsychotic medication (Stelazine).

TABLE 13.3 Medical Diagnosis (10 [N = 27]
patients [37.04%])

1. Cancer of jaw (partially removed), heart disease
2. Brain tumor
3. Parkinson's, UTI, bilateral hip fractures
4. Chronic COPD requiring oxygen at home
5. Stroke right with hemiparesis
6. CHF, stroke, anorexia, OBS
7. HTN, COPD, recent mastectomy
8. Stroke, HTM, peptic ulcer
9. CVA with leg brace
10. Asthma

EOP Intervention: Following discharge from an acute-care hospital for stabilization of her hypertension and delusional activity through reinstitution of an appropriate medication regimen, D.Y. was encouraged to attend a local adult day-care center where she would continue to receive her medications regularly. To decrease her social isolation, arrangements were made through a local civic group to provide her with a telephone, and a nursing student from a nearby college was assigned to visit D.Y. on a weekly basis. D.Y.'s adult daughter, who lived in a nearby community, was given information on the need for medication compliance and provided with support through referral to a mental health advocacy group. Finally, further plans were addressed in terms of eventual placement in a county care facility with a rehabilitative focus.

M.H. is a 75-year-old widow who was first referred for outpatient treatment following the death of her husband several years earlier. Her diagnosis at the time of referral to the EOP was "major depressive episode with mood congruent psychotic features." At this time M.H. had stopped attending day-care activities, had essentially refused to leave her home, and refused all offers for medical services. She did accept services from home-delivered meals and a homemaker. At the time of referral, M.H. was openly delusional to mental health staff, whom she accused of being "snake detectives" as well as to the neighbor lady who visited regularly. Of immediate concern was M.H.'s recent weight loss; she weighed 82 pounds at the time of referral. M.H. felt her food was "synthetic" and that she had "rabies" and was going to die soon.

EOP Interventions: The frequency of M.H.'s home-delivered meals was increased to twice daily, as her impaired eyesight (cataracts) compromised safety in the kitchen. She had started several fires trying to cook on her old gas-burning stove and was clearly a danger to herself in terms of food preparation. Further, M.H. refused attempts to get her to see an opthamologist for evaluation of her vision. Other EOP interventions included instituting Friendly Visitor and Phone-A-Friend programs through referrals to Council on Aging. Other efforts to increase her social support network, such as getting M.H. back into day-care activities have thus far proved unsuccessful. Very "task-oriented" approaches (e.g., getting her dog needed veterinary services, helping M.H. recover money from a credit union account in her dead husband's name, purchasing warm clothing, etc.) have helped establish trust and rapport so that M.H. may eventually agree to needed mental health and physical health services. Continuous nutritional and weight monitoring remains an important function of the outreach team in light of M.H.'s delusions.

H.B. is a 66-year-old female who currently resides with her elderly husband. At the time of referral to EOP, H.B. had a 20+ history of depression and histrionic personality disorder. She had been seen as an outpatient at a local CMHC until such time as her COPD forced her to become oxygen-dependent and tied her to an oxygen tank at home, thus interferring with her mobility and outpatient treatment status. Over the long course of her emotional difficulties, H.B. had made multiple suicide attempts (primarily by drug overdose) and had undergone numerous surgeries for gastrointestinal maladies. The crisis that precipitated referral to the EOP was the hospitalization of her husband for cancer. Outreach team interventions focused on enhancing the marital dyad in light of the physical problems of both parties, through increased communication and assertiveness skills for H.B. designed to promote her overall self-esteem. A further issue has been to decrease her cigarette smoking through behavioral interventions so that she may fulfill a lifelong dream to see her son married in the Mormon church (which prohibits smoking). The two significant features of this case are that outreach programs are often the *only* service delivery mechanism available to immobile or homebound elderly such as H.B. and that the crises of physical illness in a spouse or other caretaker can precipitate exacerbation of preexisting mental illness in the elderly.

Recently, Walz, Craft, and Walters (1987) conducted a secondary analysis of data collected in a statewide survey of the CMI in Iowa ($N = 9,151$). Their comparative study included both institutionalized and community based samples and focused on differences between the younger CMI group (18–55) and the geriatric CMI group (age 55 and over). Results are summarized next.

Of the 9,151 cases studied, 45% were over age 55. In the younger cohort, 48% of the CMI population are female, in contrast to 67% of the elderly cohort. Females are somewhat underrepresented in the younger group compared to the general population in Iowa. The percentage of females in the older group is approximately the same as in the general population. In keeping with the racial mix of the state, 95% of the CMI population is white, 4.7% black, and 1.2% Hispanic. Younger CMI groups are more apt to be living on their own, with family or friends, or in a residential care facility. As depicted in Table 13.4, the older CMI group live more in institutional settings, especially intermediate care facilities and skilled nursing facilities.

Over 20 diagnostic categories were included in the state questionnaire. Depressive and schizophrenic disorders were more frequently associated with younger CMI, while organic brain disorders were the primary diagnosis for the older CMI (see Table 13.5).

TABLE 13.4 Living Arrangements

	18–55	55+
Alone	20.8%	7.7%
Family or friends	44.1	10.6
RCF	16.2	28.7
Nursing home ICF	2.7	43.5
SNF	0.1	3.1
MHI	8.3	4.4
Other[a]		

[a]Iowa has no appreciable foster care or board/care living arrangements.

TABLE 13.5 Primary Diagnosis

Type of disorder	18–55	55+
Conduct disorder	1.2%	0.8%
Bipolar depression	11.7	6.3
Major depression	13.1	8.8
Paranoid schizophrenia	19.8	13.0
Personality disorder	9.9	2.1
Undifferentiated schizophrenia	22.3	16.2
Other mental health	14.3	12.8
CBS	27.0	31.1

Over half of the persons studied carried multiple diagnoses. A large percentage (21.4%) of the younger CMI group were diagnosed as also having a personality disorder, and 16% carried a dual diagnosis of mental retardation, compared to only 4.2% of the older group. Of the younger group, 17.4% also had a diagnosis of chemical dependency (only 4.9% for the older group). Among the secondary diagnoses, 30.7% of the younger group had physical health problems, compared to 47.7% of the older group, of whom 57% required daily to 24-hour access to medical care. Of the younger group, only 15% required such an intensive level of medical services. In terms of physical health status, as expected, the elderly CMI group had far more problems with vision (25%) and hearing (16.7%) than the younger group. Similarly, the health status of the CMI population declines rapidly after age 55 (see Tables 13.6 and 13.7).

Regarding aggressive behaviors toward self, others, or property no appreciable difference appeared between the two age cohorts, representing less than 10% of the CMI population. The services received by the CMI groups follow their age and functional status patterns. Younger CMI persons receive more treatment-related services such as information and referrals, diagnosis and evaluation, case management, academic and vocational training, community living skills, and cognitive/behavioral therapies. The older CMI group receive more health and functional support-related services such as support services, transportation, legal

TABLE 13.6 Health Status

Level of Impairment	18–55	55+
No impairments	83.7%	39.4%
Few or slight	11.3	29.6
Many or significant	0.5	31.0

TABLE 13.7 Level of Support Needed

Scale Level	18–55	55+
1. Dangerous (violent)	2.3%	2.1%
2. Unable to function due to psychiatric condition	12.0	19.3
3. Lack of ADL skill	9.8	42.5
4. Lack of community living skills	12.0	11.1
5. Need for role support/treatment	25.6	10.6
6. Need for role support/treatment in exceptional circumstance	25.8	9.0
7. Seeks treatment to maintain/enhance personal growth	10.3	3.0
8. System independent	2.2	2.4

and self-care training services, physical therapy and medical services (see Table 13.8).

This finding is somewhat troubling in that the elderly are not receiving adequate case management or psychosocial treatments, suggesting that they are perceived as "beyond help" and must settle for only basic supportive tangible services such as transportation. Indeed, the elderly CMI group in Iowa appear to have considerable functional limitations with a high degree of dependency. Although only 7% of the elderly population in Iowa are institutionalized, half of the elderly CMI population surveyed were living in an institutional setting.

Data from this large statewide survey complement findings from the Elderly Outreach Project. Together, they suggest a profile of a chronically mentally ill rural

TABLE 13.8 Services Received

Type of Service	18–55	55+
Information and referral	67.2%	52.0%
Diagnostic and evaluative	79.3	74.3
Case management	64.6	53.2
Support services	52.7	70.1
Transportation	34.6	62.5
Legal	22.6	29.8
Academic	23.0	29.8
Vocational training	34.1	12.6
Community living	43.7	36.5
Self-care training	37.5	51.6
Cognitive-behavioral treatment	77.7	58.5
Physical therapy	27.2	53.4
Medical treatment	78.9	87.0

population that is physically frail and dependent, with a high degree of functional limitations. And yet this population is not receiving adequate community-based psychiatric treatment. In many cases, this lack of services may result in premature and inappropriate institutionalization of the CMI.

IMPLICATIONS FOR HEALTH SERVICES RESEARCH

As we look to the future for older adults in these United States, two factors stand out—the growing numbers of older citizens in need of a range of health and social services and the inadequacy and fragmentation of our present system for delivering such services. What must be developed is a continuum of adequate, available, acceptable services for all older adults, appropriate to their needs at any given time. (Winston, 1978)

CMI elderly and their families must be evaluated against the overall criterion of continuity of care, a concept that mandates the need for access to a variety of medical and supportive services over a potentially unknown, unpredictable, and changing clinical course. If possible, the elderly patient and the family should be treated together because change in status of one affects the other.

Currently, continuity of care is more an ideal than a reality. Most service delivery systems are fragmented and characterized by unrelated agencies variously involved in the care of the CMI elderly patients and their families. And yet, as Bachrach (1986) notes, continuity of care can be achieved "only when there exists true access to needed services" (p. 171). She sets forth four dimensions that are essential to continuity of care and relevant to our understanding of the applied services research needs with regard to the CMIE population in rural areas: (1) longitudinal access—because of the long-term nature of many psychiatric illnesses, services must be available over long periods of time; (2) psychological access—systems of care must be easily accessible, helpful, and leave elderly patients and their families with positive feelings about their use; (3) financial access—elderly patients and their families must be able to pay for needed services; and (4) geographical access—elderly patients and their families must be able to get to places where needed care is provided, or the services must be taken to them, as is the case with the rural outreach model described in this chapter. Treatment for chronic mental illnesses must be "multidimensional, multidisciplinary, and long-term" (Bellack & Mueser, 1986, p. 178) and should integrate patient and family needs with treatment programs (Shern, Wilson, Ellis, Bartsch, & Coen, 1986, p. 191). A chronic illness model, one that focuses more on symptom management and quality of life, rather than an acute disease model with its more curative focus is therefore most appropriate when considering health services for the CMI elderly.

But even in those rare situations where there is an integrated continuum of services, health-care providers often remain uncertain about what specific treatments and services are best for particular patient symptoms or family problems. Thus, applied services research on the CMI elderly must be broadly focused on needs, costs, quality, and access issues, as well as on the elderly patients themselves and their families throughout the sometimes unknown and unpredictable course of a psychiatric illness over time. We also need to evaluate models of care critically. Only through systematic and coordinated research efforts can we hope to improve care for CMI elderly patients and their families.

RESEARCH RELATED TO DISCHARGE PLANNING IN ACUTE-CARE HOSPITALS

Discharge planning and continuity of care are important elements in the delivery of health care that have recently received more attention because of increased concerns regarding utilization costs, the rigorous monitoring of the health care industry by regulatory agencies, and increased emphasis on quality of patient care. Discharge planning is fundamental to effective health-care delivery for the elderly and involves a complex assessment of patient needs and the integration of hospital and community support services. This integration establishes crucial links between the elderly patient, her family, and the community, and facilitates reentry (Kennedy, Neidlinger, & Scroggins, 1987).

And yet there is ample evidence that the current health-care system in the United States does not promote discharge planning based on individual needs (McClelland, Kelly, & Buckwalter, 1985). This may be particularly true for the CMIE who, because of the potential for high comorbidity of physical illness, may interface with acute-care hospitals on a frequent basis. Smooth and effective movement of the elderly from one level of care to another is no easy task. For the CMIE especially, preparation for discharge should include assessment of their values and health perceptions, support networks, and the home setting, with the goal of enabling them to regain or maintain optimum health and maximize their personal resources and level of independence. To achieve this goal, the CMIE, the family when available, and health-care providers from a variety of disciplines and settings must be brought together in an ongoing coordinated effort. It is critical that CMIEs and their families be exposed to all the available health-care options and allowed some choice in their disposition. Persons who have no part in decision making about their location and care have been shown to feel powerless, insignificant, and manipulated (Leibowitz, 1974).

Effective discharge planning and its end product, continuity of care, require that the CMIE have access to a variety of community-based services, services that provide for both sustenance and growth. Some examples of mental health related services include (1) social clubs; (2) drop-in centers; (3) foster care and residential services; (4) day hospitals; (5) day treatment with skills training programs; (6) case management; (7) family advocacy and respite; (8) outpatient services, both individual and group; and (9) crisis and emergency services. But perhaps most important for this frail population are the essential supportive services necessary to foster independent community living for the CMIE, including information and referral, transportation services, nutrition services, recreational services, handyman and chore services, and homemaker services.

The availability and accessibility of these services for the CMIE in rural settings are limited. Research needs to be conducted on the utilization of these services where available, alternative modes of service delivery in rural settings, and reluctance (barriers) to utilization of services by the CMIE. If resistance to service utilization is widespread, this problem must be addressed and innovative delivery mechanisms developed and tested for this population.

Although in 1981 the White House Conference on Aging *Report on Long Term Care* noted that "the long term care system . . . should encourage support services in the least restrictive environment, preferably at home or in community settings, . . ." at present long-term home health care and other nonhospital services are not sufficiently available, nor are the funds to meet the needs of the Medicare population (Kelly, Shea, & Ross, 1987). These inadequacies contribute to increased morbidity and recidivism rates among psychogeriatric patients discharged from acute-care settings. Services research needs to be directed toward discovering whether the CMIE and their families would use in-home long-term care services if those services became more widely available and less costly. Further, would these home-care services help to delay or prevent institutionalization? How can we best assure quality of care for home-care services for the CMIE? Finally, to what extent do home-care services support informal caregiving and thus add to the financial burdens of local, state, and federal governments (Haber, 1986)?

The CMIE are at particularly high risk for relocation stress or translocation trauma—mental and physical problems associated with moving from one setting to another. Older persons with severe mental and social impairments are most likely to suffer relocation stress, in part because of their poor coping mechanisms. Thus, the CMIE may react more adversely to dischrage from the hospital because it is perceived as a threatening event that can potentially overwhelm their adaptive capacities. As Kasl (1972) has noted, the elderly who are particularly vulnerable to the stress of the translocation are those who are "older, and in poor health; living alone and having few contacts with friends and kin; in poor financial circumstances and of lower social class; having lived in an old neighborhood a long time; of low morale and life satisfaction, reacting to the move with depression, giving up, and hopelessness-helplessness" (p. 381).

Research is sorely needed to determine ways to decrease the impact of change and thus minimize the trauma and anxiety often generated by translocation for the CMIE.

RESEARCH ON THE MENTAL HEALTH ASPECTS
OF PHYSICAL ILLNESS

As data from both the state survey of the CMIE and the Elderly Outreach Project indicated, chronically mentally ill persons in rural environments suffer from a high degree of physical as well as mental impairment. Cohen (1987) has noted a number of important clinical concerns and research questions that arise from the impact of mental health status on the course of physical health. Cohen's work poses some interesting research questions for the CMIE within the domain of health and behavior with aging. For example, what role does physical disability play in the institutionalization of the CMIE? Similarly, what is the influence of the CMIE's social situation, that is, the availability of family or friends to help out? Cohen (1989) has set forth four models or paradigms for examining relationships between mental and physical health that are potentially fruitful sources of research questions related to the chronically mentally ill elderly residing in rural settings: (1) the impact of severe psychological stress, leading to physical health consequences; (2) the effect of physical disorder that leads to psychiatric disturbance; (3) the interplay of co-existing physical and mental disorders; and (4) the impact of psychosocial factors on the clinical course of physical health problems.

Researchers are thus challenged to find ways to identify and treat the CMIE in rural environments and to understand more about the interaction between mental and physical health in this underserved population. These research findings should then be translated into the development and testing of service delivery programs that are relevant and accessible to the special needs of the rural elderly.

REFERENCES

Bachrach, L. (1986). The challenge of service planning in chronic mental patients. *Community Mental Health Journal, 22*(3), 170–174.

Bellack, A. S., & Mueser, K. T. (1986). A comprehensive treatment program for schizophrenia and chronic mental illness. *Community Mental Health Journal, 22*(3), 175–189.

Cohen, G. D. (1989). The interface of mental and physical health phenomena in later life: New directions in geriatric psychiatry. *Gerontology & Geriatrics Education, 9,* 27–38.

Haber, D. (1986). In-home and community-based long-term care services: A review of recent AOA projects involving self-determination. *Journal of Applied Gerontology, 5*(1), 37–50.

Heffernan, W. D. (1985). Testimony prepared for a hearing of the Joint Economic Committee of the Congress of the United States. Washington, DC, September 19.

Kahn, R., & Tobin, S. (1981). Community measures for aged persons with altered brain functions. In N. Miller and G. Cohen (Eds.), *Clinical aspects of Alzheimer's disease and senile dementia aging* (Vol. 15). New York: Raven Press.

Kasl, S. V. (1972). Physical and mental health effects of involuntary relocation and institutionalization of the elderly—a review. *American Journal of Public Health, 62*(2), 377–383.

Kelly, J. T., Shea, M. A., & Ross, J. E. (1987). Implications of Medicare hospital utilization trends for long-term care health care. *Pride Institute Journal, 6*(2), 14–18.

Kennedy, L., Neidlinger, S., & Scroggins, K. (1987). Effective comprehensive discharge planning for hospitalized elderly. *The Gerontologist, 27*(5), 577–580.

Lazarus, L. W., & Weinberg, J. (1979). Psychosocial intervention with the aged. *Psychiatric Clinics of North America, 5,* 215–227.

Leibowitz, B. (1974). Impact of intra-institutional relocation. *Gerontologist, 14,* 293–295.

McClelland, E., Kelly, K., & Buckwalter, K. C. (1985). *Continuity of care: Advancing the concept of discharge planning.* Orlando, FL: Grune and Stratton.

National Institute of Mental Health. (1977). *Staffing differences between federally-funded CMHCs located in metropolitan catchment areas* (Memorandum #21). Rockville, MD: Division of Biometry and Epidemiology.

Palmer, C. M., & Cunningham, S. T. (1983). Rural mental health delivery: An imperative for creativity. In Jacobsen and Kelley (Eds.), *Issues in rural mental health practice* (pp. 2–12). Iowa City, IA: University of Iowa.

President's Commission on Mental Health. (1978). *Task panel on rural mental health* (Vol. 3, Appendix). Washington, DC: U.S. Government Printing Office.

Raschko, R. (1985). Systems integration at the program level: Aging and mental health. *The Gerontologist, 25*(5), 460–463.

Raskind, M., Alvarez, C., Pietrzyk, Westerlund, K., & Herlin, S. (1976). Helping the elderly psychiatric patient in crisis. *Geriatrics, 31,* 51–56.

Reifler, B. V., Kethley, A., O'Neill, P., Hanley, R., Lewis, S., & Stenchever, D. (1982). Five year experience of a community outreach program for the elderly. *American Journal of Psychiatry, 139,* 220–223.

Rosen, C. D., Coppage, S. J., Troglin, S. J., & Rosen, S. (1981). Cost effective mental health services for the rural elderly. In Kim & Wilson (Eds.), *Toward mental health of rural elderly* (pp. 165–186). Washington, DC: University Press of America.

Scheidt, R. J., & Windley, P. G. (1982). Well-being profiles for small-town elderly in differing rural contexts. *Community Mental Health Journal, 18,* 257–267.

Shern, D. L., Wilson, N. Z., Ellis, R. H., Bartsch, D. A., & Coen, A. S. (1986). Planning a continuum of residential/service settings for the chronically mentally ill: The Colorado experience. *Community Mental Health Journal, 22*(3), 190–202.

Toseland, R. W., Decker, J., and Bliesner, J. (1979). A Community outreach program for socially isolated older persons. *Journal of Gerontological Social Work, 1,* 211–224.

Walz, T., Craft, J., & Walters, K. (1987). *Chronically mentally ill older adults: Need assessment.* Unpublished manuscript, University of Iowa School of Social Work, Iowa City.

Wasson, W., Ripeckyj, A., Lazarus, L. W., Kupferer, S., Barry, S. & Force, F. (1984). Home evaluation of psychiatrically impaired elderly: Process and outcome. *Gerontologist, 24,* 238–242.

Winston, E. (1978). Continuum of care: The wave of the future. *Perspective on Aging, 7,* 28–29.

14

Spokane Community Mental Health Center Elderly Services

Raymond Raschko

BACKGROUND AND PHILOSOPHY

The Spokane Community Mental Health Center (CMHC) is a comprehensive mental health center providing services to residents of Spokane County, Washington. This includes all services mandated by the National Institute of Mental Health (NIMH) with particular emphasis on target groups.

According to the 1980 census of population, there are 341,058 persons living within Spokane County, and of that number, 54,000 (almost 16%) are 60 years of age and older, and 95% are living in their own homes or apartments.

Since 1978 the Spokane CMHC has manifested a strong commitment to serving the elderly population of Spokane, those in their own homes as well as those in long-term care facilities. The Spokane CMHC has had a special concern for those persons over 60 whom the Federal Council on Aging calls the frail or vulnerable elderly and whom we in mental health call the moderately to severely dysfunctional. The Spokane CMHC, through a very close working relationship with the Eastern Washington Area Agency on Aging and the Washington State Division of Mental Health has operationally blended the mandates from both the

Administration on Aging (AOA) and the National Institute of Mental Health (NIMH).

The moderately to severely impaired elderly who live in their own homes have been traditionally grossly unserved by community based agencies. Prior to 1978 only 4% of the active clients of this CMHC were 60 and older. In November of 1989, however, 24% of the active clients of this CMHC were 60 and older.

There are several reasons why the elderly are unserved and underserved. First, health and social service agencies have not understood and/or appreciated the community organization (gatekeepers) effort necessary to identify and locate this large subpopulation of isolated, resistant, high-risk elderly—especially those who have no family or personal support system to act on their behalf (Knight, Reinhart, & Field, 1982). Second, community-based agencies continue to expect members of target populations to have sufficient insight and motivation to access needed services. The myriad single-service agencies makes it extremely difficult even for the highly functional to accomplish this (Wylie & Austin, 1978). Third, for some years now we have heard that the reasons high-risk elderly are unserved and underserved lie at the door of the "system." It has been fashionable to explain lack of service as problems of access, physical barriers, bureaucratization of agencies, specialization of agencies, fragmentation of human problems, etc. As important as these "system" problems are, they fail to take into account other highly related factors, the most important of which is the at-risk population's resistance to intervention (Cantor & Mayer, 1978). This resistance to use needed services results from reactions to the multiple losses they experience and is often a symptom of the problems they experience. As many elderly experience physical, cognitive, emotional, social, and economic loss and subsequent decline in function, they tend to minimize and/or deny the existence or severity of these problems. This denial of loss reinforces any isolation they may be experiencing, and many also have feelings of fear, suspicion, shame, anger, and depression, which then lead to further isolation and resistance to anyone's intervention, especially agency intervention. Many of these elderly individuals fear that if someone should discover how poorly they are functioning, what little control they do maintain over their lives will be taken away, and they will be removed from their home and placed in a nursing home (Hayslys, Ritter, Ottman, & McDonnell, 1980).

We believe that there is a complex relationship between "system" problems and the resistance of the at-risk population and that this interrelationship has contributed much to the lack of services to this group (Comptroller General, 1979; Toseland, Decker, & Bliesner, 1979).

Lastly, it has been our experience that moderately to severely impaired older adults do not self-refer for community-based services. During program year 1989, only 1% of all persons admitted to our in-home clinical case management program were self-referred. If at-risk elderly are accessed to services, it is because someone else does it for them.

CHARACTERISTICS OF POPULATION SERVED

Of the 588 elderly admitted to the multidisciplinary in-home evaluation, treatment, and clinical case management program in 1989, 67% were female, 33% male, and 5% were members of minority groups. Only 4% had had any prior outpatient or inpatient psychiatric care, which provides some evidence of late-life onset of mental illness (Cohen, 1982; Rosen & Rosen, 1982).

During the intake process, clients were assessed to determine if any significant problems are present. These problems include all areas of functioning and are taken from a list of 52 possibilities. The 588 clients presented such problems as chronic physical illnesses (79%), social isolation/support system (72%), personal care/ activities of daily living (73%), emotional depression (59%), environmental/social stress (66%), denial of illness/problems (71%), and memory impairment (61%).

One large group brought to our attention consists of older persons presenting with signs and symptoms of dementia but who live alone and have no caregiver or support system.

In December of 1987 a total of 67 persons were admitted to the multidisciplinary evaluation, treatment, and clinical case management program. A review of the presenting problems reveals that the major reasons for referral included 45% ($n = 30$) for signs and symptoms of dementia; 30% ($n = 20$) for symptoms of major depression; and 25% ($n = 17$) for all other reasons. Of the 30 clients referred with symptoms of dementia, 47% had a family or caregiver support system. Of the 20 clients referred with symptoms of major depression, 65% had a family or caregiver support system.

The above is further evidence of the multiple and interrelated nature of the problems experienced by at-risk elderly (Gurian, 1982).

The chronically mentally ill elderly, exclusive of dementia, comprise a large number of community-based elderly being seen in their homes by this program. Four diagnostic subgroups—schizophrenia, major depression, bipolar affective disorder, and late-life paraphrenia or paranoid disorders—have been identified, and the clinical charts for a sample of each subgroup have been surveyed. The demographic and clinical data for these subjects appear in Tables 14.1 and 14.2.

PROGRAM STRUCTURE AND FUNDING

The Spokane Community Mental Health Center's elderly services is composed of two highly integrated component programs: telephone information and referral; and multidisciplinary in-home evaluation, treatment, and clinical case management. Each component program receives approximately 52% of its funding from the Eastern Washington Area Agency on Aging. The remaining funds come from a Washington State Mental Health Grant-in-Aid.

TABLE 14.1 Chronically Mentally Ill Elderly Maintained in the Community by Elderly
Services Demographic Characteristics of Diagnostic Subgroups

	Schizophrenia $N = 20$	Major depression $N = 20$	BiPolar $N = 20$	Paraphrenia $N = 20$	Total $N = 80$
Sex:					
Male	15%	25%	35%	5%	20%
Female	85	75	65	95	80
Age:					
60-64	30	5	30	10	19
65-69	30	25	20	15	23
70-74	35	15	15	15	20
75-79	—	40	30	45	29
80-84	5	15	—	5	6
85 and older	—	—	5	10	3
Income:					
$301-$400	60	10	25	30	31
$401-$500	15	20	20	25	20
$501+	25	70	55	45	49
Source of income:					
SSI	60	10	25	30	31
SSA	30	50	25	20	31
SSA and vets	5	5	10	5	6
SSA and retirement	5	35	40	45	32
Race:					
Caucasian	95	100	100	90	96
Black	5	—	—	10	4
Living situation:					
Lives alone	70	65	50	85	68
Lives with spouse	10	35	25	10	20
Lives with adult children	10	—	10	5	6
Lives with other relative	10	—	15	—	6
Marital status:					
Married	10	40	20	10	20
Divorced	40	15	40	5	25
Never married	15	5	—	30	13
Widowed	35	40	40	55	42
Source of Referral:					
Gatekeeper	30	5	40	45	30
Relatives/Friends	15	25	15	10	16
Hospital/Physician	50	60	40	15	41
Public agency	—	5	—	20	6
Voluntary agency	5	—	—	5	3
Self	—	5	5	5	4
Family/Informal support system	35	65	50	10	40

TABLE 14.2 Chronically Mentally Ill Elderly Maintained in the Community by Elderly Services Clinical Characteristics of Diagnostic Subgroups

	Schizophrenia $N = 20$	Major depression $N = 20$	BiPolar $N = 20$	Paraphrenia $N = 20$	Total $N = 80$
Psychiatric hospitalizations:					
None	5%	25%	10%	45%	21%
One	5	35	25	40	26
Two	15	10	20	10	14
Three	25	25	10	—	15
Four	15	—	5	5	6
Five	5	5	10	—	5
Six	15	—	5	—	5
Seven or more	15	—	15	—	8
Functional limitations:					
None	20	25	20	25	23
Speech	5	—	—	—	1
Hearing	5	20	35	20	20
Vision	25	20	35	35	29
Walking	5	25	5	35	18
Activities of daily living	60	50	55	55	55
Needs assistance to leave home	30	45	45	25	36
Physical illness/conditions:					
None	10	10	10	25	14
Arthritis	35	15	10	15	20
Hypertension	30	25	25	30	28
COPD	25	25	20	20	23
Heart disease	45	30	25	40	35
Vascular disease	25	20	25	15	21
Cancer	20	25	15	25	21
Diabetes	20	15	20	25	20
Seizure	5	5	15	5	8
Obesity	—	—	20	25	11
CVA	10	10	15	5	10
Alcohol abuse	25	15	25	10	19
Prescription drug abuse	—	5	5	—	3
Glaucoma/Cataracts	20	10	15	20	16
Tardive dyskinesia	—	—	5	—	1
Hernia	10	15	10	15	13
Thyroid	—	5	15	10	8
All others	30	30	25	15	25
Length of psychiatric illness:					
1–5 years	10	35	15	45	25
6–10 years	—	15	10	50	19
11–20 years	10	25	25	5	16
21–30 years	35	20	35	—	23
31–50 years	45	5	15	—	16

TABLE 14.2 (*continued*)

	Schizophrenia N = 20	Major depression N = 20	BiPolar N = 20	Paraphrenia N = 20	Total N = 80
No. of prescription medications:					
None	5	5	5	25	10
One	5	20	15	20	15
Two	15	10	15	10	13
Three	20	30	30	10	23
Four	25	5	20	10	15
Five	30	5	15	15	16
Six or more	—	25	—	10	9

Telephone Information and Referral

The telephone information and referral component, staffed by three and one-half telephone screeners, is highly visible on a countywide basis and provides telephone information and referral services targeted at *higher-functioning* older adults. It is *only* this I & R component that is advertised via posters, brochures, and the local media. Calls are diverted to Community Mental Health Center Crisis Services after 5:00 P.M. weekdays and on weekends to provide 24-hour service. This also provides 24-hour access to the in-home clinical case management component.

The telephone information and referral component directly serves those elderly persons who are experiencing no dysfunction or mild dysfunction, or persons who have support systems willing and able to act on behalf of an elderly person in need who is not experiencing moderate to severe psychiatric and/or cognitive impairment. Some home visits are made by staff of this component.

Multidisciplinary In-Home Evaluation, Treatment, and Clinical Case Management

The in-home clinical case management component is mandated to maintain the independence of the elderly, to prevent premature and/or unnecessary institutionalization, and to improve their quality of life. The staff of this component consists of the following:

- Eighteen clinical case managers who are trained as generalists and carry primary case responsibility;

- Six team leaders;
- One nurse consultant;
- Two psychiatrists who rotate through the teams and provide 40 hours a week of in-home evaluation and treatment;
- Resident physicians from Family Medicine of Spokane (a residency program of the University of Washington) who provide 4 hours a week of in-home evaluation and treatment;
- One clinical coordinator;
- One practicum students' supervisor; and
- One program director (see Table 14.3).

Use of Gatekeepers to Locate High-Risk Elderly

In addition to education, the public school system has long been identifying troubled children. The workplace, through employee assistance programs, increasingly assumes the role of identifying troubled adults. Gatekeepers attempt to create a system that functions for high-risk isolated elderly living in the community as the schools and the workplace function for younger people. Gatekeepers also overcome the problems of delivery that are so much a part of contemporary social and health services.

Gatekeepers are organized nontraditional referral sources trained to identify and locate high-risk elderly living in the community who do not self-refer and who do not have relatives or others to act on their behalf. They are corporations, businesses, and other organizations that have contact with the most isolated elderly in the community, who are often living alone.

Establishing a gatekeeper system requires a systematic community organization effort. We have found these corporations and organizations eager to allow regular access to their employees once it is understood how important such organizations are to a community-based long-term care system. Ongoing scheduled training, communication after referral, and the ability to work effectively with those who are referred are essential to maintaining a gatekeeper system. Also, the gatekeeper system must belong to the system of care.

The gatekeeper system that was established includes meter readers, credit office workers, and repair personnel from the electrical and natural gas utility; residential property appraisers from the county assessor's office; trust officers and other bank personnel; apartment and mobile-home court managers; postal carriers and postal workers; water-meter readers from the city of Spokane; fuel-oil dealers; police and sheriff's departments; fire departments; pharmacies; and ambulance companies.

As an index of success, gatekeepers now account for 4 out of every 10 admissions to the in-home clinical case-management component (see Table 14.4).

TABLE 14.3 Spokane Community Mental Health Center Elderly Services Organization Chart

239

TABLE 14.4 Elderly Services—Spokane Community Mental Health Center Admissions to Multidisciplinary In-Home Assessment, Treatment, and Case Management Program, 1985–1989

Source of Referral	1985	1986	1987	1988	1989	TOTAL	%
Gatekeepers	261	213	238	292	274	1278	41%
Physicians & Hospitals	69	37	117	139	148	510	17%
Relatives, Friends and Neighbors	114	68	96	120	78	476	16%
Other Community Social & Health Agencies	139	64	64	118	63	448	15%
Area Agency on Aging Funded Programs	95	58	64	71	21	309	10%
Self	14	5	10	6	4	39	1%
Yearly and Five Year Total	692	445	589	746	588	3060	

In-Home Assessment/Evaluation

After an at-risk older adult has been admitted to the in-home clinical case management component, the first task is to provide that person with a comprehensive in-home assessment of his or her functioning (Wasson et al., 1984). Staff members have become highly skilled in establishing positive relationships with the elderly and overcoming the initial resistance expected from older persons who are fearful, suspicious, or hostile. It is this relationship that provides the conduit for the assessment, services plan, and continuity of care.

The case manager and team leader jointly conduct the initial home- visits, begin the evaluation, and, as needed, the following also make home visits with this staff and provide additional evaluation and treatment: staff psychiatrist, nurse consultant, and physicians from family medicine. These staff members, with the clinical case managers, compose the in-home multidisciplinary team approach we have developed.

The six team leaders have a very special role vis-à-vis the clinical case managers. Each supervises three case managers on a full-time basis and does not maintain a separate caseload. They field-train the clinical case managers, accompany them on home visits to assist in the assessment process, and provide daily backup measures to resolve the difficult issues inherent in serving this population.

Treatment/Service Plan

Based on the comprehensive assessment of functioning, a detailed service/ treatment plan is developed for each person. Elements include medical, psychiatric, socioeconomic, environmental manipulation, and medications. When support systems exist, they are used to their full potential. Family conferences are held whenever appropriate and feasible (Reed, 1980). A system of caregiver support groups for families caring for a member with a dementing illness has also been developed in conjunction with the Alzheimer's Association—Greater Spokane Chapter.

Because of the relationship with the Eastern Washington Area Agency on Aging and written agreements with other agencies funded by that organization, a network of preventive, supportive, and rehabilitative in-home services can be delivered. The services most often utilized and believed to be indispensable to the mission include chore-homemaker services, visiting nurses and nurse aides, day health/day care, home-delivered meals, and respite care. Elderly Services is the "front door" or "dynamic focal point" in this system.

The interrelated elements of the clinical case management approach we use include identification and location of the target population (gatekeepers); crisis intervention; assessment/evaluation; a service/treatment plan; family work; supportive therapy; coordination of services (networking); advocacy; and continuity of care.

Primary ongoing case responsibility is maintained for all persons admitted to the program. Forty-nine percent are offically terminated after long periods of stabilization, 20% because of death, 12% after placement in a long-term care facility and where future discharge home is ruled out, 11% due to moving from the community, and the remaining 8% for a variety of reasons. Follow-up after official termination of those stabilized clients is maintained by telephone and/or the network of in-home supportive services initially established by the clinical case manager.

Relationship with Other Agencies

Fourteen written coordination and referral agreements with other agencies, most of which are funded by the Eastern Washington Area Agency on Aging, have been negotiated. These agreements detail each agency's role, referral mechanisms, methods of resolving problems, and how training and other resources are shared.

The core agency in a community-based long-term care system depends on other community agencies for the implementation of much of the treatment/ service plan (O'Brien & Wagner, 1980). Some examples of assistance:

1. All agencies involved in the cases presented at weekly case staffings held by elderly services are asked to attend those meetings.
2. Chore workers, who perform housekeeping, meal preparation, and other duties, and spend more time interacting with high-risk elderly than other agency persons, are trained to reinforce the case plan and to report any decline in client functioning. A specially trained and higher paid group of 25 chore workers is selected by the contracting agency in cooperation with elderly services to work with behaviorally disturbed clients. Elderly services staff members provided 20 hours of classroom training on such subjects as dementia, depression, mental status, and medications. These chore workers are part of a multidisciplinary effort, participate in case staffings, are provided individual case conferences, and are placed in the homes of the most at-risk elderly.
3. Whenever an active elderly services client is admitted to a hospital, the social services department of the hospital is notified so that it can be involved in discharge planning and provide proper follow-up care.
4. The Adult Day Health/Day Care Program is a rehabilitative and supportive program operated by Holy Family Hospital and is essential to our mission. Elderly services accounts for 73% of all the referrals received by the Adult Day Health Program. Joint home visits are made by staff members, and the psychiatrist treats referred day-health clients.

PROGRAM RESULTS

Community mental health centers throughout the United States have tradition-ally underserved persons 60 and older in proportion to their percentage of the general population. The national average has been approximately 4% (Pratt & Kethley, 1980). As of January 1, 1990, 24% of the Spokane Community Mental Health Center's active clients were 60 or older. These are elderly people often living alone in their own homes or apartments.

Minority elders constitute 1.5% of Spokane's elderly population. Five percent of the active clients in our in-home multidisciplinary clinical case management program are minority elders.

Immediately before 1980 and during the early inception of this program, there was a critical shortage of nursing home beds in Spokane County. Persons were being transported to other parts of the state in order to secure a bed. During the last 5 years there has been no shortage of nursing home beds in Spokane County. We believe this is at least partly due to the existence of this program and the aging services network that supports it.

The Spokane Community Mental Health Center enjoys a funding and working relationship with the Eastern Washington Area Agency on Aging. This relation-ship is unique among mental health centers throughout the country. Because of this, mandates from both the National Institute of Mental Health and the Admin-istration on Aging have been effectively blended.

This program has developed a unique method of locating and identifying high-risk elderly who do not self-refer for community-based services and who constitute the population most likely to find itself under institutional care if intervention does not occur. The gatekeeper approach of using meter readers, postal carriers, apartment managers, and so on has been invaluable in identifying high-risk elderly.

The heart of the program is its in-home multidisciplinary approach. Staff psychiatrists and physicians from family medicine make home visits with clinical case managers for the purposes of evaluation, diagnosis, and treatment. Without this, it would not be possible to maintain many elderly in their own homes.

REFERENCES

Cantor, M. H., & Mayer, M. J. (1978). Factors in differential utilization of services by urban elderly. *Journal of Gerontological Social Work, 1,* 47–61.

Cohen, G. D. (1982). The older person, the older patient, and the mental health system. *Hospital & Community Psychiatry, 33,* 101–104.

Comptroller General. (1979). Report to the Congress of the United States; conditions of older people: National information system needed.

Gurian, B. (1982). Mental health outreach and consultation services for the elderly. *Hospital & Community Psychiatry, 33,* 142–147.

Hayslys, B., Jr., Ritter, M. L., Ottman, R. M., & McDonnell, C. (1980). Home care services and the rural elderly. *The Gerontologist, 20,* 192–199.

Knight, B., Reinhart, R., & Field, P. (1982). Senior outreach services: A treatment-oriented outreach team in community mental health. *The Gerontologist, 22,* 544–547.

O'Brien, J. E., & Wagner, D. L. (1980). Help seeking by the frail elderly: Problems in network analysis. *The Gerontologist, 20,* 78–83.

Pratt, C. C., & Kethley, A. J. (1980). Anticipated and actual barriers to developing community mental health programs for the elderly. *Community Mental Health Journal, 16,* 205–216.

Reed, W. L. (1980). Access to services by the elderly: A community research model. *Journal of Gerontological Social Work, 3,* 41–52.

Rosen, C. E., & Rosen, S. (1982). Evaluating an intervention program for the elderly. *Community Mental Health Journal, 18,* 21–33.

Toseland, R. W., Decker, J., & Bliesner, J. (1979). A community outreach program for socially isolated older persons. *Journal of Gerontological Social Work, 1,* 211–224.

Wasson, W., Ripeckyj, A., Lazarus, L. W., Kupferer, S., Barry, S., & Force, F. (1984). Home evaluation of psychiatrically impaired elderly: Process and outcome. *The Gerontologist, 24,* 238–242.

Wylie, M., & Austin, C. (1978). Policy foundations for case management: Consequences for the frail elderly. *Journal of Gerontological Social Work, 1,* 7–17.

15

Research and Program Experience in Residential Care Facilities: Implications for Mental Health Services to Elderly and Middle-Aged Clients

Leonard E. Gottesman, Ellen Peskin,
Kathleen M. Kennedy

Persons living in residential care facilities (RCfs) are not all equal beneficiaries of care and services that encourage growth and rehabilitation and living at the maximum level of everyday life of which they are capable. This chapter discusses programs and policy options that would help residential care for middle-aged and elderly mentally ill persons approach the success of programs for the retarded. The authors urge the nationwide adoption of individual care plans,

245

closely monitored programs, case management, psychosocial and rehabilitation services.

Residential care facilities include places that provide room and board along with a variety of supportive services short of medical and nursing care. Some of their residents seek a retirement place with some supportive care and are able to pay for the care they need out of their own or their family's resources. The majority of RCF residents are poor and mentally retarded, mentally ill, and/or physically disabled. Many of these residents went to RCFs because they were having difficulty managing their lives independently. They needed help with essential activities of daily living, could not get the services and protection they needed from other places, or found the supportive services they needed inadequate or unaffordable.

RCFs are a component within long-term care. They typically offer more support and services than is available to persons living alone. They also offer more care than single-room-occupancy hotels, boarding homes, or a foster family. RCFs are analogous to continuing-care retirement communities but differ from them in that their residents, while at risk, generally lack the private resources for care. Some RCFs approach the types and levels of personal support offered by intermediate-care nursing homes.

RCFs are not officially part of the spectrum of long-term care *directly supported* by public funds. While they serve persons who might be clients of the health, mental health, or social service systems, RCFs are *not formally* paid for by any of these systems.

RCFs are *informally* connected to public payment and to public services because most RCF residents pay for their care using their SSI entitlements. Most residents are also eligible for publicly supported health and social services. Despite their eligibility for services, however, RCF residents are often not on the "active caseload" of public agencies.

This chapter describes the composition of the community of RCFs, including their residents, owners, and staff, the sources and amounts of funds, the communities in which they are located, the internal environments they offer, and their programs and services. As a way of evaluating the current state of care at its growing edge, the chapter briefly describes several programs for the mentally ill and the retarded, and then gives more in depth attention to a few programs, including

- The Lodge program for community-living ex-mental patients;
- The Domiciliary Care (Pennsylvania) program for mentally ill and elderly persons who need a protected familylike setting;
- The Community Care Program for the Frail Elderly (Johns Hopkins' demonstration of a model residential care facility program); and
- The Pennsylvania program for serving and monitoring services to retarded residents living in the community.

The Delco/CSI study of an enhanced support program for elderly residents of RCFs includes many ideas from these and other programs. That study (which involves the authors of this chapter) tests much that may be possible in RCFs generally. The 3-year demonstration/evaluation is partially supported by the National Institute of Mental Health (NIMH), the Delaware County (PA) Office of Human Services, and the Pennsylvania Office of Mental Health. It includes 20 RCFs, two mental health providers, and the Community Services Institute (CSI) of Narberth, Pennsylvania. CSI shares responsibility for the demonstration and is primarily responsible for evaluating the program. The study includes 77 mentally ill residents of personal care homes in Delaware County and a comparison group of 118 residents in adjacent Philadelphia County.

The literature cited is primarily the work of others. For some facts cited there is a historical vulnerability, as the major studies in the field are at least 4 years in the past (e.g., Conley & McCoy, 1984; Dittmar & Bell, 1983; Harmon, 1982; Sherwood & Morris, 1981; Sherwood & Seltzer, 1981; USOIG, 1982). The primary conclusions of these studies are sustained in research stemming from a noticeable resurgence of interest in this area as evidenced by the work of Newcomer and Grant (1988), Blake (1985, 1986, 1987), and the Center for the Study of Social Policy (1988). Their conclusions will also be drawn upon here. The most recent information included is from comprehensive studies conducted by the U.S. General Accounting Office (1989) and the Conservation Company (1989). These reports became available in early 1989.

RESIDENTIAL CARE FACILITIES: GENERAL CHARACTERISTICS

Quantity of RCFs

Even an exhaustive review of the literature is apt to turn a search for an "official" estimate of the number of RCFs and their residents into a rather frustrating task. There are several reasons for this difficulty. First, as the Institute for Health and Aging (1984) notes, no reliable database exists upon which to determine accurately trends in the growth or decline of specific segments within the RCF industry. Second, because each state creates its own typology that ultimately reflects its unique efforts to categorize the many types of RCFs that meet the diverse needs of their client populations, the definition of terms vary across state boundaries. Third, in addition to licensed enterprises, residential care is given in an unknown but significant number of unlicensed room and board facilities, adult foster care homes, specialized nonmedical residences, and large apartment hotels. The recent report by the General Accounting Office cites the same list of difficulties identifying the number of RCFs (GAO, 1989) and the continued existence of an unknown large number of unlicensed RCFs.

What is clear however, is that RCFs comprise a large body of facilities that are privately owned, operated, and supported, and their numbers are increasing rapidly (Stone & Newcomer, 1985). In 1987 the National Association of Residential Care Facilities (NARCF) found 41,000 facilities nationwide, with a total of 563,000 beds (National Association of Residential Care Facilities, 1987). The average facility in their survey has a capacity of 13 to 14 residents.

RCF Residents

The lack of a clear vision regarding where within the long-term care spectrum residential care facilities correctly fit is evident in the general lack of placement criteria. Unless a state has established a mechanism for differential reimbursement rates for RCFs which offer care to special populations, admission is often based largely on a resident's ability to pay. This dynamic is particularly true for the larger homes (30+ beds), which tend to be less selective in their resident composition.

The most commonly held trait among residents is their social marginality. Many lack immediate family to care for them, and many are financially dependent. The additional characteristic that often contributes to their living in an RCF is their self-care disability.

To understand the dynamics of RCF care, it is important to understand the disabilities of RCF residents. Many residents *are able* to perform basic activities of daily living (ADLs) such as eating, bathing, dressing, and using the toilet. However, they are disabled in activities such as cooking, doing laundry, shopping, and other skills, usually called instrumental activities of daily living (IADLs). The Denver study (Dittmar & Bell, 1983) reports that in RCFs which serve the elderly, 31% of the residents have physical impairments restricting outside activity.

Similarly, a recently completed study of a sample of 1,176 residents of 82 RCFs in Pennsylvania was conducted by The Conservation Co. (1989). That study reported that of the estimated population of 2,400 RCF residents, only 8% were moderately or severely disabled in a list of activities that included eating, indoor ambulation, transferring, dressing, bathing, and toileting. Ranges of disability varied within the state from 19% for residents of RCFs in the western part of the state to 1.4% of residents in the southeastern region.

The range of estimated degrees of physical disability reflects the wide range of populations served by RCFs and especially differences among homes that primarily serve residents with mental disabilities, others that serve primarily the elderly and physically disabled, and a few which are mainly retirement residences.

Our own study of 195 elderly mentally ill residents of 20 RCFs demonstrates the point that the major problem with RCF residents is their ability to deal with the physical and social aspects of the larger world. In our sample, 80% of residents reported themselves completely able to manage activities of daily living, but the residents' difficulties in managing life increased sharply the more that they needed to interact with others or to manage the outside world. Specifically, only 40% felt able to buy things when they had money, only 30% felt able to use public transportation, and only 30% felt able to do things with other people! In the same group of residents, 64% reported themselves able to clean their own room.

This difficulty in dealing with the larger world and with other people may be a reflection of the backgrounds and central disabilities of many RCF residents. There is considerable evidence that persons who are the most likely to have been sent to mental hospitals and who are the current residents of RCFs, have impaired coping skills and have led generally marginal lives. These persons are relatively less likely than others in their age cohort to have married and/or have had a significant long term two person relationship. They are unlikely to have close family ties or to have had successful employment histories (Talbot, 1978).

The GAO (1989), citing the 1983 Denver data, reports that about 40% of residents of RCFs serving the elderly had a family member visit them and 16.5% had a visit from a friend in the previous month. Our Delco/CSI study found only 32% who had a visit from a relative or friend in the 2 weeks preceding their interview. A possible contradiction of these findings lies in the Conservation Company study, which reports that 67% of the residents had a visit from an outside person at least monthly. "Outside person" in that study may, however, include a wider group than family members and friends, such as service professionals.

The elderly are the primary users of RCFs. In 1984 and 1989, for example, 80% and 89%, respectively, of all personal-care home residents within Pennsylvania were at least 60 years of age (Conservation Co., 1989; Office of Mental Health, 1985). The national study (Ditmar & Bell, 1983) estimates 66.5% elderly.

Regardless of their prior residential history, the elderly are more likely to be found in the larger facilities (over 25 beds) than in the smaller homes. It is suspected, however, that due to the more stringent safety codes that often govern facilities with an aged clientele, many elderly people are currently living in the very small unlicensed homes that legally avoid regulatory scrutiny. Sherwood and Seltzer (1981) identify two types of elderly residents: those who have been discharged from the state mental hospitals and those who, as a result of complications developed from aging, can no longer live independently.

To be sure, the mentally ill do comprise a substantial share of the RCF resident population. The Denver Research Institute's national study (Dittmar & Bell, 1983) reported 28% of residents in RCFs serving the elderly, and 77.9% in RCFs serving the mentally ill, had previously lived in an institution for the mentally ill. Pennsylvania estimates, in two studies made several years apart, show from 20% (Conservation Co., 1989) to over 30% (Office of Mental Health, 1985) of RCF residents have a mental illness diagnosis of some kind.

In the Pennsylvania data (Office of Mental Health, 1985), the proportion of residents who are mentally ill increased directly with age. Dittmar and Bell (1983) found that 33% of elderly individuals receiving services in personal care homes also had significant mental illness. Sherwood and Morris (1981), in an evaluation of a domiciliary-care pilot program, found that 47% of the individuals referred from mental health agencies were over the age of 60.

Sherwood and Seltzer (1981) note that with deinstitutionalization, state mental hospital beds are primarily reserved for those with illnesses in the more acute stages. Those hospitalized individuals with chronic psychiatric disorders are more likely to have been released into sheltered community living. Thus, many of those mentally ill people who in the past were chronic residents of mental hospitals are now the long term residents of RCFs (Segal & Aviram, 1978).

Sherwood and Seltzer (1981) report that studies of mentally ill RCF residents generally find that this group exhibits a relatively mild degree of psychiatric disability; thus the reason for their placement is not always initially evident to a casual visitor or to an interviewer. Indeed, they report that only between 16–20% of the residents exhibit severe symptoms of pathology. In the Conservation Co. study, 16.5% of residents with a mental problem have it interfere frequently in their life (1989).

In the Delco/CSI sample, on the nine dimensions that compose Derogatis's Basic (mental) Symptom Inventory (Derogatis & Spencer, 1982), the 195 people interviewed consistently achieved mean scores between those of "nonpatient normals" and the average scores of psychiatric outpatients. Staff ratings of the residents' level of functioning on the Multidimensional Observation Scale for Elderly Subjects (MOSES) Scale (Helmes, Csapo, & Sher, 1987) also yielded measures that are more indicative of a nursing home population than of those who are psychiatrically institutionalized.

The role of psychotropic medications in stabilizing the former mental hospital patient should not be underestimated in this regard. The Blake (1985/1986) and the Segal and Aviram (1978) studies found approximately 80% of the residents they studied were taking psychoactive drugs. The Conservation Co. (1989) reports that 83% of residents with a mental problem are taking prescribed psychotropic drugs.

The Milieu of RCFs

The ambiguity of vision regarding what a residential-care facility ought to be or what services they should provide is reflected in the diversity of facilities that compose the current milieu. While some homes house four residents or less, other RCFs have a bed capacity in excess of 250. Nationally, small residences (1–30 beds) account for two-thirds of all facilities and between one-quarter to one-third of all beds (Newcomer & Grant, 1988).

The Delco/CSI study suggests that the experiences, concerns, and problems encountered by the facility's management largely differ by facility type. A heuristic model devised by CSI divides facilities into three groups. In the first category is the small home, often a family operation, that is unaffiliated with any medical or social agency. Operators frequently reside within facilities of this type, and there is a skeletal support staff who primarily assist with housekeeping, cooking, and laundry duties.

The second category is the medium or large size home (30+ beds), usually a corporately owned and operated entity that is not associated with any skilled nursing or intermediate care facility. These homes tend to be more institutional in character than their smaller counterparts and often serve residents who are supported by SSI.

The third group of personal care homes is also composed of larger facilities, but these are affiliated in some way with medical agencies such as nursing homes and hospitals. Often, the residents of these facilities are somewhat older, have more chronic conditions, and are more physically disabled than those housed by the other RCFs, and many are ultimately transferred to the associated skilled nursing units when their medical needs extend beyond the capacity of the personal care providers or when the residents fail to meet the mobility requirements mandated by the state regulatory agency. This group of RCFs is similar to some types of continuing care communities, except that the residents of RCFs are poor.

The Physical Environment

Residents of RCFs are often regarded as "socially undesirable" by the general public. As a consequence, it is common for residential care facilities to confront neighborhood resistance when upscale suburban communities learn of their plans to operate there. Likewise, RCF charges do not generally support the costs of real estate in "better" neighborhoods. Consequently, RCFs tend to be concentrated in poor, socially transitionally urban areas or in mixed residential and commercial districts (Dittmar & Bell, 1983). Most of the homes from which the Delco/CSI sample is drawn are in economically depressed, urban areas. Indeed the Denver study (Dittmar & Bell, 1983) reported that nearly one-fourth of board and care homes for the elderly and one-third of those that serve the mentally ill are in environments described above.

Such locations often impede vulnerable residents from venturing outside of the facility as residents are often concerned for their physical safety. In reality, this reticence may be well founded. Lehman and Linn (1984) discovered that one-third of the discharged mental patients in board and care homes in Los Angeles had been victims of violent crime in the year preceding their interview. This compares with 3.5% in the general population and 23% among non-mentally ill RCF residents.

Although the mentally ill are easy targets, those that are elderly are particularly vulnerable. It is no surprise, therefore, that Dittmar and Bell (1983) report that despite their fairly high level of physical functioning, only two-thirds of the aged residents left the facility one or more times per week and that one-half of them did not go more than four blocks away from the building at least one time per week. This inhibition ultimately serves to compound the isolation these residents encounter and thus detracts from any serious effort to integrate them into the surrounding community.

Often, even within the neighborhoods the facilities eventually join, it is rare that relationships are developed between the residents and members of the larger community. While neighbors tend to avoid personal contacts with residents due to their resentment and fear of their presence, many providers may respond to community pressure and surveillance by being disinclined to encourage residents to leave the facility, fearing that their unpredictable or bizarre behaviors may serve to rock the somewhat shaky community boat.

In general, residential care facilities are located in dwellings which are no longer desired for typical residential use, and they are sometimes in need of major repair. Compounding this problem is the fact that these homes were not built to be congregate living structures but are older single-family dwellings modified for this new purpose. Consequently major structural renovations are often necessary—modifications with prohibitive price tags that can preclude their completion. For example, all of the small facilities in the Delco/CSI sample were originally row or twin homes, which involved extensive renovations for their new function.

These structural hurdles are often magnified by safety regulations that can be blind to the financial realities of small facilities and the funds available for this type of residential care. While resident safety must take priority over the interests of financial solvency, owners of the smaller homes report that they are often seriously threatened by the high costs of renovations they must undertake to meet the ever changing local and state regulations. In some instances, the cost of fire alarm systems exceeds the initial cost of the home.

A provider of one of the smaller facilities participating in the Delco/CSI project reports that she purchased her home for $15,000 and recently installed a $10,000 fire alarm system to comply with local regulations. She then incurred an additional $5,000 expense in order to meet local health codes. Another home, in compliance in other domains, is currently under threat of closure due to the owner's inability to afford a sprinkler system that is required by local law. Larger homes are not without their problems either, however, as the renovation costs for these facilities are often proportionately larger.

Internally, RCFs in the Delco/CSI study are clean in appearance. While some facilities provide their residents with private rooms, it is not uncommon for three people to share a single bedroom. In all of the homes, the personalization of the bedrooms with the individual's own furniture or effects is encouraged.

Particularly within larger homes, resident autonomy is low. In an environment in which large numbers of psychiatrically troubled people are the responsibility of a relatively small number of untrained staff people, daily activities tend to be highly routinized, and individuals become indistinguishable from their fellow residents. Goffman (1961) has documented the tendency of large programs with clear ingroups and outgroups to develop strong and restrictive rule structures. The consequence of this can be seen in Blake's (1985/1986) observation that in many RCFs residents move collectively through the home to receive medications, eat meals and watch television, a situation that obviously violates the spirit of normalization, which ought to be conceptually at the center of these programs.

RCF Owners

The issues of ownership, management, and staffing of residential care facilities cannot be separated from differences in facility type. There have been several studies that have described the service providers in these dwellings (Blake, 1987; Dittmar & Bell, 1983; Harmon, 1982; Zweben, 1979). In general, the vast majority of homes, particularly the smaller facilities, are family enterprises, primarily operated by a female relative. Blake reports that 80% of the providers of the boarding homes he studied in New Jersey were married women whose husbands had only peripheral involvement in the home's operation.

In these small facilities, it is common for operators to live on the premises, along with other family members. Often, these owners are middle-aged people (40-60 years) who have little or no previous entrepreneurial experience. These residences are the result of an investment of a family's life savings; consequently, less than one-third of these proprietors own more than one facility (Newcomer & Grant, 1988). The small facilities in the Delco/CSI project also reflect these trends, although three of these family operations represent the enterprises of one loosely related group of families.

The minimal educational requirements that exist in most states with regard to persons who operate an RCF is evidenced in the diverse levels of experience of the service providers. As one would expect, these different backgrounds translate into very dissimilar conceptions among operators regarding what a residential care facility ought to be and yield an assortment of perspectives about the role, rights, and responsibility of those who reside within it. For example, Zweben (1979) found that providers with previous employment experience working in institutional settings were more likely to entrust deinstitutionalized residents with assorted tasks related to daily living and to include them in various events that can help to develop, promote, or maintain residents' social skills.

As the residential care facility has become more established in the long-term care continuum and accepted as a viable service option, the operators of homes are becoming more trained and ownership of homes attracting more educated persons. While Sherwood and Seltzer (1981) report that by the early 1980s only about one-third of RCF operators have an education beyond a high school diploma, 40% of Blake's (1987) sample of 10 boarding home owners had a college degree.

Larger residential care facilities (30+ beds) are generally owned by a corporate entity. Often, the principals in the company have holdings in real estate, other RCFs, and/or are associated with one or a chain of nursing homes. These owners often also operate businesses that are affiliated with the RCF establishment. These may include laundry and janitorial services, pharmacies, and private social service enterprises. In general, corporate owners are rarely on-site. The administration and daily operations of the facility are entrusted to a director who often has extensive decision-making authority in areas of programming.

Differences also exist in the degree to which facility management involve residents in the daily responsibilities of operating a home. Zweben (1979) found that older providers were less inclined to encourage residents to perform a variety of routine tasks and allowed them to hang around the home more than did the younger providers. However, many operators may be understandably ambivalent about assigning tasks to residents because they do not want to be accused of exploiting them (Blake, 1987). This is an area in which operator training and individualized service plans would lessen the ambiguity and uncertainty of appropriate role expectations that exist at the residents' expense.

RCF Staff

Limitations on a maximum resident/staff ratio exist in only 28% of the states (Newcomer & Grant, 1988). This carte blanche, coupled with the small size of many facilities, the low fees they can realistically charge, and the limited societal expectations regarding the level of care they provide all contribute to the propensity of these facilities to be understaffed. Among the staff members who are present, few have specialized treatment skills in the areas of nursing, social work, or other therapeutic domains.

Dittmar and Bell (1983) report that in 1980 the highest ratios existed among facilities that primarily serve the elderly (3.2 residents to 1 staff person), followed by the homes for the mentally ill (3.0 to 1) and the residences for the mentally retarded (2.3 to 1). The six homes within the Delco/CSI study, regardless of size, all report a much higher resident to staff ratio of 7 to 1. It should be noted however, that the ratios for the Delco/CSI homes, while high, represents only those workers who provide personal care or direct services to residents and exclude those who provide only housekeeping functions. These homes do meet the limit required by state law.

Smaller homes tend to be staffed primarily by the operator with only minimal assistance from part-time employees or family members who assist with housekeeping functions. The presence of volunteer help is rare. In larger facilities there are more part-time staffers; however, these individuals are generally assigned to laundry, cleaning, or cooking detail rather than charged with providing direct services to residents. In nine out of ten boarding homes he studied, Blake (1987) found no staff people employed to provide psycho/social therapeutic activities for residents and virtually no professional staff members.

Facility size appears to have little impact on the characteristics of the staff members below the managerial levels. In general, employees have limited formal education. Among the homes in the Delco/CSI sample, the only training received in addition to on-the-job instruction is that which is periodically provided by an area agency which provides medical or psychiatric services to some of their residents.

The staff with whom we have contact demonstrate a commitment to the well-being of the residents and have a clear understanding of the clients and what is "normal" behavior for them. Despite this understanding, the lack of professional sophistication that characterizes many providers, and their staff has some negative consequences that may impact residents in subtle ways.

Some facility owners in the Delco/CSI sample have expressed concern about their inability to communicate their personal knowledge of a client's condition to outside service providers, particularly those involved with crisis intervention. Their inability to use the standard professional jargon, their lack of formal knowledge, and the low esteem with which they see themselves as viewed in professional circles often results in what they experience as a denial of access to specific procedures and a general disregard of their opinions.

For example, one client in the Delco/CSI project who attends a partial hospitalization program was observed by the program staff to be exhibiting signs of decompensation. The RCF staff was alerted and advised to contact the treatment facility if the client's condition declined. RCF staff did eventually notice that the resident was very well dressed and groomed, a condition atypical for her, and they notified the facility that a crisis was imminent. No action was taken in response. The following night the client experienced a manic crisis and ultimately required a month of hospitalization.

Such occurrences compound the frustration felt by facility staffers and decrease their confidence in community service providers. Consequently, they are less likely to communicate with professionals to prevent crises and are daunted in their efforts to view these providers as sources who can offer regular services to their clients.

Accordingly, critics of deinstitutionalization (see Plum, 1987) express concern that the exodus from the state mental hospitals has created a new "indigenous" nonprofessional who, without special training or credentials, has been called on to alleviate the increase in demand that has strained the resources of the community mental health centers. Thus ironically, the most severely disabled individuals are often cared for by the least specifically trained service providers. It should be reiterated, however, that studies have consistently demonstrated that these staff are, in general, caring, trustworthy, and conscientious persons who attempt to offer the best possible care with the limited resources available to them (see Dittmar & Bell, 1983; Sherwood & Seltzer, 1981, for a good discussion of this).

Payment Sources and Cost of Residential Care

Nationally, RCF providers report operating under a severe financial strain despite the fact that much of the care provided is indirectly supported by a mixture of federal and state SSI financing. Total government expenditures for this type of community care is very small, especially when compared with other forms of long term care. For example, the 1985 National Nursing Home Survey determined that public support for intermediate care in a nursing home, the next higher level of care to that received by RCF residents, averages $1185 per month (American Association of Homes for the Aged, 1988). That rate is more than double the national monthly average of $525 for RCF care (Center for the Study of Social Policy, 1988). In stark contrast, the typical cost of residential care for the retarded in ICF/MRs is about $2,897 per month! (Lakin, Hill, White, & Write, 1987).

This figure ($525), which represents the national average monthly income for residents dependent on SSI, falls far short of the $776 per month that the National Association of Residential Care Facilities (NARCF) estimates is the cost of providing residential care (Center for the Study of Social Policy, 1988). Typically, homes respond to this shortfall of reimbursement by a variety of means. Some limit the number of SSI residents. Others seek to become larger so that they may benefit from economies of scale. Some cut corners and stay within the bare limits of the regulations they must follow. Few offer on-site social activity programs for their residents.

Although many facilities do endeavor to balance the proportion of their residents who are SSI recipients with the number who are able to pay with their personal funds, this goal is extremely difficult to accomplish. The Center for the Study of Social Policy (1988) in a national study estimates that SSI recipients comprise at least 75% of all RCF residents. Not all states provide supplements to this federal entitlement, and while the actual number of individuals receiving state supplemental SSI payments for residential care is not known, the Center for the Study of Social Policy (1988) calculates that roughly 58% of all people in RCF beds receive such payments.

Not surprisingly therefore, the availability, cost, and quality of services accessible to individuals who need them change across state borders in a manner which reflects differences in *state* policies concerning supplemental SSI payments, nursing home reimbursements, and RCF regulations—state decisions that ultimately affect the cost of operation (Newcomer & Grant, 1988). For example, state supplements to the basic federal monthly SSI payment of $340 to recipients living in RCFs are simply not offered in eight states and the range of payments among those states that do provide such supplements spans a continuum from

$1.70 to $634.50 per month (Center for the Study of Social Policy, 1988). The availability and quantity of state supplements is of considerable importance, as $2.5 billion, or 21% of the total $11.8 billion spent on SSI payments in fiscal 1987 was of state origins. Thus owners may find themselves forced to choose between vacant beds, admitting additional SSI residents, or closing their doors. With increasing frequency some RCF operators, given the opportunity to fill beds with private pay residents, are deciding against admitting residents supported by SSI.

In general, the rates facilities ultimately charge for services do conform to the funds available from publicly supported residents in the state. However the range of fees, even within states, is rather large. In Pennsylvania alone, for example, rates fluctuate between $450 and $3,000 per month when both publicly supported and privately paying residents are included (PADPW, 1987). SSI recipients pay for their care by using virtually all of the income that they receive from SSI. Except for a small personal allowance that they are entitled to retain, often as little as $25 dollars per month, SSI residents are left with little financial resources (Center for the Study of Social Policy, 1988).

Services and Activities within RCFs

Theoretically, being paid in large part directly from their residents' income, RCFs are subject to consumer wishes. However, because they serve individuals whose disabilities often reduce their assertiveness or impair their judgment and who are not organized into a consumer group, consumer influence on the care provided is not usually high.

Many government programs address the physical environment of the RCF as it relates to fire safety and other health hazards. There are, however, few governmental regulations and also few treatment programs of community agencies that offer care in RCFs. The chronic and often passive elderly ex-mental patient generally has a history replete with failures, both rehabilitative and personal. Consequently, the prevailing notion among local mental health professionals is that aged RCF residents are the "lost causes"—the residents assessed to have the least likelihood for long-term improvement.

There are few states that require individualized care plans for the elderly or mentally ill residents within RCFs. Operators are left to provide whatever services their small staffs and strained budgets will allow. In many instances, it is literally left to the individual provider to take the initiative of contacting mental health agencies on behalf of their residents. Rather than a comprehensive care plan designed to enhance their physical, emotional and psychological welfare, most residents ultimately are left to exist on a program of maintenance alone.

Mental health needs often do not get necessary attention. Dittmar and Bell (1983) report that within their sample, over one-half of the elderly and one-third of the mentally ill who were assessed as needing mental health services did not receive them during the year preceding their interview.

In this regard, the Delco/CSI residents within one county are atypical in that nearly 48% of the elderly and mentally ill people do attend some partial hospitalization or day program. Prior to the implementation of a county outreach program that occurred in the fall of 1987, this figure was closer to 10%. The lower level of participation is more consistent with the participation level of the residents of the other counties and with the residents observed in other studies (see Dittmar & Bell, 1983; Faulk, 1988). Some of this results from the providers' lack of familiarity with the resources available to their clients, and it partially reflects the frustration and difficulty they often encounter when attempting to navigate the professional service network in the community.

The promise of social integration that accompanies the concept of community residential care has failed to materialize for the deinstitutionalized mentally ill patient. And for the elderly, this insulation and isolation is particularly acute. Despite the fact that the mentally ill do leave the facility during the day and thus enter the community environs, there is very little evidence to suggest that actual friendships are forged with neighbors. The several factors which impede these residents from developing linkages with their neighbors and with community services include the residents' illnesses and deficits, neighborhood distrust, and provider resistance.

Generally, while physicians do regularly provide physical examinations at the facility, more detailed medical workups are often long overdue, thereby making the early detection of serious conditions difficult. The need for medical and dental care is extreme within these facilities as demonstrated by Sherwood and Gruenberg's (1979) finding that 99% of the elderly residents examined by clinicians were found to need physician services and/or hospital care. Although some of the larger homes that are associated with skilled nursing facilities do have pharmacists who regularly monitor the medications of residents, this connection is rare; in general, there is very little comprehensive review of the residents' prescription drugs.

The most critical unmet physical needs exist in the areas of hearing, dental care, and eye exams. Much of this results from gaps in the protection offered through Medicaid coverage. In Pennsylvania, for example, while Medicaid will cover the cost of an eye or hearing exam, glasses and hearing aids are left to the individual recipient to fund. Because dentures are reimbursable only every three years, the residents in the Delco/CSI sample have grown accustomed to ill-fitting or broken dentures, or simply forgo them. Thus, providers are placed in the unenviable predicament of either absorbing the cost of these necessities for their needy residents, or allowing them to go without these aids.

Dietary problems are also common. While all residents receive three hot meals each day, many operators express a lack of knowledge about the special dietary needs of the elderly or those with diseases requiring special nutritional attention. Consequently, it is not surprising that Faulk (1988) found many meals in the board and care homes he studied to be nutritionally inadequate.

One factor that limits RCF residents' participation in programs is the difficulty they often encounter in arranging for transportation. For those residents who are functionally able to negotiate the public transit system, the cost is often prohibitive. Many RCF residents are eligible for special transportation services for the elderly and disabled, but using the services is often problematic. Many services are so backlogged that riders must reserve a ride weeks in advance. In most situations, this is impractical. In addition, many companies impose rules which further stymie efforts to access needed services. For example, some transportation companies stipulate that an aide must accompany a RCF resident. For the typical RCF with few staff people, this provision is often impossible to comply with. Finally, both providers and residents frequently cite the fees charged by these services to be excessive.

This issue of transportation is crucial. In one home participating in the Delco/CSI project the mental health center's partial hospitalization program that many residents attend provides door-to-door transportation. This rare but essential service helps ensure a high rate of participation. Although some of the middle- and larger-size facilities own a van in which they can transport their residents, most do not. Thus, unlike other adults in the community, many residents are unable to participate in normal activities which can decrease their level of boredom, slow the process of deterioration, and reduce their dependency.

It is not clear that if transportation problems were to be somehow overcome, however, that there would be many community agencies who would willingly accept RCF residents into their programs. This is particularly relevant for programs designed for the elderly. In the Delco/CSI intervention for example, some senior centers and geriatric programs expressed reservations about the inappropriate behaviors sometimes exhibited by RCF residents and strongly stipulated that they would welcome them only if they were properly medicated and groomed.

Thus, the release of mentally ill patients from hospitals has, in reality, more often resulted in a transinstitutionalization. In terms of day-to-day living, long-term prognosis, and integration into the surrounding community, the resultant qualitative improvement is seldom obvious, particularly for the elderly. Although the facility doors do not have locks, which prohibit residents from entering the neighborhood, they appear to have increased difficulty accessing psychiatric services that were integral during their hospitalization. Ironically, the increased use of residential-care facilities occurred when many community mental health systems were trying to offer services to such a wide range of citizens (and with such limited funds) that the "difficult to treat" chronically mentally ill within the community were often overlooked. The vacuum caused by this isolation from the community is not compensated for by an increase in activities or services available within the home itself. Rather, the relentless and all-consuming responsibility of an understaffed operation to provide personal care services generally precludes much expenditure of effort in providing regular organized social or rehabilitative activities within the facility.

Other than the occasional celebration of a resident's birthday, Faulk (1988) found that 90% of the homes he studied did not provide any regular stimulative type activities. Among the homes within the Delco/CSI study, there is little evidence of organized activities. Major holidays are celebrated in all the homes and some of the smaller facilities do plan an annual outing. Although a few facilities have religious services conducted on the premises, social activities are generally limited to a few homes with bingo and one facility in which a violin player entertains the residents on a volunteer basis. Unfortunately, this is of short duration and occurs sporadically.

The Denver study (Dittmar & Bell, 1983) reported that 20% of the residents in board and care homes for the mentally ill and the aged did not participate in any social activities even within the facility, and similar patterns are found within the Delco/CSI sample. It is no surprise, therefore, that according to reports filed by the Delco/CSI specialists who provide direct services to the sample participants, residents frequently complain of extreme boredom and restlessness. This situation becomes particularly acute on weekends, when the few programs that are offered by some facilities are not generally conducted.

TREATMENT VARIATIONS AND APPROACHES
Programs for the Mentally Ill

In general, services to the mentally ill reflect the degree to which the public harbors serious doubts regarding the ability of mentally ill people to improve. Often, the unsuccessful past of a mentally ill person has been the basis for others in his/her environment to anticipate continued limited performance. Unfortunately, this limited expectation of significant others has often been fulfilled. A body of experience and research is available that demonstrates that it is possible to raise the expectations for normal behavior of both former mental patients and the significant others in their environment. These raised expectations are often met with improved behavior of the former patient.

Gottesman and Brody (1975) have suggested that raised expectations are central to the effectiveness of milieu therapy which fosters ego growth for the mentally ill by increasing the demand (i.e., expectations) placed on mental patients. The same point of view has been elaborated by Test and Stein (1976, 1977), who advocate in vivo teaching of life skills in noninstitutional environments. Their studies and those of Gottesman (1974) and Gottesman and Bourestom (1974) describe the negative effects of environments which support former patients more than is absolutely necessary and the positive effects of training these people to meet demands of less protected environments.

It is especially hard to stimulate residents because many residents, having led marginal lives, expect little. The facilities' limited resources sometimes encourage staff to accept low expectations as the norm. Yet, studies of residents' life satisfaction (Faulk, 1988; Lehman, Reed, & Possidente, 1982) consistently demonstrate that many residents express desires to improve their lives in the areas of personal growth, social affiliation, and independence and would give a high priority to social service programs designed to address these needs.

Programs That Provide Community Supports in Independent Housing

There is some limited experience with programs that provide supports directly to former mental patients who are living on their own. One report brings together perspectives on implementing apartment living programs and discusses both the theoretical basis and the actual experiences of a number of approaches (Goldmeier, Mannino, & Shore, 1978).

One program, in southwest Denver, takes social supports directly into the homes of persons who are in mental crisis and attempts to help the person and those with whom they are involved or live to deal with each crisis and to develop approaches that will avoid future episodes. If removal from the home is necessitated, they are placed in small private homes with existing families (Office of Mental Health, 1986).

A new project in Philadelphia, funded by the Robert Wood Johnson Foundation, provides a variety of respite and emergency housing. This program is targeted at street people or persons experiencing acute psychiatric emergencies. Workers provide as much support as needed during a crisis period, but do so in the actual living situation of the client. For example, sitters are available to stay 24 hours a day with a client in crisis.

Other programs include the provision of support to the former mental patient through the use of advocates or ombudsmen, through the sponsorship of client-run cooperative residences, and through subsidizing private housing in existing apartment developments. Of particular interest here are programs that provide both residential supports and services.

The Lodge Program

In one notable series of programs called Lodges, discharged mental patients occupy residences with other former patients and staff. In addition to their participation in the democratic governance of the household, they perform some business/work enterprise in the community. Frequently, this employment consists of some sort of food service, small assembly work, or household maintenance and minor repair tasks. Residents were able to carry on these activities successfully. As of 1980, there were more than 50 ongoing Lodge programs nationally. The number of former mental patients who have achieved total independence is small. However, it should be noted that with continued living in the unit, 67% of former mental patients were still in successful community residence after three years. This rate of success can be contrasted with the nearly 75% of discharged patients generally who returned to the hospital during that same period of time (Fairweather, 1980).

Two exemplary programs that are at least partially focused on the elderly mentally ill, and which have been systematically evaluated, are the Pennsylvania Domiciliary Care program and the Community Care Program, a foster care project for the frail elderly developed by the Social Work Department of the Johns Hopkins Hospital. Unlike the active treatment goal of employment and independent living which exists for the younger mentally ill resident in residential rehabilitation facilities, the goal of these programs is to support or increase participants' levels of independence and their physical and mental status. Positive outcomes in both studies are critically related to a needs assessment, goal setting, a plan of care, and an independent monitor.

Domiciliary Care

Pennsylvania's Domiciliary Care Program began in August 1976 and serves a broad target population of elderly and nonelderly people who are either physically impaired, chronically ill, mentally ill, or mentally retarded. New permanent regulations have recently been published for public comment. The goal of the program is to furnish a supportive, homelike, community-based living arrangement for adults who cannot live independently. In the first reporting period of 1988–89 the program served 2,308 residents, most of whom receive both federal and state supplementary security income. Approximately 50% of all residents served are over the age of 60. They include 20% who are physically disabled, 17% who are mentally ill, and 12% who are mentally retarded. Of the remaining 50% who are younger than 60, 17% are mentally ill, 30% are mentally retarded, and 2% are functionally disabled. A total of 1,225 certified homes have participated, and 86% of these homes had between one and three residents. Because of a grandfather clause in the newly proposed regulations for the program, homes already certified have a maximum allowable size of 13 residents. Due to the program's emphasis on small facilities, it more closely resembles an adult foster care model than group-living situations.

The Domiciliary Care Program (Dom Care) is an integrated program which places central administration in the state Department of Aging. Placement and case management functions are vested in Area Agencies on Aging (AAA) at the local level as are recruiting and regulating of facility providers.

The program is noteworthy in that placement in a home is connected with a systematic broad-based standardized assessment of each client and the preparation of a plan of care developed with the client and the receiving home. Plans are monitored semiannually, and reassessment is required at least annually. Homes are inspected and certified by the AAA. The major requirements placed on buildings relate to the possibility of safe escape in case of fire. In general, requirements are fewer than in larger residential care facilities since the intention is that private homes and families be the context of care. Almost all residents are supported by SSI and receive an income supplement to pay for Dom Care. Rates are set by the central administration and are generally below that for residential care in larger settings. Residents receiving SSI retain about 18% of their benefit for personal use.

Case managers are integral agents of the Dom Care Program and have as their primary functions client placement and extensive follow-up and monitoring activities. The placement process consists of (1) client intake; (2) medical and psychosocial assessment for functional eligibility determination; (3) client-provider matching; and (4) facility placement. Once a client is placed with a provider, both assist the case manager in drafting a service plan.

Although the case managers do not provide direct treatment, they act as brokers in acquiring appropriate services for clients' needs. The case manager continues to monitor the client, and therefore the home, for the duration of the placement. In addition, a joint team composed of representatives of state agencies for the mentally retarded and mentally ill advises and monitors the placement agencies.

Provider responsibilities include meeting the shelter and nutrition needs of residents as well as assistance in the provision and maintenance of self-care skills, aid in the taking of medication, help in accessing transportation to needed services, and where necessary, assist in financial management.

Shortcomings of the program appear to be (1) the absence of limits on worker case loads; (2) that training of case managers and staff, while mentioned in the program regulations, is required only "as needed"; and (3) that residential providers are expected to help residents with ADLs, medications, transportation, and financial management, but few other activities related to client goals are required of them. Instead, the case manager is expected to obtain services needed by the client from outside the home and to "keep the provider informed." Furthermore, there is no expectation that residents participate in any regular activities outside the home. These program characteristics appear to incline the program toward less resident opportunity than may be optimal. This lack of emphasis on client participation in activities is a major difference between the Dom Care program and the Delco/CSI intervention.

There have been no recent formal evaluations of the Dom Care program, but an evaluation of client outcomes was included in the pilot phase. With regard to service provision, the elderly and mentally ill groups received more counseling and social services than the control group. They also obtained more transportation and escort assistance, received more recreational therapy, and were more likely to participate in social activities in the community. Although the elderly did improve in well-being, they deteriorated in performance of activities of daily living.

This last finding led evaluators to suggest that maintenance or slowdown in deterioration is a more appropriate goal for persons with progressive chronic illnesses than rehabilitation (Sherwood & Morris, 1981).

Community Care Program for the Frail Elderly— Johns Hopkins Hospital Program

The Community Care Program was developed in 1978 with support from the Robert Wood Johnson Foundation. Its goals were to experimentally compare foster care settings with nursing homes regarding the quality and costs of care provided for elderly persons with no viable family supports and who needed nursing care that would have required admission into a nursing home. All residents qualified for nursing home placement according to PSRO criteria. The program offered the combined efforts of nursing, medical, and social service professionals. The program sought to prevent inappropriate institutionalization, minimize utilization of acute care, and provide a living environment that would meet the clients' social, emotional, and physical needs. Residential providers were paid between $350 and $450 per month (Lawrence & Volland, 1988).

The total health care team included a nurse practitioner, a social worker, the residential caregiver, and a consultant physician. The professional team (1) recruited, screened, and trained caregivers; (2) evaluated and selected prospective clients; (3) monitored the clients' placement in the foster care home; (4) provided personal care and skilled services to the client; and (5) provided long-term case management services.

Once accepted into the program, caregivers were trained in several areas related to providing services to elderly persons and dealing with their own stress. Although most residents had multiple health problems, the most common primary diagnoses were mental disorders, injuries or poisonings, and disorders of the circulatory system. Upon admission into the program, a plan of care was formulated and put in place for each client (Sylvester & Sheppard, 1988).

Both the nurse practitioner and the social worker visited the home at least once a month to monitor the resident's condition and the quality of service provided. Referrals for professional services were made, but many of the in-home services were provided directly by the nurse practitioner and the social worker on a 24-hour basis.

The nurse practitioner treated acute conditions that might otherwise require emergency room admission and also monitored routine care of chronic conditions. Direct services were also provided by the social worker to both the caregiver and the resident. Their services included counseling and help in resolution of conflicts among caregivers and families. The social worker also coordinated needed services and equipment, helped negotiate financial matters, evaluated residents for senior day care inclusion, and encouraged caregivers to include the residents in out-of-home activities. Evaluation of the program supported this type of active intervention. Patients in foster care did better on functional measures, nursing goals, discharge, and mortality. Patients in nursing homes did better on life satisfaction, perceived health, and social recreation activities. Foster care residents were highly satisfied with their placements—praising them for the family environment, the food, their flexibility, and the homelike atmosphere (Oktay, Horwitz, & Volland, 1988). Costs of the program, including both payments to providers and treatment team professional services, were $855 per month. The project concluded that even including the costs for external health and social services, the total cost of the program was below the $1,163 estimated for nursing home care (Oktay et al., 1988; Volland, 1988).

Other programs in current operation focus on improving the use of residential-care facilities to offer support to former mental patients. California, for example, provides additional reimbursements to operators of RCFs that provide programmatic supports to mentally ill residents. Programs in Pennsylvania have offered additional training and technical support to residential care home operators.

PROGRAMS FOR MENTALLY RETARDED RESIDENTS

Treatment provided by facilities serving the mentally retarded represents the most successful approach to returning the individual to the community. As a result of national legislation, aggressive intervention approaches that include extensive community supports and a system of monitoring were developed in each state. These factors have frequently been identified as significant contributors to positive outcomes (Braddock, 1987). Active treatment of the client is initiated with an individual habilitation plan which assesses physical health, functional abilities, psychosocial skills, the need for special and/or vocational education, as well as any mobility and sensory needs. Goals are formulated for each client and can range from the mastery of a single ADL skill to obtaining employment. Residents are referred to the appropriate community service provider who can meet their needs, or the service is provided in the home. In order to attain established goals, behavioral modification techniques have been broadly adopted and refined. Residential staff receive training in physical care and in teaching activities in daily living and more advanced social skills. Monitoring by private nonprofit agencies evaluates not only the physical site and safety features but also the habilitation plan, service provision, goals, and general tone of the home.

Over time, as approaches to the care of the retarded have become more established, there has been a refocusing toward community care in small dwellings and away from larger community facilities (15+) and institutions. This shift is demonstrated by a decrease nationwide in the average daily census of institutionalized retarded people between 1977 and 1986 (149,176 and 100,421 residents, respectively) (Braddock, Hemp, & Fujiura, 1987).

Receipt of needed services as an outcome reflecting this level of care is striking. In their study of board and care homes for the mentally retarded, the mentally ill and the elderly, Dittmar and Bell (1983) found dramatic differences in the amount of services received by residents in these three type of homes, as shown in Table 15.1.

This survey confirmed that personal care needs were being met for most residents of all types of facilities. Support services such as transportation, planned outings, parties and get-togethers, shopping, and managing residents' spending money, were more commonly provided by the facilities serving the mentally retarded than by facilities serving the mentally ill and elderly (Dittmar & Bell, 1983).

Care provided in community facilities (ICF/MR) is very expensive, particularly for those facilities with less than 16 beds. Lakin et al. (1987) estimate that the costs of support in these small residences was close to $90 per day in 1986. Even as the cost of community programs has been growing, the national average per diem reimbursement of $127 for MR/DD care in larger institutions in 1986 has been increasing. Cost for institutional care in 1986 represented an *increase* (in constant dollars) to 150% of the 1977 rate.

One model program of residential services (Karp, 1986) is the Lynch Homes in Pennsylvania, which serves 118 people, many of whom are profoundly retarded and medically fragile. This program includes nearly 50 homes, each of which have fewer than 8 residents who were refused by other agencies as being "too handicapped." Even with these persons of profound retardation and accompanying mental illness, Lynch Homes has been able to maximize day-to-day performance. Support services to the small homes is provided by a mobile core team employed by the overall organization.

In some jurisdictions, private nonprofit agencies which monitor program performance can evaluate individual programs against nationally developed

TABLE 15.1 Proportion of Residents Receiving Various Types of Help in RCFs

Type of assistance	Type of facility		
	Retarded	Elderly	Mentally Ill
Getting med/dental/MH care	93.0%	64.6%	64.4%
Planned outside activities	92.2	32.9	54.5
Planned inside activities	90.8	49.1	59.1
ADL training	89.7	5.9	18.1

standards. For example, an independent monitoring team which is affiliated with the Temple University Developmental Disabilities Center is employed by the Commonwealth of Pennsylvania to monitor the state-funded program for the mentally retarded and to report on the progress of class members of the Pennhurst Class Action Suit which contributed to the initial impetus for the growth of ICF/MR programs nationally.

Of importance to understanding possible goals for residential care facilities that serve the mentally ill elderly, the monitors have groups of "red and pink flags" which guide them in their discovery of potential problems. Any red flag indicator is the basis for immediate corrective action by the local base service unit toward the specific community living unit (Conroy, Feinstein, & Lemanowicz, 1986).

The following list, which provides some examples of what constitutes a red or pink flag, indicates some priorities set forth in the program's development.

Red Flags:
1. Resident has no day program.
2. Resident needs glasses/hearing aid/wheelchair/helmet.
3. Resident has no Individual Habilitation Plan (IHP).

Pink Flags:
1. Medication error occurred in last 3 months.
2. Day program is provided at the residence.
3. More than 12 months have elapsed since medical exam.
4. Person receives four or more prescribed meds daily.
5. Case manager has not visited residence in last 4 weeks.

As is evident, these standards address not only the medical care needed by residents but convey the need for active, goal-oriented care both inside and outside the residential care facility. Simply by the monitoring activity itself, the facility and service providers in the community are induced to work cooperatively and to provide active care to residents. Overall, a successful program is expected to demonstrate outcomes that include such results as individual happiness and comfort, family satisfaction and increased acceptance, higher status, and integration of the developmentally disabled individual within our society.

The success of programs for the retarded may be partly attributed to the characteristics of the majority (80%) of the residents who, during the times of the studies, were young adults, moderately retarded, and capable of some type of employment. At the present, however, the average age of retarded persons in residential placements has risen. The impact of this change is not known. There is also increased interest in programs which provide services to retarded persons of all ages living alone or with family members.

There are also problems implicit in the current MR/DD program. First, the heavy reliance on an educational model and on the educational system itself creates problems of program continuity during the nonschool months. Second, the emphasis on children has put programs for adult and elderly persons into the background. This issue is particularly important now as the enhanced level of care provided to the mentally retarded has kept them alive longer and is therefore increasing the proportion of retarded people approaching advanced years. In fact, as the population in the homes ages, there is a shortage of places for new residents. Third, there are ongoing staffing problems in smaller noninstitutional settings where a great deal of day-to-day care is in the hands of relatively poorly paid workers. Fourth, Braddock et al. (1987) also cite as a problem the continued disparity between the large expenditures for institutional care as compared to community residential care. Finally, the costs of residential programs for the retarded far exceeds that of other groups.

THE DELCO/CSI STUDY

The Delco/CSI program is an attempt to integrate some of the successful aspects of previous programs for the mentally ill and the retarded into a program targeted at the mentally ill elderly in residential care homes. Prior to the beginning of this study, the Delaware County (PA) Office of Human Services and two of its mental health service agencies had already begun targeting personal care programs in the County for added mental health services. That program, funded by the state Office of Mental Health, had provided some training to personal care home operators, made crisis support services available from a base service unit, and had employed two case managers to work directly with some clients in personal care homes. The intervention of this study represents an intensifying of the program, adding a particular emphasis on residents over the age of 50, and the addition of an evaluation of the program.

The intensified program includes an on-site case management approach with moderate and low functioning elderly, mentally ill residents of six personal care homes. For the resident, the goals of the intervention include the maximum development of their potential and the prevention of a decline which would result in rehospitalization. Concurrent goals for the RCF provider are the broadening of a knowledge and practie base upon which they can rely in recognizing the needs of their residents and increasing the degree to which they can access community mental health services for them. Critical components that have demonstrated success in previous studies of comparable populations (Gottesman & Brody, 1975; Gottesman, Ishizaka, & Macbride, 1979) have been adapted to the special needs of these residents and include case management, psychosocial rehabilitation, counseling, and advocacy. To facilitate goal fulfillment for the RCF owner, an additional component of the intervention provides regularly scheduled training sessions, which represents a collaboration between CSI and Horizon House Rehabilitation Institute, the affiliated psychosocial rehabilitation agency.

The Sample Selection

For inclusion in the Delco/CSI study, a convenience sample was drawn from residents of personal care homes in Delaware County, Pennsylvania, and within particular neighborhoods of Philadelphia that met the following criteria:

1. at least 50 years of age;
2. a known history of mental illness;
3. a current diagnosis of mental illness; *or*
4. currently in need of mental health services (in the opinion of the RCF provider).

Because these preadmission criteria immediately precluded a substantial proportion of the overall RCF population, this sample was not designed to be representative of the general RCF resident group but rather a simulation of a specialized segment, specifically the middle-aged and elderly mentally ill. All participants were given an opportunity to learn about the project and were informed that refusal to participate would not in any way affect the services and care they receive. Residents who were thought by the interviewer or the RCF staff to be too confused to give informed consent were not approached; thus the sample was biased toward more functional residents. To be included in the sample, residents had to consent to and complete successfully a standardized personal interview with an interviewer trained by CSI staff and to agree to have a staff member discuss them with study personnel. An interview with a staff person was conducted in which additional information was gathered about the resident along with Cohen and Struening's (1962) Opinions About Mental Illness (OMI) scale.

Among the 20 participating facilities in the experimental and the comparison groups, there is a combined capacity of 1,007 residents. Providers targeted 279 residents as potential candidates, and baseline interviews were successfully completed with 195 of these individuals. One-third of those not included in the study were too confused to complete the questionnaires, one-third refused to complete the interview, and the final third was not available in the facility when interviewers arrived. In this last group some had been discharged, some were physically ill, and a few had died. Six RCFs and 77 residents in Delaware County comprise the experimental group. The remaining 14 homes and 118 residents, all in adjacent Philadelphia County, composed the comparison group.

Sample Demographics

An analysis of the client and staff interviews failed to produce a single composite of sample members. The average age of the 195 residents in this study was 68, the youngest member was 50, and the oldest 93. This age distribution differs from that typical of personal care homes. Although the board and care population is reported to have a higher proportion of the very old than what exists in the general population (Bradshaw, Vonderhaar, Keeney, Tyler, & Harris, 1976; Sherwood & Gruenberg, 1979), only about 15% of the current group is aged 80 or above. This probably reflects the self-selectivity of the sample in that those that were too ill or confused to participate were not interviewed and that group was also most likely to be very old.

In general, among elderly RCF residents, women compose a 60% majority (Newcomer & Grant, 1988). In our sample, females only slightly outnumbered males, 53% to 47%, respectively.

It has been reported elsewhere that RCFs have an under representation of ethnic minorities (Newcomer & Grant, 1988), and this trend has been similarly found in this sample. Over 60% of the group is white, only 33% is black, and less than 4% are Hispanic.

Nearly half the men (47%) and almost one-third of the women (32%) were never married. In addition, nearly one-quarter (23%) were divorced or separated (24% of men and 23% of women), and 30% were widowed (18% of men and 41% of women). On the average this sample completed about 10 years of schooling; almost 70% did not complete high school.

About one-third of these residents indicated that they lived alone prior to admission to the RCF. Type of prior placement was obtained from the residents themselves, and 61% report that they lived in a private dwelling before coming to the current facility. A little less than 10% reported that their last placement was a state hospital, and 28% moved from another personal care home, boarding house/hotel, or other nonprivate placement.

The Short Portable Mental Status Questionnaire (Duke University, 1978) was administered, and the mean score of 5.7 indicates a moderate degree of intellectual impairment throughout the sample. The median MSQ score for both men and for women was six correct out of nine items. There was a statistically significant relationship between age and intellectual impairment, with older residents having greater impairment.

DELCO/CSI INTERVENTION
The Intervention Team

The intervention is executed by four case managers. Two half-time workers are supported by research funds, and the third is on the staff of a hospital-affiliated (Crozer Chester Medical Center) mental health base service unit. A staff member of the affiliated psychosocial rehabilitation agency is the fourth worker. All are at least bachelor prepared and have worked a minimum of two years with the mentally ill in the community.

The structure of the supervisory and/or consultation team is similar to the health team of the Johns Hopkins Community Care Program (Lawrence & Volland, 1988) described earlier. Three professionals provide supervision and consultation to the four case workers. The professionals include a supervisor in the rehabilitation agency, the director of geriatric services for the medical institution and a public health nurse (on CSI's staff) who takes overall responsibility for managing the intervention program. Each case manager meets weekly with a supervisor for case reviews, while the entire team convenes monthly to discuss more general issues.

The Case Management Component

Under the supervision of the consultants, a comprehensive health and social assessment is initiated by the case worker for each resident in the experimental group. Overall, the diversity of service needs identified revealed three resident groups who can be classified according to their age and the severity of their mental illness.

A small proportion (20%) of the sample exhibit aggressive acting-out and noncompliant behaviors. Consequently the case manager assigned to them devotes much of his time to crisis intervention and prevention. He routinely intercedes in incidents that result from substance abuse, noncompliance with medication regimens, arguments with other residents or the RCF staff, and runaway situations.

The majority of the residents are passive and have problems related to medical, functional, as well as social needs. For this group, an important role is played by the RN as part of the outreach team. For example, in a review of a particular assessment the client reported that he had not attended the senior center recently because he suffered bouts of alternating constipation and diarrhea. The source of this problem, the dosage of a prescribed medication, was identified by a review of his medications by the nurse, and was ultimately discontinued by the alerted treating physician. A more frequent occurrence is the discovery of a medical diagnosis such as diabetes or epilepsy with no arrangement to provide the requisite special care. In meeting these needs, the RN uses these events to teach the staff preventive health measures, common disorders of the elderly, and implications of commonly prescribed geriatric medications.

For approximately 10% of this group, lack of glasses and poor eyesight prevent their participation in recreational activities. Ten percent (sometimes the same people) needed hearing aids. While public monies will provide for both eye and hearing exams in Pennsylvania, eyeglasses and hearing aids are not reimbursable. Through the efforts of the case managers an out-of-state nonprofit agency was located which will provide glasses from participating private firms for indigent individuals. Another agency was located which will provide hearing exams and reconstructed hearing aids.

Advocacy

The personal and social circumstances which lead to the placement of an individual in a RCF also lessen his/her ability to navigate community agencies and resources for his/her own benefit. Case managers play an advocacy role in negotiating for receipt of financial benefits for some medical services and also in securing placement in community programs. For example, when residents were encountering difficulty participating in the senior citizen center, a visit to the facility by a supervisor revealed that the residents were welcome if they did not have special physical or behavioral needs, as the understaffed center lacked the expertise to manage people exhibiting strange or nonconforming behavior. As a result, the case managers are now acting as liaison between the center's administrators and the RCF operators to ensure that the client is stabilized on medication and is properly attired when attending the senior center.

Traditionally, advocates for the mentally retarded have routinely and successfully solicited community support in the form of volunteer service and monetary donations. This type of additional direct support to the client is typically absent in RCFs. As part of the community outreach aspect of the intervention, case managers have solicited local churches and volunteer agencies for the purpose of "adopting" residents of a specific RCF for Christmas sponsorship. These efforts will be expanded to year-round support for needed clothing and nonessential amenities.

Psychosocial Rehabilitation

Approximately 50% of the residents have some functional limitation carrying out instrumental activities of daily living (IADL) like shopping, working with others, or using public transportation. Nearly all also need support with good hygiene. To address these needs, psychosocial rehabilitation is provided by the case managers and three community mental health agencies. The service includes on-site group counseling and skill building, and for 15 residents of one rural home, partial hospitalization services and transportation which is crucial for these residents' participation.

In contrast to the long-term goals of employment and independent living consistently set for mentally ill residents in CRRs and higher functioning mentally retarded residents in CLAs, independent living is an unlikely goal for this population of RCF residents. Cognizant that these people will require long-term supported living, the content of the three community group programs strongly emphasizes basic skills such as personal hygiene, the use of money, the use of public transportation, and doing things with others. Decision-making processes and goal setting are discussed and demonstrated with practical application.

These groups also provide a forum in which social skills are developed. Through group discussion and role-playing, participants are helped to assess which of their behaviors foster relationships with others. In one group, for example, when members discussed their regrets about lost relationships with former friends and relatives, the case manager suggested a project in which participants wrote letters to one person with whom they had lost contact. Four of the six residents involved ultimately received return letters which initiated a renewed relationship.

Case managers have initiated social programs in an attempt to fill the void caused by fiscal limits and the absence of regulations regarding social and recreational activities. In two of the homes in which bingo was introduced, residents who were previously indifferent to the case manager's visits now assist with setups and inquire about the prizes and refreshments. After the initial bingo session the residents were asked what other prizes they would prefer, and their response was particularly revealing of their indigence—they requested tooth-brushes.

A small proportion (15%) of the sample is composed of more withdrawn individuals who are more limited by mobility, degree of continence, or periodic confusion, and do not choose to participate in group situations. For these, the most impaired residents, case managers adopted the very individualized approach seen with the moderately mentally retarded.

An unusual example of this approach occurred with a withdrawn physican who has great difficulty walking, spends most of his day sitting in the day room, and responds monosyllabically when addressed. When the case manager asked him about his interests, he related that classical music and art masterpieces had been his hobbies. The case manager promised that she would bring a tape and library books on subsequent visits. Several minutes later, the resident came to her and very simply stated, "I like poetry too."

Counseling

Counseling includes a broad range of activities which focus on the specific needs of the client which aren't addressed in a group situation. To date, only a few individual resident gains have been achieved, due to the chronicity of the client's disability and the fact that the intervention has been operational for only 1 year.

There are some indications of changes however. One resident who is a constant bed wetter with no organic etiology was deemed by the facility staff to be simply lazy. In fact, the resident was apprehensive about leaving her room during the night. The case manager is now encouraging night contin-ence by suggesting the resident limit liquids before bed and use a urinal in the room.

A case manager for a second resident, who exhibits alternate aggressive and withdrawn behavior, has worked intensely to encourage this resident to attend group sessions as prescribed. The case manager gradually reduced the resident's discomfort in groups by taking him into public restaurants for coffee and arranged meeting in smaller groups of two and three. The resident has progressed so that he participated in an award outing with other group members who had the most hours of group attendance.

Many clients (30–40%) are frail elderly who present a profile of diminishing acute mental symptoms accompanied by initial appearances of sensory and cognitive losses. Individual counseling with these people can at times resemble "friendly visits" which convey an interest and a sense that the case manager is available to them on a regular basis. Variations of remotivation therapy and reminiscence techniques have been adopted with this subgroup.

Increasing Expectations

A subtle characteristic of the program design is to encourage the residents and the staffs of both RCFs and service agencies to set higher goals for clients than that which is currently typical. In the RCF, residents often appear to be equally down-and-out, and equally impaired with little hope of improvement. This hopelessness is contagious and affects staff, residents, and service providers alike.

In the demonstration/evaluation project, workers encourage the resident to discuss both their current and former interests. When possible, case managers use this information in an attempt to engage the residents by providing them with a current challenge. Discovering the past occupations of three residents and providing each materials to support current engagement is a case in point. For each resident, case managers and RCF staff people attempt to identify an activity within the facility or outside the RCF that will activate some ability or enthusiasm on the part of the resident. Often, this is not easy because the range of possible activities in the RCF is limited and many residents have given up after a succession of failures and/or of illnesses that have been evaluated by society as failures.

Thus the project attempts to establish what are typically small goals with each resident. In reality, large gains are not likely, would be viewed by all as unrealistic, and setting these might precipitate a breakdown of either the resident or the performance of caregivers by applying undue pressure.

Program success is likely to be seen in the achievement of these small goals, as evidenced by changes in resident affect or increased daily engagement rather than large changes in mental illness symptoms. The measurement of these or other program outcomes is scheduled twice during the remainder of the project. Increased interest by service providers in the county mental health system has already occurred, and the likelihood that the program will be permanently adopted is good, even based on the small impact which already seems to be occurring.

IMPLICATIONS

The jury is still out regarding the best use of sheltered community residence for the mentally ill. There is considerable evidence cited above that programs focused on transitional rehabilitation have had spotty success. There is substantial evidence as well, however, that it may not be possible to provide enough support at the right time and within budgets that society will accept to ensure that persons continue to reside in private dwellings indefinitely.

Certainly the argument in this chapter that programs for the retarded represent an ideal toward which RCFs generally and those servicing the elderly mentally ill in particular should strive must be tempered by two considerations. First, at the cost of $4,000 or more per month, society could provide a wide range of in-home services. Second, even within programs for the retarded, younger people are now often remaining in their family homes and going to day programs only. Entry into a residence has been occurring later and later in life, in recognition of the fact that even small residential programs for the retarded are often less desirable than continuing to live at home.

For all the groups discussed in this chapter, and particularly for the elderly mentally ill person on whom we have focused, residential care continues to apear both necessary and desirable. Many RCF residents as well as some of their significant others want it, and it should thus remain available as an option.

It would be of value to understanding residential care if both the composition of residents in a setting and the size of the setting were made the subject of systematic study. The evidence from MR programs suggests that many small programs in which persons with different types of needs are mixed have a higher success rate than large establishments with similar populations. In large institutional-type facilities where most of the elderly residents are found, there is little opportunity for individuals to distinguish themselves. It is clearly unacceptable for the staff to assume that all individuals in the home are mentally ill, and it is upsetting to elderly residents to have daily exposure to many persons with periodic psychiatric episodes.

In general, residential places for the retarded have been getting smaller. While some of the data reported here cite 13 beds as the division between large and small homes, Homans (1950) long ago suggested that eight persons were the limit that could function as a small group without splintering into two smaller units as far as interaction among members was concerned. McCoin (1987) and Volland (1988), among others, also argue for the increased use of small, foster care arrangements in private homes in the care of the elderly.

As others have noted (see Beyer, Bulkley, & Hopkins, 1984; Harmon, 1982; Randolph, Laux, & Carling, 1987), placement in a residential facility is not, in itself, a sufficient long-term goal. In addition to encouraging the development of residences within communities that are able to deliver services, systems must be implemented to guarantee that providers are acquainted with these resources and that state and local authorities ensure that agencies negotiate formal agreements with board and care providers either to finance or offer services to clients.

An essential element of quality programming is systematic assessment and care planning. As the authors of the Model Act (for board and care facilities) point out, appropriate placement can be made only after each resident's needs have been properly identified (Beyer et al., 1984). They argue that since placement in a facility is the provision of a service, the assessment for that service should be used to assure that the right persons have the right service at the right time. This assessment should include discovering whether the supportive services needed by the person is available in the surrounding community, whether the particular home can provide the personal assistance required in an environment that is compatible with the resident's needs, and if the facility is located in an area in which the prospective resident has family and friends. Resident assessments can only be made by a trained case manager who is then charged with the responsibility of developing and implementing a plan of care. It is equally essential that residents have the opportunity to provide their input into the selection process and retain the right to reject placement in facilities they deem unacceptable.

Although it is clear that a satisfactory quality of life cannot be achieved without first meeting basic material needs, it is only when the higher "human" needs are met, such as the desire for independence, autonomy and self esteem that quality of life is significantly impacted (Cohen, 1987). Among the policymakers for the mentally retarded in community residential facilities, this was recognized long ago, and the commitment that has been demonstrated in their efforts to attain these higher goals has been met with impressive success. It is clear, therefore, that future policy initiatives for RCFs must recognize the importance of fulfilling these higher-level demands rather than remain concerned with simply meeting the residents' basic material requirements.

At a minimum, every resident should have an active plan of care that involves both internal and external engagement. Every resident should receive the necessary glasses, hearing aid, up-to-date prescriptions, current medical exams, and whatever other appliances are needed to do things, get about, and go out.

The current lack of activity that characterizes the lives of these residents becomes particularly troublesome when one considers that in most cases, their functional level is fairly high. Thus, a deficiency in physical ability cannot account for their inertia. Rather, there is a prevalent perception that mentally ill or elderly people cannot do many things; therefore, there is little that should be expected of them. This notion, is, ironically, often shared by the residents about other occupants of the facility. Indeed, in the CSI survey, even residents who rated themselves to be very capable of doing things with other residents qualified their response with the comment that there was no one around to do anything with.

Certainly, assuring community contact for elderly mentally ill residents of RCFs would be a reasonable goal for AAA involvement with RCFs. A corp of volunteers organized by the area agency on aging or by the community mental health associations could contribute in this effort.

A condition in which residents have done for them things that they are able to do independently not only perpetuates a pattern of passivity but also denies them one of the major bases for self esteem. Residents do express interest in playing a productive role in their environment. Yet the baseline interviews conducted by CSI found only minimal instances of residents being expected to help with chores around the facility, despite the fact that most respondents indicated a willingness to do so if asked. The lack of environmental expectations for playing productive roles is of particular concern since Lamb and Goertzel (1972) and Gottesman and Brody (1975) all found that an environment with high expectations for residents is ultimately more therapeutic despite the additional pressures such responsibilities ultimately accompany.

The aggressive monitoring of programs is an important element in maximizing program quality (see Volland, 1988, for a good discussion on this). Certainly the costs of monitoring a large number of small programs might be high. In Pennsylvania, the monitoring of the Pennhurst graduates (i.e., residents returned to the community when the institution was closed by court order) costs $250 per resident each year. The same monitoring team has found that $100 covers the cost of a somewhat differently organized monitoring program in Connecticut. A systematic evaluation of the organization and effects of program monitoring is also warranted.

While this discussion of the current state of the RCFs has been rather harsh, the intention has not been to either discount or ignore the positive services that these facilities offer to their clients. Many residents in the Delco/CSI study indicate that their fellow lodgers are like a family to them and that there is someone within the facility they can trust. Similarly, three-quarters of the residents Lehman et al. (1982) spoke with reported that they interacted with both the staff and other residents on a daily basis.

The overwhelmingly majority of providers with whom CSI has interacted have been extremely dedicated to providing the best level of care possible for their residents. They have consistently demonstrated an enthusiasm for acquiring additional training and frequently lament the existence of economic constraints which prevent them from offering more services for those within their care. Particularly in the smaller homes, it is evident that the providers are quite familiar with the residents on an individual basis, and are knowledgeable about changes in their physical and emotional status.

Certainly there is a self-selection bias at work in that providers who agreed to be in the Delco/CSI provider group may not be representative of their colleagues. It is also true, as Blake (1987) notes, that the reliability of residents' responses concerning their opinions about their environment may be questionable due to legitimate fears of reprisal if their complaints are publicly exposed. However, simply to dismiss these observations and responses would be unduly prejudicial

The formation of several provider associations around the country is evidence of efforts at self-monitoring, enhanced professionalism, higher industry standards, and consistency and advocacy on behalf of themselves and their residents.

To the extent that the success of deinstitutionalization is, for better or for worse, traditionally measured by the rate of recidivism, a systematic and sensitive matching between residents and homes is critical. Linn, Klett, and Caffey (1980) discovered that environmental characteristics of the facilities were better predictors of relapse or nonrelapse than was the individual resident's psychological profile. An environment that fails to provide the requisite therapeutic and supportive needs only perpetuates a cycle of failure, despair, and hopelessness for a vulnerable group of individuals. For the mentally ill elderly RCF resident, the elements of success may indeed be like those which work for retarded persons, namely, aggressive interventions that are specified by legislation, accompanied with extensive community supports and a mandated system of monitoring and enforcing performance.

REFERENCES

American Association of Homes for the Aged (AAHA). (1988). Personal communication, based on analysis of data tape from the 1985 Nursing home survey, National Center for Health Statistics, U.S. Department of Health and Human Services.

Beyer, J., Bulkley, J., & Hopkins, P. (1984). A model act regulating board and care homes: Guidelines for states. Rockville, MD: Project Share.

Blake, R. (1985-86). Normalization and boarding homes: An examination of paradoxes. Social Work in Health Care, 11(2), 75-86.

Blake, R. (1987). The social environment of boarding homes. Adult Foster Care Journal, 1(1), 42-55.

Bradshaw, B., Vonderhaar, W., Keeney, V., Tyler, L., & Harris, S. (1976). Community based residential care for the minimally impaired elderly: A survey analysis. Journal of the American Geriatric Society, 24(9), 423-429.

Braddock, D. (1987). Federal policy toward mental retardation and develop mental disabilities. Baltimore: Paul H. Brookes.

Braddock, D., Hemp, R., & Fujiura, G. (1987). National study of public spending for mental retardation and developmental disabilities. American Journal of Mental Deficiency, 92(2), 121-133.

Center for the Study of Social Policy. (1988). Completing the long term care continuum: An income supplement strategy. Washington, DC: Center for the Study of Social Policy.

Cohen, E., (1987). History of services for memory impaired elderly. In L. Hiatt, N. Merlino, & J. Ronch (Eds.). Innovations in the care of the memory impaired elderly (pp. 9-16). New York: New York State Department of Health.

Cohen, J., & Struening, E. L. (1962). Opinions about mental illness in the personnel of two large mental hospitals. Journal of Abnormal and Social Psychology, 64(5), 349-360.

Conley, R., & McCoy, J. L. (1984). Board and care: An overview of department of health and *human services research findings.* Washington, DC: U.S. Department of Health and Human Services, Social Security Administration.

Conroy, J., Feinstein, C., & Lemanowicz, J. (1986). *Principles of quality assurance: Recommendations for action in Pennsylvania.* Philadelphia: Temple University Developmental Disabilities Center.

Conservation Company. (1989). *A study of characteristics and condition of personal care home residents in Pennsylvania* (Vols. 1 & 2). Philadelphia: Pennsylvania Departments of Public Welfare, Health and Aging.

Derogatis, L. R., & Spencer, P. M. (1982). *The Brief Symptom Inventory (BSI) Administration, Scoring & Procedures Manual—1.* Baltimore: Clinical Psychometrics Research.

Dittmar, N. D., & Bell, J. C., (1983). *Board and care for elderly and mentally disabled populations* (Vols. 1-4). Denver: Denver Research Institute, University of Denver.

Duke University Center for the Study of Aging and Human Development. (1978). *Multidimensional functional assessment: The OARS methodology.* Durham, NC: Duke University.

Fairweather, G. (Ed.). (1980). The Fairweather Lodge: A twenty-five Year Perspective. *New Directions in Mental Health Services, No. 7.* San Francisco: Jossey-Bass.

Faulk, L. E., Jr., (1988). Quality of life factors in board and care homes for the elderly: A hierarchical model. *Adult Foster Care Journal, 2*(2), 100-117.

Goffman, E. (1961). *Asylums: Essays on the social situation of mental patients and other inmates.* New York: Doubleday.

Goldmeier, J., Mannino, F., & Shore, M. (Eds.). (1978). In *New directions in mental health care: Cooperative apartments 5.* (DHEW Pub. No. [ADM]), 78-685. Washington, DC: U.S. Government Printing Office.

Gottesman, L. (1974). Nursing home performance as related to resident traits, ownership, size and source of payment. *American Journal of Public Health, 64,* 269-276.

Gottesman, L., & Bourestom, N. (1974). Why nursing homes do what they do. *The Gerontologist, 14*(6), 501-506.

Gottesman, L., & Brody, E. M. (1975). Psychological intervention programs within the institutional setting. In S. Sherwood (Ed.), *Long-term care: A handbook for researchers, planners, and providers* (pp. 455-509). New York: Spectrum.

Gottesman, L., Ishizaka, B., & MacBride, S. (1979). Service management-plan and concept in Pennsylvania. *The Gerontologist, 19,* 379-385.

Harmon, C. (1982, June). *Board and care: An old problem, a new resource for long term care.* Washington, DC: Center for the Study of Social Policy.

Helmes, E., Csapo, K. G., & Shor, J. A. (1987). *A survey of psychological functioning in the institutionalized elderly in Ontario.* Bulletin #8605 ISBN # 0711-0612, London, Ontario: Department of Psychiatry, The University of Western Ontario.

Homans, G. C. (1950). *The Human Group.* New York: Harcort Brace.

Institute for Health & Aging (IHA). (1984). Data from 1983 Residential Care Facility Telephone Survey. San Francisco: IHA, University of California.

Karp, N. (1986). *Programs demonstrating model practices for integrating people with severe disabilities into the community* (mimeo). Syracuse, NY: Center on Human Policy, Syracuse University.

Lakin, K. C., Hill, B. K., White, C. C., & Write, E. A. (1987). *Medicaid's intermediate care facility for the mentally retarded (ICF-MR) program: An update* (Report No. 25). Minneapolis: Department of Educational Psychology, University of Minnesota.

Lamb, H. R., & Goertzel, V. (1972). High expectations of long term ex-state hospital patients. *American Journal of Psychiatry, 129,* 131–135.

Lawrence, F., & Volland, P. J. (1988). The community care program: Description and administration. *Adult Foster Care Journal, 2*(1), 26–37.

Lehman, A. F., & Linn, L. S. (1984). Crimes against discharged mental patients in board-and-care homes. *American Journal of Psychiatry, 141*(2), 271–274.

Lehman, A. F., Reed, S. K., & Possidente, S. M. (1982). Priorities for long term care: Comments from board and care residents. *Psychiatric Quarterly, 54*(3), 181–189.

Linn, M. M., Klett, J., & Caffey, E. M. (1980). Foster home characteristics and psychiatric patient outcome. *Archives of General Psychiatry, 37,* 129–132.

McCoin, J. M. (1987). Adult foster care: Old wine in a new glass. *Adult Foster Care Journal, 1*(1), 21–41.

National Association of Residential Care Facilities. (1987). *1987 Directory of residential care facilities.* Richmond, VA: Author.

Newcomer, R. J., & Grant, L. (1988). *Residential care facilities: Understanding their role and improving their effectiveness* (Policy Paper No. 2 [1]). San Francisco: Institute for Health & Aging, University of California at San Francisco.

Office of Mental Health. (1985, November). *Mental health bulletin: Characteristics of personal care home residents in Pennsylvania.* Harrisburg, PA: Department of Public Welfare, Commonwealth of Pennsylvania.

Office of Mental Health. (1986, June). *Pennsylvania adult concept paper* (mimeo). Department of Public Welfare, Commonwealth of Pennsylvania.

Oktay, J. S., Horwitz, K., & Volland, P. J. (1988). Evaluation of the quality of care and the cost of the community care program. *Adult Foster Care Journal, 2*(1), 52–71.

Pennsylvania Department of Public Welfare (1987). *Interdepartmental task force report on long term care.* Unpublished paper.

Plum, K. C. (1987). Moving forward with deinstitutionalization: Lessons of an ethical policy analysis. *American Journal of Orthopsychiatry, 57*(4), 508–514.

Randolph, F. L., Laux, B., & Carling, P. J. (1987). In search of housing. In *Creative approaches to financing integrated housing.* Rockville, MD: National Institute of Mental Health.

Segal, S. P., & Aviram, U. (1978). *The mentally ill in community-based sheltered care: A study of community care and social integration.* New York: Wiley.

Sherwood, C., & Seltzer, M. M. (1981). *Task III report—Board and care literature review, evaluation of board and care homes.* Boston: School of Social Work, Boston University.

Sherwood, S., & Gruenberg, L. (1979). *Domiciliary care management information system* (mimeo). Boston: Hebrew Home for the Aged, Department of Social Gerontological Research.

Sherwood, S., & Morris, J. (1981). *Pennsylvania's domiciliary care pilot program.* Boston: Hebrew Home for the Aged, Department of Social Gerontological Research.

Stone, R., & Newcomer, R. J. (1985). The state role in board and care housing. In C. Harrington, et al., *Long term care of the elderly: Public policy issues.* Beverly Hills, CA: Sage.

Sylvester, C., & Sheppard, F. (1988). Health and social service in the community care program. *Adult Foster Care Journal, 2*(1), 38–51.

Talbot, J. A. (Ed.). (1978). *The chronic patient: Perspectives from the 29th institute on hospital and community psychiatry.* Washington, DC: American Psychiatric Association.

Test, M. A., & Stein, L. I. (1976). Practical guidelines for the community treatment of markedly impaired patients. *Community Mental Health Journal, 12*(1), 72–82.

Test, M. A., & Stein, L. I. (1977). Special living arrangements: A model for decision making. *Hospital and Community Psychiatry, 28*(8), 608–610.

U.S. General Accounting Office (GAO). (1979). *Identifying the disabled: A major step toward resolving a national problem.* Report to the Congress by the Comptroller General of the U.S. Washington, DC: U.S. General Accounting Office.

U.S. General Accounting Office (GAO). (1989). *Board and care: Insufficient assurances that residents' needs are identified and met.* Report to Congressional Requesters by the Comptroller General of the U.S. Washington, DC: U.S. General Accounting Office. GAO/HRD-89-50.

U.S. Office of the Inspector General. (1982, April). *Board and care homes: A study of federal and state actions to safeguard the health and safety of board and care residents.* Washington, DC: U.S. Office of the Inspector General.

Volland, P. J. (1988). Foster care for the frail elderly. *Adult Foster Care Journal, 2*(1), 72–82.

Zweben, A. (1979). Family care for the mentally ill: A new perspective. *Social Work in Health Care, 5*(2), 205–217.

PART V

Methodological and Research Resources Issues

16

Methodological Issues in Long-Term Follow-Up Studies of Chronic Mental Illness

John A. Toner, Ann C. Stueve

The purposes of this chapter are to discuss what can be learned about chronic mental illness in old age from follow-up investigations of schizophrenia and other psychiatric disorders, to review some of the problems associated with long-term follow-up studies, and to suggest practical strategies for conducting such studies with the chronically mentally ill elderly. Although many of our comments pertain to the course and outcomes of schizophrenia (a major contributor to chronic mental illness among the elderly), much of the discussion is relevant to other diagnostic and age groups. Most of the problems described, along with the practical approaches taken by investigators to solve these problems, are typical of those encountered in large-scale follow-up studies of any age group, with or without psychiatric disorders.

Perhaps the most challenging aspect of any follow-up study is the problem of tracking subjects, especially when the time interval is long and recontact was not anticipated in the initial study design. There are also problems associated with interviewing elderly respondents, who are more likely than other age groups to be physically frail and/or cognitively impaired. Follow-up studies also present organizational problems, especially if staff responsible for conducting follow-up interviews are kept blind to baseline information since baseline information is essential for relocating subjects. Since many subjects may be deceased, uncooperative, or too impaired at follow-up to be interviewed, questions arise about whether and how to obtain information from proxy informants.

These issues, along with a host of related concerns, are discussed in this chapter. However, because the success of longitudinal work hinges on the successful tracing and reassessment of subjects, we give primary attention to strategies for organizing data collection and relocating respondents. Before turning to methodological considerations, we begin with discussions of critical questions that are best addressed with longitudinal research.

ISSUES FOR LONGITUDINAL RESEARCH

Longitudinal studies, especially those covering a decade or more, are generally more difficult and costly than cross-sectional studies, raising the question why embark on this form of research?

First, long-term follow-up studies are necessary for accurate descriptions of the courses of mental disorders, as demonstrated by the findings of Bleuler (1978a, 1978b), Ciompi (1980, 1985), Harding, Brooks, Ashikaga, Strauss, and Breier (1987a, 1987b), Tsuang and Dempsey (1979), and others. Each of these studies challenges the commonly held view of schizophrenia as a necessarily deteriorating condition with the observation of sizable numbers of once schizophrenic individuals who are largely asymptomatic and/or functioning quite well at follow-up. In addition, what looks to be a deteriorating condition early in the course of the disorder may turn around or stabilize with time (Bleuler, 1978a; Harding et al., 1987a). Fluctuating courses also characterize some individuals with schizophrenia, as seen in the typologies developed by Bleuler (1978b), Ciompi (1980), and Huber, Gross, Schuttler, and Linz (1980). Less optimistic results reported by McGlashan (1984c) and Stone, Stone, and Hurt (1987) serve as powerful reminders that not all cases of schizophrenia improve over the life cycle, however, and Huber et al. (1980) and Vaillant (1978) show that some who improve initially eventually take a turn for the worse.

Such a variety of courses are easily missed with cross-sectional snapshots of hospital populations or consecutive admissions, where subjects of all ages are likely to be quite debilitated. They also risk being missed in longitudinal studies of short duration and in follow-up studies that assess outcome only at one point in time. Harding and colleagues (1987a) report, for example, that the profile of patients tracked in the Vermont Study changed substantially (and for the better) between the 10- and 20–25-year follow-ups. To complicate the picture further,

Strauss and Carpenter (1972, 1974, 1977, 1978) demonstrate that single global indicators of outcome are conceptually and empirically inadequate and emphasize the importance of tracking multiple components of outcome (see also Harding, 1986). They report only moderate associations among hospitalizations, social, occupational, and symptom measures at both two- and five-year follow-ups of persons with several psychiatric disorders.

While the variety of courses reported in the literature in part reflects differences in sample composition, diagnostic criteria, choice of outcome measures, etc., our understanding of the relationship between such factors and courses of schizophrenia remains incomplete (Westermeyer & Harrow, 1988). The same can be said of other psychiatric disorders. For example, Coryell and Winokur (1982) conclude from their review of longitudinal research on affective disorders: "The prognosis is quite good for a large proportion of patients, but many others experience marked long term impairment. Results of outcome comparisons between unipolar and bipolar illness are inconsistent" (p. 103). They also note that "nosological variations across existing follow-up studies severely limit firm conclusions" (p. 103). Indeed more may be known about the natural history of schizophrenia than of other disorders that contribute to the population of chronically mentally ill elderly. (For research on the course and outcomes of affective disorders, we refer the reader to Angst, 1986; Coryell & Winokur, 1982; Keller et al., 1984; Lavori, Keller, & Klerman, 1984; Prien, 1984; Tsuang & Dempsey, 1979).

Second, in addition to providing descriptive information on the range and relative frequency of different courses and outcomes (which serve as guides in clinical management), long-term follow-up studies inform our conceptualization of psychiatric disorders insofar as disorders (or their subtypes) are expected to manifest different courses. They also inform the refinement and validation of diagnostic criteria by permitting investigations of which criteria—e.g., Feighner, Research Diagnostic Criteria, DSM-III, DSM-III-R, first-rank symptoms (for schizophrenia)—identify the most homogeneous case groups with respect to outcome or course. The development of diagnostic criteria has consumed considerable time and energy on the part of the American research community in recent years, and debates about concepts and criteria persist both within the American community and between American and European traditions. For example, controversy continues over the relative utility of broad versus narrow conceptions of schizophrenia. Whether or not late-onset schizophrenialike conditions merit a separate diagnosis also warrants further investigation, as does the validity of the various paraphrenia subtypes that have been suggested by Post and others (Gurland, 1988). Westermeyer and Harrow (1988) also point out that many early longitudinal investigations of schizophrenia failed to include non-schizophrenic comparison groups, yet "a comparison of different diagnostic groups is of value to disentangle the relative predictive merits of various diagnostic and prognostic criteria, and to justify schizophrenia as a disease-specific concept" (p. 230). Inclusion of "normal" groups is also needed in long-term follow-up studies to separate disorder-specific changes from normative responses to the aging process and old age.

A third use of long-term follow-up studies lies in the identification of prognostic variables. For example, several studies indicate that early onset, insidious onset, poor premorbid personality and functioning, absence of affective symptoms, and absence of precipitating factors are associated with poorer outcomes in adult onset schizophrenia (Stephens, 1978; Strauss, Kokes, Carpenter, & Ritzler, 1978; Westermeyer & Harrow, 1988). Not only do these call for replication using different conceptualizations and diagnostic criteria, but long-term follow-up studies would also shed light on whether similar factors predict poor outcome in cases of paraphrenia as well as other psychiatric disorders. Indeed, a core question in the field of chronic mental illness is whether a common set of prognostic factors, identifiable early in the disorder, predict chronic impairments or poor outcomes across a range of diagnoses. This question also speaks to the validation issues discussed earlier insofar as predictors of course are expected to be disorder specific. In a two-year follow-up of first admission schizophrenic (DSM-III) and nonschizophrenic subjects, Strauss et al. (1978) report that the same variables predicted outcome in the two groups. Whether these results hold for narrower definitions of schizophrenia and over longer time intervals are important topics for follow-up research. Toner, Gurland, and Leung (in press) also note the large numbers of elderly psychiatric patients with severe deficiencies in communication and suggest the hypothesis that early-life deficits in communication skills may predict severe impairments in old age. McGlashan's (1986a) longitudinal work also raises the question of whether prognostic variables remain constant over the duration of the disorder: his data suggest that at least some predictors of short, medium, and long-term outcomes in schizophrenia are not the same.

Finally, follow-up studies provide a vehicle for chronicling many other changes in the lives of psychiatric patients. For example, little is known about how individuals' experiences of mental illness change over the course of the disorder, although Gurland and Toner suggest that such a phenomenological change is central to the transition from acute to chronic illness (see Chapter 1, this volume). Similarly, little is known about long-term changes in symptom content and configuration, quality of life, and coping strategies, and how they are jointly shaped by both normative age-related changes and the disease process. Long-term follow-up studies also provide an opportunity to record how changes in mental health policy are played out in the lives of individuals. For example, it would be enlightening to track what has become of individuals who were caught up in the state hospital system at the start of the deinstitutionalization movement as well as individuals with psychiatric disorders who came of age after the movement had taken hold. In short, we believe that long-term follow-up studies, especially those with repeated assessments at frequent intervals, hold great promise for enhancing our understanding of the evolution and experience of chronic mental illness among the elderly and other age groups.

METHODOLOGICAL ISSUES IN AND ALTERNATIVES TO FOLLOW-UP STUDIES

There are two basic types of follow-up investigations: prospective studies and retrospective cohort designs (Kelsey, Thompson, & Evans, 1986). In a prospective study, the researcher defines a sample on the basis of current characteristics and follows the sample forward in time. In a retrospective design, the investigator defines a sample on the basis of some past characteristic or exposure (e.g., first admission to hospital during some specified prior interval, or participation in an earlier study) and then reconstructs their subsequent course up to some later point in time. Retrospective follow-up studies require less time to complete than prospective cohort studies of similar duration and are the focus of the rest of this chapter. However, the issues we discuss apply to both types of studies, especially when the studies span a decade or more.

Although we strongly advocate follow-up investigations of chronic mental illness, such studies entail considerable investment of time and resources and are subject to practical and methodological difficulties. Thus, before deciding to undertake such a venture, several issues and problems that recur in this type of research should be weighed.

First are issues concerned with the representativeness of the baseline sample and the extent to which results can be generalized. Many long-term investigations of psychiatric disorders begin with samples of hospitalized patients, yet patient samples are often not representative of individuals with a particular disorder, especially if most affected individuals are not hospitalized. Even if the baseline sample is truly representative of a well-defined population, as Rutter points out, "the longitudinal sample can only be representative of the population as it was constituted some years ago" (1981, p. 326). If a geographic area has undergone substantial changes due to migration, as is the case for the elderly in many central cities, findings from the follow-up of a community sample may not reflect the experiences of current residents. The same applies to patient populations. Results from the follow-up of pre-deinstitutionalization patient samples, for example, may not apply to current psychiatric patient populations. Rutter suggests ways of combining cross-sectional samples with longitudinal investigations to minimize this problem.

More significant is the problem of sample attrition, due to death, refusal or inability to participate, or inability to trace. Many studies indicate that individuals who agree to participate tend to differ systematically in terms of outcome and/or baseline characteristics from nonrespondents, and those who refuse may differ systematically from those who are never successfully traced (Criqui, Barrett-Conner, & Austin, 1978; Greenland, 1977; Kelsey et al., 1986; Rutter, 1981). While the availability of baseline data allows one to assess better the type and extent of differences between responders and nonresponders in follow-up compared with cross-sectional studies, nevertheless, as Kelsey et al. point out, "the only way to ensure that differential losses to follow-up have not biased study results is to hold all losses to an absolute minimum" (1986, p. 137). This means that the feasibility of locating follow-up data on the vast majority of the baseline sample must be determined. This entails considering not only the composition of the baseline sample (since some groups are more difficult to trace than others) but also the adequacy of "leads" to relocation provided by baseline data, the resources that can be devoted to follow-up efforts, access to interim records and other informational sources that can aid in sample retrieval, and the acceptability of one's procedures to relevant Institutional Review Boards (IRBs).

The adequacy and timeliness of baseline measures must also be considered. Scientific interests, theories, and instrumentation change over time, so that the selection and measurement of baseline variables may not be adequate by current standards (Harway, Mednick, & Mednick, 1984). Even if resources are allocated to recoding or supplementing baseline data (e.g., rediagnosis of subjects' psychiatric status at baseline using current criteria), the extent to which baseline raw data are sufficiently complete across respondents must be determined. Some variables, of course, cannot be recaptured, such as those based on new technologies.

There is also the difficulty of filling in the gaps between baseline and follow-up. For many questions, the longer the timespan between baseline and follow-up, the more likely that intervening events play an important role in shaping the outcomes of interest. Many of these events may be particular to the lives of subjects; others may stem from more global changes in treatment modalities, public policies, and the like. Problems posed by memory failure and biases introduced by differential recall of past experiences are well documented (Gutek, 1978; Powers, Goudy, & Keith, 1978; Raphael, 1987) and call for creative approaches to reconstructing and corroborating the past (see below).

Given the difficulties entailed in locating respondents, there is an understandable tendency to collect as much data as possible, often from records and significant others as well as the subjects themselves. The sheer volume of data collected calls for numerous staffing, quality control, data management, and storage considerations (Gruenberg & Le Resche, 1981, p. 323). Follow-up studies may also call for extensive political connections and networking to gain access to data and the nurturing of "goodwill" on the part of many individuals.

Ethical considerations also loom large in long-term follow-up studies, particularly in light of the techniques often needed to relocate subjects. Unlike prospective studies, where one informs participants at baseline of the longitudinal nature of the study, follow-up studies are often undertaken as an afterthought. This can create a chicken-and-egg problem, insofar as records generally considered confidential (at least by the public) are needed to relocate subjects, but subjects cannot grant permission to release records or even be informed of their use until they are traced. Given the stigma associated with mental illness, follow-up studies are particularly problematic. Not only is there a risk that letters and phone calls targeted to subjects will be seen or overheard by relatives, but relatives and neighbors are often approached directly for information on study subjects. Even if care is taken not to reveal the psychiatric focus of the study or history of the subject (as is the case for the studies discussed later in this chapter), there is always the potential for slips and mistakes.

Finally, it is important to underscore that not all questions about chronic mental illness require long-term follow-up studies, and those that do may not require new data collection. For example, Harway and Mednick (1984) have compiled information on 380 longitudinal projects undertaken in the United States that are potentially suitable for secondary analyses; selected projects are described by the original investigators in the two-volume *Handbook of Longitudinal Research* (Mednick, Harway, & Finello, 1984). While these studies encompass a wide range of age groups and research interests, some are clearly relevant to the study of aging and chronic mental illness (see especially chapters by Harding & Brooks, Srole & Fischer, and Tsuang).

In addition, many datasets concerned with aging, adult development, and health are easily available for secondary analysis through the National Archive of Computerized Data on Aging (NACDA). Funded by the National Institute on Aging and housed within the Inter-university Consortium for Political and Social Research (ICPSR) at the University of Michigan, NACDA supplies most data and documentation free of charge to individuals affiliated with ICPSR member institutions; analogous services are available for a fee to unaffiliated individuals. Information on NACDA holdings can be found in *Data Collections from the National Archive of Computerized Data on Aging* (ICPSR, 1988); this and other information on ICPSR are available in single copies without charge by writing ICPSR/NACDA, P.O. Box 1248, Ann Arbor, MI 48106.

A final alternative to mounting a full-scale follow-up study is to limit the study to information available from records. Research on differential mortality, for example, can be conducted using the National Death Index (see below). Hospitalization records have also been creatively used. Goldstein (1988), for example, investigated gender differences in the course of schizophrenia by linking data from the New York State Department of Mental Health on number and duration of hospitalizations with information abstracted from the hospital records of a sample of first and second admission patients. Engelhardt, Rose, Feldman, Engelhardt, and Cohen (1982) challenged the "revolving door" thesis of current hospital admissions practices by tracing the hospitalization records of 646 schizophrenic outpatients over a 15-year period. While access to and use of records can itself be problematic (see especially Robins, 1986), records searches often provide more expedient investigations of research hypotheses and may entail less intrusion into the lives of individuals.

DATA COLLECTION STRATEGIES

In this section we describe specific strategies for relocating subjects and organizing the data collection effort. In the course of doing so, we also touch briefly upon strategies used to protect subjects' rights of privacy and confidentiality and issues that arise in the assessment process. We draw on three sets of information. First are methodological texts that discuss the design and conduct of follow-up studies, especially chapters from *Methods in Observational Epidemiology* (Kelsey et al., 1986), *Handbook of Survey Research* (Rossi, Wright, & Anderson, 1983), and *Handbook of Longitudinal Research: Volume One* (Mednick et al., 1984). Second are published descriptions of the history and methodology of individual projects, especially those focusing on mental health. These include both classic texts such as Robins's *Deviant Children Grown Up* (1966) and Myers and Bean's *A Decade Later: A Follow-up of Social Class and Mental Illness* (1968), as well as descriptions of recent and ongoing follow-up studies. Several excellent accounts of follow-up strategies with adolescent and adult American populations are included in Volume 2 of the *Handbook of Longitudinal Research* (especially chapters by Brunswick, Harding, & Brooks, and Steel, Wise, & Abeles); several European studies are described in Mednick and Baert's (1981) edited volume; additional references are listed in Table 16.1. Follow-up studies outside the field of mental health were also selectively consulted (e.g., Boice, 1978).

Our final source of information comes from informal interviews with investigators who have successfully conducted long-term follow-up studies of psychiatric patients or community samples (or short-term studies with special populations; e.g., the homeless). Several of these individuals also provided unpublished documentation or instruments from their studies.[1]

We have tried to incorporate studies that cover a variety of settings and populations and that emphasize psychiatric or mental health outcomes. We do not pretend to have systematically reviewed all of the long-term longitudinal studies that could have provided information for this chapter, nor have we limited our coverage to studies focused on the chronically mentally ill elderly. We do, however, highlight studies that include subjects that were elderly or in late middle age by follow-up.

Relocating the Sample: It Can Be Done!

Perhaps the most important point to make about long-term follow-up studies is that with time, effort, ingenuity, and perseverance, most subjects (or their significant others) can be relocated. Table 16.1 summarizes the retrieval record, length of follow-up, sample characteristics, and major publications of several recent American longitudinal studies whose subjects were middle-aged or older at follow-up. All involve interviews with subjects or their significant others; studies relying exclusively on records are not included. Five of the studies—the combined Iowa 500 and non-500, Maine, Vermont, Chestnut Lodge, and PI 500—focus on psychiatric patient samples. The Iowa 500 and non-500 (the two companion studies are combined in Table 16.1) include patients with dianoses of schizophrenia, mania, depression, or atypical schizophrenia and a control group of surgical patients from the same period. The Maine and Vermont studies represent a collaborative effort. The Vermont study focuses on back-wards patients who were released to a "hospital-run comprehensive community aftercare program between 1955 and 1962" (Harding et al., 1987a, p. 718); 79% received DSM-I baseline diagnoses of schizophrenia, and 44% of the total sample were rediagnosed as DSM-III schizophrenia at baseline (Harding et al., 1987b). The Maine sample was selected to match the Vermont patients on length of hospitalization, sex, and age in order to assess the effects of the aftercare program on outcome; the Vermont instruments and procedures were used (DeSisto, personal communication). The PI 500 followed patients admitted for long-term "psychoanalytically oriented psychotherapy" to the General Clinical Service of the New York State Psychiatric Institute (Stone, 1987, p. 187); nearly 30% were rediagnosed as having DSM-III schizophrenia at baseline, and 54% had DSM-III borderline personality disorder. The Chestnut Lodge study followed patients from this private psychiatric hospital in Rockville, Maryland. Chestnut Lodge "specializes in the long-term residential treatment of severely [and usually chronically] ill patients" (McGlashan, 1984b, p. 573). Clausen (1986), by contrast, focused on the families, mainly spouses, of first-admission patients, most of whom were psychotic; 35% were rediagnosed as definitely or probably schizophrenic by Research Diagnostic Criteria and 28% as possibly schizophrenic at baseline. Srole's study is a 20-year follow-up of the now classic community survey of Midtown Manhattan residents; unlike the other studies, it does not focus on a psychiatric population but charts changes in role functioning and mental health of a community sample.

Only the Vermont study was initially planned as a longitudinal study, yet as Table 16.1 indicates, in each case two-thirds or more of the subjects were relocated (though not always reinterviewed) 10 or more years after initial contact. Four studies—Iowa 500 and non-500, Maine, Vermont, and PI 500—traced over 90% of the original sample to their death or current address and, drawing upon multiple sources of information (e.g., interviews with patients, their significant others, medical records), were able to rate outcomes for over 85% of the original subjects (DeSisto, personal communication; Harding et al., 1987a; Stone, 1987; Tsuang & Fleming, 1987). Clausen (1986) relocated and interviewed either the

TABLE 16.1 Design and Retrieval Characteristics of Selected Long-term Follow-up Studies

Study references[1]	Diagnostic profile of baseline sample[2]		Duration & timing of follow-up	Sample selection & baseline characteristics	Retrieval record[3]	
Iowa 500 and Iowa non-500 (combined)	Schizophrenia	200	30–40 yr.	Psychiatric cases selected from 3800 consecutive admissions to the	baseline sample N = 1171	
Coryell & Tsuang, 1986;	Mania	100	Index admission or baseline: 1934–1945	University of Iowa Psychiatric Hospital between 1934 and 1945.	%traced (of baseline)	97%
*Morrison et al., 1973; Tsuang, 1984, 1986;	Depression	225		Control group of 336 appendectomy and herniorrhaphy patients	%rated[4] (of baseline)	92%
Tsuang & Dempsey, 1979; *Tsuang & Fleming, 1987;	Atypical schizophrenia	310		admitted to the surgical department of the University of Iowa's	%dead (of traced)	45%
*Tsuang & Winokur, 1975; Tsuang & Woolson, 1978;	Surgical controls	336		general hospital between 1938 and 1948. Proportionate to case groups	%living (of traced)	55%
Tsuang, Woolson, & Fleming, *1979, 1980;				on age range at admission, sex ratio, and mode of payment.	% Ss interviewed[5] (of traced & living)	71%
Tsuang, Woolson, & Simpson, 1980, 1981; Tsuang, et al., 1981.				Mean age at index admission & follow-up:	% Ss interviewed[5] (of baseline)	38%

	ADM	FU
Schizophrenia	28.6	64+7
Mania	34.2	65+10
Depression	43.8	72+10
Atypical schizophrenia	27.7	—
Surgical controls	29.8	61+11

Study references[1]	Diagnostic profile of baseline sample[2]		Duration & timing of follow-up	Sample selection & baseline characteristics	Retrieval record[3]	
Family Impact Study	Schizophrenia (RDC, definite or probable)	35%	15–20 yr.	Families (spouses) of 63 married white persons, 20–49 yrs. first admitted to a public mental hospital	baseline sample N = 80	
Clausen, *1975, 1983, 1984; *1986;			Index admission or baseline: 1950s	in the Washington, D.C. area in the 1950s;	%traced (of baseline)	92%
Clausen & Huffine, 1979; *Clausen & Yarrow, 1955;	Schizophrenia (possibly)	28%			%rated[4] (of baseline)	82%

294

References	Sample description	Follow-up	Diagnostic / outcome distribution		Tracing / follow-up status	
*Sampson, et al., 1964.	Plus, 17 married women first admitted to a California state mental hospital in the late 1950s (initially studied by Sampson, Messinger & Towne).		Affective disorder	18%	%dead (of traced)	15%
			Non-psychotic psychiatric disorders	19%	%living (of traced)	85%
			Other	1%		
Midtown Manhattan II *Fischer, et al., 1979; Srole, 1985; Srole & Fischer, 1984; *Srole, Fischer, & Biel, 1985; *Srole, et al., 1962.	Probability sample representative of the resident Midtown Manhattan population between the ages of 20 and 59 in 1954. N = 1660. Non-institutional, white, urban sample, heterogeneous with respect to other demographic variables.	20 yr. Index interview: 1954	Baseline mental health impairment profile:		baseline sample N = 1660	
			Well	22%	%traced (of baseline)	68%
			Mild impairment	43%	%dead (of traced)	24%
			Moderate	21%	%living (of traced)	76%
			Marked	9%	% Ss interviewed[5] (of traced & living)	81%
			Severe	4%	% Ss interviewed[5] (of baseline)	42%
			Incapacitated	0.6%		
Chestnut Lodge Dingman & McGlashan, 1986, 1988; McGlashan, *1984a, 1984b, 1984c, 1986a, 1986b, 1986c.	All patients without organic brain syndrome hospitalized at Chestnut Lodge more than 3 months and discharged between 1950 and 1975 (N = 582); Plus, patients admitted to Chestnut Lodge between 1945 and 1975 and still in residence in 1975 (N = 34). White, upper socioeconomic brackets; 4/5 ill more than two years at index admission & averaged 3 prior hospitalizations. Mean age at admission to Chestnut Lodge = 29 yr.	2–32 yr.; average = 15 yr. Index admission or baseline: 1950-1975	Retrospective rediagnosis of 532 Ss from the baseline sample:		baseline sample N = 616	
			Schizophrenia	35%	%traced (of baseline)	87%
			Schizophreniform psychosis	3%	%rated[4] (of baseline)	72%
			Schizoaffective psychosis	16%	% Ss interviewed[5] (of rated)	63%
			Bipolar disorder	4%	% Ss interviewed[5] (of baseline)	46%
			Unipolar disorder	11%		
			Schizotypal personality	6%		
			Borderline personality	18%		
			Other	6%		

(continued)

TABLE 16.1 continued

Study references[1]	Duration & timing of follow-up[1]	Diagnostic profile of baseline sample[2]	Sample selection & baseline characteristics	Retrieval record[3]
Vermont Longitudinal Research Project *Chittick, et al., 1961; *Deane & Brooks, 1967; Fenton & McGlashan, 1987; *Harding & Brooks, 1984; Harding, 1986; Harding, et al., *1987a, 1987b; Harding, Zubin, & Strauss, 1987.	20–25 yr. Index admission or baseline: 1955–1965	(DSM-III): Schizophrenia 44% Schizoaffective 12% Affective disorders 17% Atypical psychosis 7% Other 12% Organic disorders 8%	269 patients from the back wards of Vermont State Hospital who were referred to a comprehensive rehabilitation program between 1955 and 1960 and released to a comprehensive community after-care program between 1955 and 1965. All were disabled for one year or more before referral. At time of program referral, Ss were characterized as middle-aged, poorly educated, lower class, with repeated and prolonged hospitalizations (eg., Ss averaged 6 years of continuous hospitalization prior to selection into the rehabilitation program). Mean age of Ss at last follow-up = 59 yr; 2/3 of Ss were 55 yr. or older.	baseline sample N = 269 %traced 97% (of baseline) %rated[4] 97% (of baseline) %dead 27% (of traced) %living 73% (of traced) % Ss interviewed[5] 93% (of traced & living) % Ss interviewed[5] 66% (of baseline)
Maine Project Manuscript preparation in progress	20–25 yr. Index admission or baseline: 1956–1961	Data not available	269 patients from the Augusta State Hospital between 1956 and 1961. Computer matched with the Vermont sample in length of hospitalization, sex and age. Patients with	baseline sample N = 269 %traced 94% (of baseline) %rated[4] NA (of baseline)

296

Study	Sample	Diagnosis[2]		Outcomes[3]	
PI 500 Stone, 1987; *Stone, 1988; *Stone, in press; *Stone, Stone, & Hurt, 1987.	10–23 yr. average = 16 yr. Index admission or baseline: 1963–1976	Schizophrenia (DSM III)	30%	%dead (of traced)	48%
		Schizophreniform	6%	%living (of traced)	52%
		Affective psychosis	7%	% Ss interviewed[5] (of traced & living)	89%
		Other psychosis	.5%	% Ss interviewed[5] (of baseline)	44%
		Borderline personality (DSM III)	41%		
	onset of arterio-sclerotic brain disease after age 69, with a primary diagnosis of substance abuse, or admitted for legal reasons were excluded.	Other "at borderline level"	14%	baseline sample N = 550	
		Other	2%	%traced (of baseline)	95%
	550 patients screened for amenability to long-term psychoanalytically oriented psychotherapy, admitted to the general Clinical Service of the New York State Psychiatric Institute, and treated at least 3 months. Patients over 40 yrs. at admission or with verbal IQ scores less than 90 were excluded. Mean age at admission = 22 Mean IQ = 119 97% Caucasian Mean socioeconomic status - 2.7			%rated[4] (of baseline)	95%
				%dead (of traced)	12%
				%living (of traced)	88%
				% Ss interviewed[5,6] (of traced & living)	87%
				% Ss interviewed[5,6] (of baseline)	73%

[1]References with asterisk contain detailed information on the study sample and design.
[2]Based on retrospective rediagnosis of baseline data; criteria and procedures vary by study.
[3]Figures are taken or calculated from data provided in referenced articles.
[4]Adequate information obtained from subjects, informants, and/or records to rate at least some outcomes.
[5]Refers to interviews conducted by phone or in person with subjects (not proxy informants).
[6]Estimated figures.

patient or a family member for 82% of his sample. McGlashan (1984b) traced the whereabouts or death of 87% of his sample and obtained sufficient information from interviews with patients or significant others (and in a handful of cases, from records) to rate 72.4% of the baseline group. Srole relocated 67.7% of the original Midtown cohort ($N=1660$) and reinterviewed 81% of those located and still alive (695 of 858) (Srole & Fischer, 1984). Given the different focus of his study and sample composition (Srole did not interview significant others about deceased or "uncooperative" subjects), there are follow-up data on only 42% of the original sample. When one compares the proportion of baseline subjects who were personally interviewed at follow-up, however, the 42% reported by Srole compares favorably with that of several other studies.

General Components of Successful Follow-up Studies

Before launching into specific procedures for tracing subjects, it is instructive to ask what made the studies listed in Table 16.1 so successful? What emerged first in our discussions with researchers and in published documents is the utility of including significant others as informants. As Table 16.1 indicates, one can expect substantial proportions of older samples to be deceased at follow-up and that others will be too ill or mentally disturbed to complete interviews or unwilling to participate. Since survivors and participants tend to differ systematically from nonparticipants, it is critical to locate other sources of information on nonparticipants. It is also important to recognize that information provided by relatives and records may differ systematically from that provided by subjects and thus require strategies for addressing this potential source of bias. Collecting and comparing data from multiple sources on at least a subset of interviewed subjects is one possible strategy. Another entails stratifying the sample on the basis of who provided the data (subject vs. informant), conducting separate but parallel analyses, and recombining the sample only if results are similar. A thorough discussion of the problem along with design and data analytic considerations can be found in Walker, Velema, and Robins (1988).

Second, with the exception of the Midtown Manhattan project, all of the follow-up studies had access to very rich baseline material that provided leads to respondents' current whereabouts. For example, in addition to identifying demographic data about the subject, hospital records on the patient samples tended to include identifying information on relatives and visitors, detailed psychiatric and social histories, and handwritten progress notes by physicians, nurses, social workers, and the like. In addition to records, Clausen had access to multiple in-depth interviews with spouses that were conducted as part of the baseline study. As an aside, DeSisto notes that early records tend to provide many more clues to the location of former patients than the more problem-oriented computerized records often kept today. Stone also notes that emerging concerns about patient confidentiality limit the amount of peripheral information maintained in patient records.

Third, in several cases, members of the research staff were familiar with many of the subjects and their families, through either their involvement in the baseline study or their affiliations with the attending hospital or as residents of the same community. The two individuals who abstracted records in the Maine Project, for example, had worked in the state hospital and mental health system for many years, were intimately familiar with the records system, and knew many of the research subjects personally. In the Vermont project, Brooks conducted both the baseline and 10-year follow-up studies and had kept in touch with many of the former patients (Chittick, Brooks, Irons, & Associates, 1961; Deane & Brooks, 1967). In other cases, researchers were acquainted with subjects even though they had not kept track of their status and whereabouts. Stone, for exmple, was on staff at the New York State Psychiatric Institute during the baseline years of the PI 500 Study. He knew all of the psychiatric residents who served as the subjects' therapists and was acquainted with most of the subjects and their parents. He reports, "it was easy to trace the first 100 patients through their therapists, many of whom were still seeing one or two of their 'PI' patients 10-15 years later" (1987, p. 236). As principal investigator, Clausen was also acquainted with many of the baseline families in his series.

It is also notable that three of the four studies with the highest retrieval records—the Iowa 500 and non-500, Maine, and Vermont projects—are based in more rural communities. A constellation of factors may account for this phenomenon, none of which is inherently limited to rural areas. One is the relative geographic stability of subjects and/or their significant others. Harding and associates (1987a), for example, report that only 17 of the 191 nondeceased and traced subjects (9%) were residing outside Vermont at follow-up. By contrast, Chestnut Lodge draws patients from across the nation, making McGlashan's sample (and their significant others) geographically dispersed (McGlashan, 1984b). Srole reports that while approximately 50% of those located alive still resided in Manhattan, nearly 16% lived more than 100 miles from New York City (Srole, Fischer, & Biel, 1985), and one wonders what proportion of the 536 untraced respondents were lost to follow-up as they moved from place to place. Most of the patients and families traced by Clausen initially resided in the Washington, D.C., area, a city that changed from a predominantly white to a predominantly black population between baseline and follow-up. Although many of the study families remained within the larger metropolitan area, such population turnovers clearly render follow-up efforts more difficult (Clausen, 1975). Fleming also notes that compared with kinship networks in Iowa (a largely rural site), family members in the urban area where he is now working seem less informed about their patient-relatives (personal communication).

In addition to the advantage of a relatively proximate and stable sample, DeSisto identifies three other factors that facilitated their follow-up efforts: a "compact" mental health service system where personnel know one another, a research team with long-standing and collegial ties to the service system, and a research team operating under state auspices. When records were needed, there were relatively few hospitals and agencies to contact; personal relations between the research team and local service providers meant that access to records and other information was often only a phone call away; knowing the "lay of the land" facilitated the use of bureaucratic channels (both DeSisto and several of his staff have held a number of positions within the mental health system); and although the muscle of state sponsorship never had to be wielded, acting under state auspices lent credibility and authority to requests for help. By contrast, interim medical records of McGlashan's geographically dispersed sample were not concentrated in a few state hospitals, nor were they generally available. He reports that requests for information from out-of-state medical institutions usually resulted in letters indicating that such records are confidential and that access requires prior consent of the patient or family.

Ties between the research institution and wider community can also be critical. For example, Fleming notes that the excellent reputation of the University of Iowa Hospital not only opened doors with the service establishment but also helped motivate subjects and their families to participate. Brunswick (1984) also emphasizes the importance of nurturing community relations when the study focuses on what might be viewed as politically sensitive issues—in her case, a study of drug use among more than 500 urban black adolescents. Following community protests over "'black interviewers' coming around to do what 'white cops' could not," Brunswick organized a community advisory committee whose members served as local consultants, hired and trained interviewers from the economically depressed community, collaborated with local residents to convert baseline research findings into community programs, and incorporated free medical examinations and service referrals into the baseline study design (1984, pp. 291–293). Such community paybacks may have facilitated later follow-up efforts (e.g., letters of endorsement from the community advisory committee were appended to the follow-up grant application), but as Brunswick notes, "activities such as these require staff time and, therefore, can be costly. Such an expense should be considered in designing budgets for longitudinal community studies such as these" (p. 293).

Virtually everyone with whom we spoke also emphasized the importance of commitment, perseverance, ingenuity, and time as critical to the success of a follow-up study. There was near-unanimous agreement that follow-up studies are not the sort of projects that can be "run by committee"; someone must be committed to seeing the project through. Tracing subjects also calls for ingenuity and perseverance in the face of frustration. Even with efficient staffing and tracing procedures, some individuals are simply hard to find. This seems to be especially the case for geographically mobile subjects (who may be among the healthiest respondents), women who marry and change their names between baseline and follow-up, and individuals who are socially isolated and thus have no networks to help with the tracing efforts. McGlashan estimates that for every

2 hours spent interviewing, 5 hours were spent tracing. Staff spent an additional 16 to 20 hours per case abstracting records. Data collection in his study was interspersed with other activities and took approximately 5 years to complete. Time was also a factor in the other studies, with data collection generally taking between 2 and 4 years. Only Stone reports tracking his sample in less than 2 years; ironically, this data collection effort had the smallest budget and staff.

Finally, the special efforts of someone who "went the extra mile" were often noted as important to the success of a project. Goldstein, for example, recalled the staff member at the state mental health office who traced and recorded by hand the admission and discharge dates of all hospitalizations of every patient in her sample (personal communication). In addition to these general considerations, several more specific strategies were used to accomplish the research, and it is to these that we now turn.

Organizing the Data Collection Effort

The organization and staffing of the projects listed in Table 16.1 varied considerably. The PI 500, for example, was largely a single-handed effort. Stone traced and interviewed the former patients and/or their proxy informants and rediagnosed their baseline records. The project was carried out with the aid of his son in tandem with his other clinical and academic responsibilities, without benefit of external funding. Clausen also relied on a small staff for data collection. A Ph.D.-level student collaborator was based in the Washington, D.C. area, and a second post-B.A. interviewer worked in the San Francisco Bay area. These were the two locations of the baseline sample. Clausen also participated in the interviewing and tracing.

The Iowa 500 project, by contrast, entailed a considerably larger and more differentiated operation (Fleming, personal communication; see also Tsuang & Winokur, 1975; Tsuang, Woolson, & Fleming, 1979). Upper-level undergraduate and graduate students were hired to abstract records and trace respondents, with as many as five or six tracers working in two shifts. Tracers located and contacted respondents, ascertained basic information, and set up an interview time and place. Two teams of interviewers, blind to baseline information and diagnostic status, conducted the structured in-person interviews; as many as 10 clinically oriented juniors, seniors, and graduate students were hired and trained for this task. An M.B.A.-level coordinator was responsible for coordinating interviews and travel, which was considerable since in-person interviews were conducted with probands and kin regardless of location. Records and death certificates were photocopied by a clerk-administrator.

In conducting the Chestnut Lodge study, McGlashan's staff interviewed subjects first and abstracted records later, with separate teams working on the two tasks. Armed only with last known addresses found in Chestnut Lodge records, McGlashan and two social workers traced and interviewed respondents; all three interviewers were blind to subjects' prior diagnostic status and characteristics. B.A.-level psychiatric aids at Chestnut Lodge were employed to abstract medical records; as many as nine worked part-time during the most intense data collection period. A social worker/research assistant rated the abstracted information; both the chart abstractors and rater were blind to the follow-up interview results. Statistical and other consultants and a project secretary rounded out the staff (McGlashan, 1948b; personal communication).

Staffing of the Maine project included two records reviewers, two interviewers, an office manager, and the project director. The data-entry, cleaning, and analysis were carried out by a Vermont-based data manager, aided by statistical and other consultants.

While the project directors of the above studies directly hired and supervised staff to carry out the data collection, other follow-up projects have contracted out the interviewing to survey research centers. Srole, for example, retained and cosupervised experienced health survey interviewers from the National Opinion Research Center (Srole & Fischer, 1984). Brunswick (1984) relied on a tracing supervisor and clerk to relocate subjects but, following a lengthy in-house pretest and feasibility study, subcontracted out the bulk of the follow-up interviews. Neither of these studies focused on psychiatric samples, nor did their instruments require clinically experienced interviewers.

To recapitulate, decisions about the size and complexity of staffing vary by project and reflect a number of considerations, many of which are not particular to follow-up studies or studies of the elderly. For example, funding constraints, access to personnel (e.g., students vs. psychiatric aids), choice of instruments (e.g., open-ended clinical interviews vs. closed-ended structured interviews), and investigators' preferences all play a role in staff size and composition. Several staffing issues and recommendations, however, did recur throughout our interviews with follow-up investigators.

First is the question of who should be blind to what information. As many have noted, both research and clinical staff (as well as the general public) tend to make assumptions about the likely course of particular disorders. These assumptions can be grounded in theory, empirical results, clinical or personal experience, and the like. As a result, in order to keep observations and ratings as objective as possible, McGlashan, Tsuang, Harding, and their associates all emphasize the importance of keeping follow-up interviewers blind to the diagnostic and baseline status of subjects and keeping coders of baseline material blind to patients' long-term outcomes (Harding et al., 1987a; McGlashan, 1984b; Tsuang & Winokur, 1975; Tsuang et al., 1979). This has obvious implications for staffing since it requires two data collection teams. It also means that those tracing subjects, if they are to be given full background information, cannot serve as follow-up interviewers. They can, of course, rate background material.

Keeping interviewers blind to past history is particularly important for investigations using data on long-term outcome and course to assess the validity of diagnostic classifications. Clausen notes, however, that it may be less important for studies focusing on other issues. His own study, for example, focuses on the implications of psychiatric disorders for family members and does not focus on diagnostic differences in course.

Second is the necessity of careful record-keeping procedures at all stages of the data collection effort. At the beginning, careful and thorough documentation of all sources and strategies used in tracing subjects is necessary to avoid duplicating efforts and to make sure no subject is forgotten or lost. This information should also be used to identify and compare groups of easy- and hard-to-locate respondents, which in turn provides clues about the likely characteristics of subjects lost to follow-up. In addition, Harding reports that log-in and log-out forms are useful for keeping track of coding sheets and instruments, especially when several individuals (interviewers, coders, raters, etc.) are handling instruments at different times. Harding and DeSisto also note that wall charts are effective for monitoring the project's progress. For example, one chart lists the study numbers of subjects on one axis and tasks and instruments on the other. As tasks and instruments are completed, they are checked off. DeSisto also uses a chart to track the progress of interviewers, with expected and completed numbers of interviews marked. Much record keeping and scheduling can also be tracked by computer, although this method cannot completely replace visual aids and written forms.

Third, Fleming strongly recommends bringing a data manager on board at the outset of the project. An experienced data manager can set up a system that is easily used by project staff. In addition, having someone knowledgeable about database programs inform the development and layout of research instruments before they are finalized greatly facilitates data entry and circumvents many potential data management problems.

Two staff-related problems repeatedly mentioned by investigators are frustration and "burnout" on the part of tracers and role conflicts for interviewers. Locating hard-to-find subjects can become demoralizing; it is easy to put aside "difficult" repondents after many false starts and dead-end trails. Fleming notes that informal contests developed naturally among tracers or teams of tracers in the Iowa projects, and the spirit of competition motivated staff to persevere in their efforts. Randomly assigning subjects to tracers may also be useful insofar as it limits the likelihood that any one person will be tracking a disproportionate number of hard-to-reach subjects; if the number of tracers is large, however, doing so may mean that no one's detective skills become finely honed.

In addition, study designs that purposely or inadvertently foster attachments between subjects and interviewers may create role conflicts for both parties while also conferring advantages. For example, Jane Plapinger notes how investigations that entail intense, frequent contact between study participants and interviewers can subtly transform the research relationship in ways that enhance the quality of data collected and provide supportive relationships to participants; at the same time, however, "these relationships [are] often emotionally difficult for both interviewers and participants. Disengaging from these relationships require[s] care and delicacy" (Plapinger, written communication; see also Barrow et al. 1989). Role difficulties are also created when needy participants request assistance that interviewers are unable or unprepared to provide (Margaret Newmark, personal communication). Several pointers for dealing with such problems were suggested, beginning with careful selection and training of interviewers. Plapinger and Newmark also suggest that interviewers be strongly counseled not to intervene directly (unless, of course, service delivery is a component of the project) and not to reveal home phone numbers. Instead, they suggest that interviewers offer to connect needy subjects with appropriate services and, if the sample is likely to comprise many such persons, that this liaison work be explicitly recognized and built into the project budget and staff. Service linkage and follow-through may be a designated part of interviewers' responsibilities (assuming they are familiar with the service system) or assigned to another member of the central office staff.

Finally, as with any project, there are trade-offs to be made in staffing decisions. The projects with larger more differentiated staffs tended to be associated with greater scientific rigor (e.g., teams blind to baseline or follow-up status; interrater reliabilities established for chart abstractors, interviewers, diagnostic assessors; more elaborate or detailed data analyses). Such checks on the data increase confidence in the findings but are costly to implement. For investigators lacking resources to underwrite a large project and for research questions not warranting such elaborate efforts, Stone (1988) points to advantages associated with his "lone operator" method. Momentum is not lost writing proposals and waiting for funding, and costs are substantially less. He estimates the total cost of his study to be approximately $4,000, excluding his donated time (which was considerable). A lone investigator who is acquainted with the subjects may find it easier to establish rapport and elicit interviews (although the studies discussed here report few refusals).

Tracing Strategies and Sources of Information

There are two basic strategies for tracing subjects. One entails assigning subjects (along with any available background information) to individual tracers and allowing tracers to pursue any and all leads until subjects are found. Researchers using this approach (e.g., Stone) emphasize the importance of thoroughly combing baseline material for leads on respondents, constructing a "genogram," "family tree," or "informational profile" that records this information, following leads suggested by the genogram, and updating the genogram as tracing proceeds. This strategy can be thought of as a grapevine or networking approach to tracing and is best described by Stone (1988).

The second strategy entails beginning with a core set of procedures that are likely to provide data on the whereabouts of many subjects before attempting more individually tailored searches. This search strategy was described by Brunswick as "start[ing] with a procedure that was likely to locate the most respondents with the least effort, then group[ing] the remaining cases according to another common procedure that might locate a large number, [and] gradually working down to the more specialized and individually tailored follow-ups" (1984, p. 301). In one of the more thorough discussions of tracing operations available, Brunswick (1984) lists 13 tracing steps she devised to relocate her sample.

Baseline or Last Available Records

Baseline (or last available) records are an obvious place to start the tracing process. Here one is looking for information on the study subject and his or her formal and informal network that may provide clues to the subject's current whereabouts. One is also looking for identifying information that can be used to access other records (e.g., the National Death Index) or to verify that subsequent records obtained in fact refer to study subjects. In addition to the full names (including maiden names) and last addresses of study subjects, other information to look for includes alternate spellings and nicknames of subjects; identification numbers such as Social Security number, hospital identification number, date and place of birth; demographic data that may be useful in searching and verifying records (e.g;, ethnicity); schools attended (especially those with alumni associations); former residences (where subjects may return or other kin may live); occupation, places of employment, and names of co-workers; organizational affiliations; names of physicians and other treatment providers; services used or recommended; and information on particular interests or skills that may provide clues about subsequent affiliations, places of work, and the like. Since it is often necessary to track members of subjects' networks in order to locate subjects (or obtain information on deceased subjects), similar identifying information on current (or former) spouses, household members, relatives, friends, visitors, and the like should be noted.

Recording this information can be time-consuming. If baseline records are easily accessible, one might decide to abstract material only as needed, especially if most study participants can be located with limited biographical information or if there are no plans to code such information for later use in data analyses. In either case it is useful to develop a form for recording information so that efforts are not duplicated.

Telephone and City Directories

Telephone and city directories are another source of information. Names of subjects and potential informants can be searched in local directories. Many libraries contain phone directories for major metropolitan areas. In completing directory searches, it is useful to consider who is likely to be residentially stable and how subjects' names are likely to be listed. People who were middle-aged or older at baseline, for example, are more likely to have been geographically stable than younger subjects or network members. Women are often listed by their surname and initials or under the husband's name. Stone also notes the usefulness of examining subjects' and relatives' signatures to make sure that the spelling corresponds to that found in records; and added or dropped letter can greatly hinder tracing efforts.

Directory assistance can be used for subjects or informants whose whereabouts have been tentatively established. The number of names accepted and specificity of location needed by directory assistance operators vary by region and population density (e.g., Connecticut and Florida require the specific town). It is also useful to note that some localities routinely conduct a local census. Massachusetts, for example, requires that towns publish annual listings of all residents 20 or older; these listings are organized by street address and include self-reported information on residents' names, ages, and occupation. Such information can be used to verify phone numbers located for subjects by determining whether the demographic characteristics of the subject match those given in the census listings.

Phone books and reverse directories (which list by address rather than surname) can also be used to locate geographically proximate informants whose presence is otherwise unknown. For example, Brunswick looked for names and phone numbers of participants' neighbors that had not changed from baseline to follow-up. Faced with an out-of-date address for a subject with a common last name, Stone looked for persons with the same surname who lived in the immediate vicinity of the last known address.

Phone sweeps can also be conducted to locate hard-to-find subjects. For example, if the subject is known to have come from a small town, directory assistance (or phone books) can be used to locate the phone number of anyone with the same surname or maiden name as the subject or with the subject's mother's maiden name. One can then determine whether the potential contact is in fact linked to the study subject through telephone calls. Similarly, if the subject's surname, maiden name, or mother's maiden name is unusual, an analogous search can be conducted in urban areas. Stone, for example, conducted phone sweeps of the northeastern states as well as major metropolitan areas for subjects who eluded other tracing efforts.

In making such phone sweeps or tracking down neighbors, care must obviously be taken to protect the study subject whose psychiatric history may not be known to located family members and neighbors (see below). At the same time, for such tracing to be effective, it is crucial to allay the suspicions and anxieties of participants and their families. Clausen, McGlashan, and Stone, among others, became involved in the tracing process, making phone calls themselves to help establish the legitimacy of the research. Stone also emphasizes the importance of reviewing the genogram before placing such phone calls both to establish the researcher's "bona fides" and to establish quickly and accurately whether the potential informant is actually associated with the subject's family. Finally, while several studies suggest that phone work is the most effective technique for relocating subjects (e.g., Boice, 1978; Crider, Willits, & Bealer, 1971-1972), extensive phone sweeps can become costly toward the end of the tracing process, when efforts are directed toward the hard-to-reach (Boice, 1978).

General Mailings and Use of the U.S. Postal Service

General mailings are often used to relocate subjects. Although generally less effective than telephone tracking (Boice, 1978; Crider et al., 1971-1972), the lower cost often makes this a reasonable place to start. Brunswick (1984), for example, began her search by sending two first-class letters, spaced roughly a month apart, to the last known address of respondents. She enclosed an introductory letter, an answer form, and a stamped return envelope, and requested fowarding and address corrections from the post office. McGlashan (1984b) also initiated contact by mail with his geographically dispersed sample; a letter from the medical director explaining the study and a self-report questionnaire were enclosed. Telephone contact requesting an interview was initiated several weeks later following either a reply or a nonresponse.

Boice (1978) notes that because change-of-address cards are kept for only a couple of years, requests for address corrections are of limited utility for geographically mobile samples and subjects who moved long ago. Crider et al. (1971-1972) note, however, that visits to small-town and rural post offices can be effective since local personnel sometimes know the whereabouts of subjects or their families. Brunswick (1984) also conducted a borough by borough post office search for address corrections in New York City in addition to the general address-correction request.

Sending certified return-receipt-requested letters is another option. Although they are more expensive than first-class letters, Boice (1978) reports that many of the initial letters that were returned and stamped "addressee unknown" or "moved, not forwardable" were delivered when resent as certified mail. Brunswick (1984) also sent certified letters to addresses where telephone contact was not established and the two initial mailings were not returned.

Other Sources of Leads for Individually Tailored Searches

Before turning to records that have been used in follow-up studies, it is useful to mention other sources of leads to subjects' (or potential informants') whereabouts. For example, some families are served by self-designated genealogists who can be very helpful in locating kin (Stone, 1988). Hometown newspapers and churches are sometimes a source of information, if not on the subjects' current address then on whether relatives are still in the vicinity or where they have moved. Local banks may also give forwarding addresses, and as mentioned above, local post office personnel may be helpful. College alumni associations maintain rosters of members, as do many social and charitable organizations. Stone, for example, obtained the address of a subject's relative through a local social club after convincing a club official that his reasons for locating the person were legitimate.

If a prior place of employment is known, inquiries can be made of the employer, personnel department, or co-workers. Stone (1988) suggests asking for the employee with the longest tenure in the unit if more specific information is unavailable. In areas with relatively few large employers, major offices or plants can be contacted if they match with subjects' (or potential informants') lines of work. Robins (1986) notes, however, that many records, including much employment information, must be kept confidential and are no longer available for purposes of research.

Patients are another potential source of information. In long-term treatment programs especially, patients befriend one another and sometimes remain in contact over the years. Stone (1988) found what he calls the "old buddy system" to be sufficiently effective in locating some elusive patients that he chronologically ordered all subjects with respect to time of admission so that he would know which subjects were on the unit during overlapping periods. He notes that the more sociable borderline patients especially developed and maintained ties within the unit; schizophrenic patients, by contrast, were more likely to have been on the periphery and rarely provided leads to other subjects.

If tracers are members of therapist or other service-provider networks, these contacts may provide leads to subjects as well. Stone (1988) comments, however, that information gleaned from personal acquaintances may well not be forthcoming from therapists who are strangers to the investigator. Thus while Stone and DeSisto were able to mobilize their professional networks to help locate patients, McGlashan abandoned his efforts to locate subjects' physicians who were outside his network because they largely led to dead-end trails.

Locating subjects who live in rooming houses or SROs is particularly difficult because they tend to be isolated from family and have no listed phone numbers. Lists of licensed board and care homes can be obtained from local government, but operators are apt to be suspicious of calls from researchers, especially if they have ties to the licensing body. DeSisto suggests that once subjects are traced to boarding or nursing homes (or to a guardian), an introductory letter be sent to the residence director as well as to the subject, informing him or her that an interviewer will be contacting the subject and asking for a convenient time and place. This tends to allay operator concerns about the purpose of the visit and to elicit the cooperation of someone who may serve as an informant if need be.

Finally, Stone (1988) emphasizes the importance of intuition in locating elusive subjects. By this he means trying to get "inside the skin" of subjects in order to make educated guesses about where they (or their families) are likely to go. In part, this entails detecting commonalities in the movement of similar subjects. For example, he notes that affluent Protestants in his sample tended to retire to small towns and ranches; Jewish families were more likely to retire to Florida; Irish families stayed within a 100-mile radius. When faced by an otherwise unfound elderly subject or informant, he tried concentrating his efforts on a likely retirement region.

Death Records

Three useful resources for tracking samples of older subjects, many of whom are likely to be deceased by follow-up, are the National Death Index, the Social Security Administration Master Beneficiary Record File, and state Departments of Vital Statistics. Each of the three records systems leads to the retrieval of death certificates and has its advantages and limitations.

The National Death Index (NDI) is a recently established computerized index of death records compiled from data on death certificates and maintained by the National Center for Health Statistics (NCHS) (Wentworth, Neaton, & Rasmussen, 1983). The NDI is readily available for record linkage and can provide qualified researchers with information on whether, where, and when anyone matching study subjects on a number of dimensions has died in the United States, Puerto Rico, or the Virgin Islands since 1979; it also provides death certificate file numbers, which can be used to request copies of death certificates from the identified states (Stampfer et al., 1984).

Stampfer et al. (1984), Wentworth et al. (1983), and the NDI *User's Manual* discuss the use and capabilities of the NDI. In brief, NDI and study records are matched on the basis of some combination of first and last name (and for women, father's surname), month and year of birth, and Social Security number. Name matches can be made on either an exact spelling or a soundex code. Because some study subjects may be associated with multiple possible matches, the NDI also contains other identifying information (e.g., middle initials, sex, race, marital status, day and state of birth, age at death, and state of residence) that can be used to help differentiate between correct and incorrect links (Stampfer et al., 1984). Requests for data are made by submitting an NDI application form in which the research project and procedures for maintaining data confidentiality are described. Applications are reviewed quarterly, and if approved, a computer printout (or tape) is returned for a modest charge.

Investigators have assessed the sensitivity and specificity of the NDI by submitting data on cohorts of known mortality status and found the results to be excellent. Stampfer et al. (1984) submitted the names of 570 married women from 11 states and reported a sensitivity of 96.5% and a final specificity of 100% (after ruling out false positives using secondary matches). Wentworth et al. (1983) submitted the names of nearly 13,000 men between the ages of 35 and 57 years and report that the NDI correctly identified 98.4% of the known deaths. They also report a large false positive rate, however, and note that secondary matches are essential to rule out erroneously identified deaths.

Wentworth et al. (1983) note additional advantages of the NDI. For example, the service is priced on a per-record basis, making it affordable for small-scale studies. In addition, Social Security numbers are not necessary to use the system; computer processing is done by the NCHS; and several groups are more fully covered than in the Social Security Administration files (see below). However, they also note that deaths prior to 1979 are not covered, and at the time of their study, there was a considerable time lag between occurrence of death and entry into the index.

For deaths prior to 1979 two options are available. One is the Social Security Administration (SSA) Master Beneficiary Record File (MBRF). The MBRF contains a record for every person entitled to receive retirement, survivors, or disability insurance and has been maintained since 1962. Deaths resulting in lump-sum payments have been entered only since 1977; these tend to be men who die before retirement and leave no surviving children at home (Wentworth et al., 1983).

The advantages and limitations of the MBRF and NDI differ. As described by Wentworth and associates, both produce similarly accurate results for post-1978 death ascertainment, but the MBRF produces fewer false positives (i.e., erroneous deaths). The MBRF covers a longer time period and is updated on a monthly basis but may not be adequate for preretirement-age samples prior to 1977. There is evidence of a slight underreporting of deaths among rural and Southern residents, and a notable underreporting for unmarried males (and presumably others) who are less likely to be survived by SSA-eligible family members. Social Security numbers are essential for any matching algorithm, and SSA does *not* process the information in-house. Instead data from the MBRF are duplicated onto magnetic tapes and supplied at cost to approved users. Wentworth et al. report that their request for data from 1962 through June 1981 resulted in about 26 million records. While relatively inexpensive for large-scale projects with adequate computer facilities, such files can prove daunting to small-scale studies. Finally, the only data provided by MBRF are last names, Social Security numbers, and dates of death. Information is not provided on place of death, making death certificates hard to locate without additional sources of information. Wentworth et al. add that a death master file is being developed by the SSA that will include additional identifying information and should improve coverage of younger decedents.

The third source of mortality data is state Departments of Vital Statistics. McMahon (1983) points out that in order to obtain a death certificate on a study subject, it is generally necessary to know that the person has died, where the death was registered, and the approximate date of death. This information must be gleaned from other sources, for example, the NDI or interviews with informants. Ann Goodman (personal communication) suggests that it is sometimes feasible and practical to conduct a search of state death records to determine which study participants are deceased. In a 3.5-year follow-up study of 1,033 psychiatric patients, Haugland, Craig, Goodman, and Siegel "ascertained which patients had died by matching their name, age, sex, and residence with mortality data obtained from the New York State Office of Biostatistics" (1983, pp. 848–849). In addition to sex and residence, they provided the state office with names and alternate spellings and a 5-year age range; after receiving from the state office the output on possible matches, they manually ruled out the unlikely ones. Such searches for persons not known to have died become impractical, however, when many states' vital statistics departments must be approached.

Three other points about tracking via death certificate should be noted. First, if the state office permits (and not all do; Boice, 1978), the names and addresses of informants listed on death certificates can be noted and may be useful in obtaining proxy follow-up data on deceased subjects. Second, when faced with an impossible-to-find subject, one can search for death records on the subject's relatives; the listed informant may provide leads to the subject's whereabouts. Finally, whether one conducts a death-record search on all subjects, hard-to-find subjects, or only those known to be deceased depends upon a number of considerations, including the time frame of the study (e.g., post-NDI), the age of the sample, and the ease of ascertaining mortality status through other channels.

Other Records

Many other records are potentially available to qualified researchers, though they may require negotiation, assorted approvals, time, perseverance, or connections to activate. Some samplewide searches may also generate data on functioning and outcomes (e.g., arrest records), even if they do not facilitate subject retrieval. In general, the more geographically dispersed the sample, the more costly and time-consuming the searches unless the record base is centralized (e.g., the NDI) or one has very specific leads and requests.

Hospitals, other treatment centers, and social service agencies are likely sources of information on psychiatric and older subjects. While detailed records may only be available from the agencies directly, some subject-based data (e.g., state hospital admissions and discharges) may be reported to state governments. Local governments also collect data on users of publicly funded programs (e.g., shelters) that may also be available for tracking subjects who were recent service recipients. In some localities, voluntary organizations may keep track of local service recipients. For instance, both Brunswick (1984) and Robins (1966) made use of records kept by the now-defunct Social Service Exchange.

What medical and service data are recorded by state and local governments varies by location and is subject to change as new regulations take effect. For example, during the 1970s, the New York State Department of Mental Health required all private and state psychiatric hospitals to provide data on admissions and discharges; today, private hospitals are exempt (Goldstein, personal communication). The extent to which early records are accessible and computerized also varies. As a result, detective work is needed to investigate the availability and record-keeping practices of relevant medical, social service, and governmental agencies in order to determine whether and how to organize a records search. For example, Fleming notes that in the Iowa 500 study, records on subjects were requested from the four other state mental health institutes directly (personal communication). In an area served by a larger number of hospitals, however, one might directly approach facilities most likely to have been used by subjects and only supplement this effort with a "wider net" records search, if necessary.

Other databases that have been used in epidemiological follow-up studies include marriage, birth, and divorce records. Searching marriage records is particularly useful for women who were single at baseline; husbands' surnames and addresses can be added to the subjects' genograms and traced. Birth and divorce records searches tend to be time-consuming but may provide more recent addresses for otherwise unlocated subjects. Also useful are computerized records maintained by state departments of motor vehicles, which contain information on names, addresses, birth dates, and often Social Security numbers; record linkage is often feasible even with large numbers of subjects (Kelsey et al., 1986) and can be a source of recent addresses. Heim and Van Dusen (1984) provide a highly informative review of the availability, content, and use of criminal-history records for samples likely to brush with the law. Although not permitted to release addresses of recipients, state Social Security offices will sometimes forward letters to study participants whose names are included in their files; state Medicaid offices may also do so.

Finally, credit and detective agencies have been used to locate subjects once other in-house methods have been exhausted. This strategy, however, tends to be quite expensive and may decrease investigators' ability to maintain confidentiality of study and patient data.

In summary, tracking subjects is an exercise in detective work. One begins with obvious leads and follows subjects' trails. Multiple strategies may be needed for any given respondent; they certainly will be needed to locate the entire sample. Stone (1988) estimates calling a minimum of 6,000 wrong numbers in his search for respondents, and one respondent required as many as 19 different contacts to locate. While not all follow-up studies and subjects require such labyrinthine efforts, the task of relocating subjects decades later remains daunting.

Ethical Considerations

Locating subjects through mailings to last known addresses, phone sweeps, record searches, grapevine leads, clearly raises a number of ethical considerations. Thus, decisions regarding procedures for locating subjects must be made in consultation with individual ethical-review boards. Several conventions that have been used to protect patients include describing the study, the institution, and patient status in broad nonpsychiatric terms. For example, when placing phone calls or sending letters, one might describe the project as a follow-up health and attitude survey of people who were once treated at the affiliated XYZ General Hospital instead of describing the study as a psychiatric follow-up of people treated for mental problems at XYZ Psychiatric Institute. Before revealing even this information (at least in phone calls), Stone recommends using knowledge of the genogram to confirm that one has reached the designated subject or informant. For example, after introducing oneself as Dr. _____ from XYZ Hospital, one might ask, "Am I speaking with Mr. Q, father of Q Jr. who was once under our care?" If yes, one proceeds to verify other genogram information: "Then your wife must be AQ and your older daughter BQ . . . ," until one is certain that the correct person has been reached. An additional safeguard entails operating under the assumption that the person contacted, even if verified, is uninformed about the subject's history of psychiatric or other problems until clear evidence to the contrary is volunteered. Even here, investigators must be careful not to add to the informant's store of information unless sure that the subject does not consider it confidential. Among other things, this means that research instruments to be used with informants must be kept sufficiently broad in their coverage that informants do not intuit the psychiatric focus of the study and history of subjects.

There are also questions about informed consent once subjects are relocated. For example, some individuals may not be competent to give informed consent to participate. Others may refuse to participate. When phone interviews are the means of collecting data, there is the problem of how to obtain and document consent. One strategy entails informing subjects of the study's purposes by letter or phone prior to the interview and sending consent forms to be signed by subjects afterward. Consent forms, however, are not always returned by subjects, even in circumstances where subjects agree to participate. An alternative strategy entails informing subjects that interview material will be used unless they specifically request otherwise and providing mechanisms (e.g., phone contacts, change-of-consent forms) for those who wish to do so.

Other issues likely to be raised by institutional review boards include how data will be stored, who will have access, how material will be published, and what procedures will be used to minimize the identification of any individual. These are not particular to follow-up studies but are questions to be considered when designing the study and preparing IRB protocols. In addition, such questions are likely to be raised not only by the review board of the sponsoring research institution but also by review boards affiliated with organizations whose records are used.

Much has been written in recent years about the rights of study participants and tensions that ensue between subject-oriented protective procedures and the pursuit of scientific research (e.g., Cann & Rothman, 1984, 1985; Fletcher, Dommel, & Cowell, 1985; Harway, 1984; Hershey, 1981; Kelsey, 1981; Pattullo, 1982; Reich, 1978; Robins, 1986; Stanley & Stanley, 1982; Taub, 1986). There is even a journal that focuses exclusively on these issues: *IRB: A Review of Human Subjects Research.* In light of disagreements and continuing developments in the area of confidentiality, privacy, informed consent, and related matters, we refer investigators embarking on follow-up ventures to this journal for guidelines and information, as well as to members of their home institution's ethics review committee.

SUMMARY

In summary, long-term follow-up studies provide opportunities for examining a range of theoretical and policy issues regarding the development, course, and consequences of chronic mental illness among the elderly; however, they raise a host of methodological problems. In this chapter we have tried to address a number of these problems and possible solutions. The best advice, however, is to approach each new data collection effort as a potential baseline study and to weigh the costs of incorporating information that would facilitate follow-up, even if no longitudinal design is planned. The types of information that are useful have been described in this chapter; in general, the more specific and extensive the biographical and network information collected, the better for future follow-up purposes.

NOTE

1. In particular, we would like to thank the following individuals for taking the time to share their experiences and recommendations: Carol Caton, John Clausen, Patricia Cohen, Michael DeSisto, Jerome Fleming, Jill Goldstein, Ann Goodman, Courtenay Harding, Thomas McGlashan, Margaret Newmark, Jane Plapinger, Carole Siegel, Michael Stone, Elmer Streuning, and Joseph Wanderling. We would also like to thank Leo Srole for providing us with an unpublished account of the Midtown Manhattan follow-up (1985; Srole, Fischer, & Biel, 1985), and Michael Stone (1988) for providing us with an unpublished manuscript documenting his tracing efforts.

REFERENCES

Angst, J. (1986). The course of major depression, atypical bipolar disorder, and bipolar disorder. In H. Hippius, G. L. Klerman, N. Matussek, with M. Schmauss (Eds.), *New results in depression research.* Berlin: Springer-Verlag.

Barrow, S. M., Helman, F., Lovell, A. M., Plapinger, J. D., & Streuning, E. L. (1989). *Effectiveness of programs for the mentally ill homeless: Final report.* New York State Psychiatric Institute: CSS Evaluation Program.

Bleuler, M. E. (1978a). The long-term course of schizophrenic psychoses. In L. C. Wynne, R. L. Cromwell, & S. Matthysse (Eds.), *The nature of schizophrenia: New approaches to research and treatment.* New York: Wiley.

Bleuler, M. (1978b). *The schizophrenic disorders: Long-term patient and family studies.* New Haven: Yale University Press.

Boice, J. D. (1978). Follow-up methods to trace women treated for pulmonary tuberculosis, 1930-1954. *American Journal of Epidemiology, 107*(2), 127-139.

Brunswick, A. F. (1984). Health consequences of drug use: A longitudinal study of urban black youth. In S. A. Mednick, M. Harway, & K. M. Finello (Eds.), *Handbook of longitudinal research* (Vol. 2). New York: Praeger.

Cann, C. I., & Rothman, K. J. (1984). IRBs and epidemiologic research: How inappropriate restrictions hamper studies. *IRB, 6*(4), 5-7.

Cann, C. I., & Rothman, K. J. (1985). Reply: Overcoming hurdles to epidemiologic research. *IRB, 7*(2), 9.

Chittick, R. A., Brooks, G. W., Irons, F. S., & Deane, W. N. (1961). *The Vermont story.* Burlington, VT: Queen City Printers.

Ciompi, L. (1980). The natural history of schizophrenia in the long term. *British Journal of Psychiatry, 136*, 413-420.

Ciompi, L. (1985). Aging and schizophrenic psychosis. *Acta Psychiatrica Scandinavica, 71*, 93-105.

Clausen, J. A. (1975). The impact of mental illness: A twenty-year follow-up. In R. D. Wirt, G. Winokur, & M. Roff (Eds.), *Life history research in psychopathology* (Vol. 4). Minneapolis: University of Minnesota Press.

Clausen, J. A. (1983). Sex roles, marital roles, and response to mental disorder. *Research in Community and Mental Health, 3*, 165-208.

Clausen, J. A. (1984). Mental illness and the life course. In P. B. Baltes & O. G. Brim, Jr. (Eds.), *Life-span development and behavior* (Vol. 6). Orlando: Academic Press.

Clausen, J. A. (1986). A 15- to 20-year follow-up of married adult psychiatric patients. In L. Erlenmeyer-Kimling and N. E. Miller (Eds.), *Life-span research on the prediction of psychopathology.* Hillsdale, NJ: Lawrence Erlbaum.

Clausen, J. A., & Huffine, C. L. (1979). The impact of parental mental illness on children. *Research in Community and Mental Health, 1*, 183-214.

Clausen, J. A., & Yarrow, M. (1955). Introduction: Mental illness and the family. *Journal of Social Issues, 11.*

Coryell, W., & Tsuang, M. T. (1986). Outcome after 40 years in DSM-III schizophreniform disorder. *Archives of General Psychiatry, 43*, 324-328.

Coryell, W., & Winokur, G. (1982). Course and outcome. In E. S. Paykel (Ed.), *Handbook of affective disorders.* New York: Guilford Press.

Crider, D. M., Willits, F. K., & Bealer, R. C. (1971-1972). Tracking respondents in longitudinal surveys. *Public Opinion Quarterly, 35*(4), 613-620.

Criqui, M. H., Barrett-Connor, E., & Austin, M. (1978). Differences between respondents and non-respondents in a population-based cardiovascular disease study. *American Journal of Epidemiology, 108*(5), 367-372.

Deane, W. N., & Brooks, G. W. (1967). *Five-year follow-up of chronic hospitalized patients.* Waterbury, VT: Vermont State Hospital.

Dingman, C. W., & McGlashan, T. H. (1986). Discriminating characteristics of suicides: Chestnut Lodge follow-up sample including patients with affective disorder, schizophrenia and schizoaffective disorder. *Acta Psychiatrica Scandinavica, 74,* 91–97.

Dingman, C. W., & McGlashan, T. H. (1988). Characteristics of patients with serious suicidal intentions who ultimately commit suicide. *Hospital and Community Psychiatry, 39*(3), 295–299.

Engelhardt, D. M., Rose, B., Feldman, J., Engelhardt, J. A. Z., & Cohen, P. (1982). A 15-year followup of 646 schizophrenic outpatients. *Schizophrenia Bulletin, 8*(3), 493–503.

Fenton, W. S., & McGlashan, T. H. (1987). Prognostic scale for chronic schizophrenia. *Schizophrenia Bulletin, 13*(2), 277–286.

Fischer, A. K., Marton, J., Millman, E. J., & Srole, L. (1979). Long-range influences on adult mental health: The Midtown Manhattan longitudinal study, 1954–1974. *Research in Community and Mental Health, 1,* 305–333.

Fletcher, J. C., Dommel, F. W., & Cowell, D. D. (1985). Consent to research with impaired human subjects. *IRB, 7*(6), 1–6.

Goldstein, J. M. (1988). Gender differences in the course of schizophrenia. *American Journal of Psychiatry, 145*(6), 684–689.

Greenland, S. (1977). Response and follow-up bias in cohort studies. *American Journal of Epidemiology, 106,* 184–187.

Gruenberg, E. M., & Le Resche, L. (1981). Reaction: The future of longitudinal studies. In S. A. Mednick & A. E. Baert (Eds.), *Prospective longitudinal research: An empirical basis for the primary prevention of psychosocial disorders.* Oxford: Oxford University Press.

Gurland, B. J. (1988). Schizophrenia in the elderly. In M. T. Tsuang & J. C. Simpson (Eds.), *Handbook of schizophrenia* (Vol. 3): *Nosology, epidemiology and genetics.* New York: Elsevier.

Gutek, B. A. (1978). On the accuracy of retrospective attitudinal data. *Public Opinion Quarterly, 42*(3), 390–401.

Harding, C. M. (1986). Speculations on the measurement of recovery from severe psychiatric disorder and the human condition. *The Psychiatric Journal of the University of Ottawa, 11*(4), 199–204.

Harding, C. M., & Brooks, G. W. (1984). Life assessment of a cohort of chronic schizophrenics discharged twenty years ago. In S. A. Mednick, M. Harway, & K. M. Finello (Eds.), *Handbook of longitudinal research* (Vol. 2). New York: Praeger.

Harding, C. M., Brooks, G. W., Ashikaga, T., Strauss, J. S., & Breier, A. (1987a). The Vermont longitudinal study of persons with severe mental illness, 1: Methodology, study sample, and overall status 32 years later. *American Journal of Psychiatry, 144*(6), 718–726.

Harding, C. M., Brooks, G. W., Ashikaga, T., Strauss, J. S., & Breier, A. (1987b). The Vermont longitudinal study of persons with severe mental illness, 2: Long-term outcome of subjects who retrospectively met DSM-III criteria for schizophrenia. *American Journal of Psychiatry, 144*(6), 727–735.

Harding, C. M., Zubin, J., & Strauss, J. S. (1987). Chronicity in schizophrenia: Fact, partial fact, or artifact? *Hospital and Community Psychiatry, 38*(5), 477–486.

Harway, M. (1984). Confidentiality and ethics in longitudinal research. In S. A. Mednick,

M. Harway, & K. M. Finello (Eds.), *Handbook of longitudinal research* (Vol. 1). New York: Praeger.

Harway, M., & Mednick, S. A. (1984). Rationale for the study. In S. A. Mednick, M. Harway, & K. M. Finello (Eds.), *Handbook of longitudinal research* (Vol. 1). New York: Praeger.

Harway, M., Mednick, S. A. & Mednick, B. (1984). Research strategies: Methodological and practical problems. In S. A. Mednick, M. Harway, & K. M. Finello (Eds.), *Handbook of longitudinal research* (Vol. 1). New York: Praeger.

Haugland, G., Craig, T. J., Goodman, A. B., & Siegel, C. (1983). Mortality in the era of deinstitutionalization. *American Journal of Psychiatry, 140*(7), 848–852.

Heim, M., & Van Dusen, K. (1984). Usefulness of official records in longitudinal research in criminology. In S. A. Mednick, M. Harway, & K. M. Finello (Eds.), *Handbook of longitudinal research* (Vol. 1). New York: Praeger.

Hershey, N. (1981). Using patient records for research: The response from federal agencies and the state of Pennsylvania. *IRB, 3*(8), 7–8.

Huber, G., Gross, G., Schuttler, R., & Linz, M. (1980). Longitudinal studies of schizophrenic patients. *Schizophrenia Bulletin, 6*(4), 592–605.

Inter-university Consortium for Political and Social Research. (1988). *Data collections from the National Archive of Computerized Data on Aging.* Ann Arbor, MI: ICPSR.

Keller, M. B., Klerman, G. L., Lavori, P. W., Coryell, W., Endicott, J., & Taylor, J. (1984). Long-term outcome of episodes of major depression. *Journal of the American Medical Association, 252*(6), 788–792.

Kelsey, J. L. (1981). Privacy and confidentiality in epidemiological research involving patients. *IRB: A Review of Human Subjects Research, 3*(2), 1–4.

Kelsey, J. L., Thompson, W. D., & Evans, A. S. (1986). *Methods in observational epidemiology.* New York: Oxford University Press.

Kraepelin, E. (1912). On paranoid diseases. *Zentralblatt Fur Die Gesamte Neurologie Psychiatrie, 11*, 617–621.

Lavori, P. W., Keller, M. B., & Klerman, G. (1984). Relapse in affective disorders: A reanalysis of the literature using life table methods. *Journal of Psychiatric Research, 18*(1), 13–25.

McGlashan, T. H. (1984a). Chestnut Lodge follow-up study: Instructions on the use/interpretation of assessment instruments. Rockville, MD: Chestnut Lodge Research Institute.

McGlashan, T. H. (1984b). The Chestnut Lodge follow-up study, 1: Follow-up methodology and study sample. *Archives of General Psychiatry, 41*, 573–585.

McGlashan, T. H. (1984c). The Chestnut Lodge follow-up study, 2: Long-term outcome of schizophrenia and the affective disorders. *Archives of General Psychiatry, 41*, 586–601.

McGlashan, T. H. (1986a). Predictors of shorter-, medium-, and longer-term outcome in schizophrenia. *American Journal of Psychiatry, 43*(1), 50–55.

McGlashan, T. H. (1986b). The prediction of outcome in chronic schizophrenia, IV: The Chestnut Lodge follow-up study. *Archives of General Psychiatry, 43*, 167–176.

McGlashan, T. H. (1986c). Schizotypal personality disorder. Chestnut Lodge follow-up study, 6: Long-term follow-up perspectives. *Archives of General Psychiatry, 43*, 329–334.

McMahon, B. (1983). The National Death Index. *American Journal of Public Health, 73*(11), 1247–1248.

Mednick, S. A., & Baert, A. E. (Eds.). (1981). *Prospective longitudinal research: An empirical basis for the primary prevention of psychosocial disorders*. Oxford: Oxford University Press.

Mednick, S. A., Harway, M., & Finello, K. M. (Eds.). (1984). *Handbook of longitudinal research* (Vols. 1, 2). New York: Praeger.

Morrison, J., Winokur, G., Crowe, R., & Clancy, J. (1973). The Iowa 500: The first follow-up. *Archives of General Psychiatry, 29*, 678-682.

Myers, J. K., & Bean, L. L. (1968). *A decade later: A follow-up of social class and mental illness*. New York: Wiley.

Pattullo, E. L. (1982). The limits of the 'right' of privacy. *IRB, 4*(4), 3-7.

Post, F. (1984). Schizophrenic and paranoid psychoses. In D. W. K. Kay & G. D. Burrows (Eds.), *Handbook of studies on psychiatry and old age*. New York: Elsevier.

Powers, E. A., Goudy, W. J., & Keith, P. M. (1978). Congruence between panel recall data in longitudinal research. *Public Opinion Quarterly, 42*(3), 380-389.

Prien, R. F. (1984). Long-term maintenance pharmacotherapy in recurrent and chronic affective disorders. In M. Mirabi (Ed.), *The chronically mentally ill: Research and services*. New York: Spectrum.

Raphael, K. (1987). Recall bias: A proposal for assessment and control. *International Journal of Epidemiology, 16*(2), 167-170.

Reich, W. T. (1978). Ethical issues related to research involving elderly subjects. *The Gerontologist, 18*(4), 326-337.

Robins, L. N. (1966). *Deviant children grown up*. Baltimore: Williams & Wilkins.

Robins, L. N. (1986). Consequences of the recommendations of the Privacy Protection Study Commission for Longitudinal Studies. In L. Tancredi (Ed.), *Ethical issues in epidemiologic research* (pp. 99-113). New Brunswick, NJ: Rutgers University Press.

Rossi, P. H., Wright, J. D., & Anderson, A. B. (1983). *Handbook of survey research*. Orlando: Academic Press.

Rutter, M. (1981). Longitudinal studies: A psychiatric perspective. In S. A. Mednick & A. E. Baert (Eds.), *Prospective longitudinal research: An empirical basis for the primary prevention of psychosocial disorders*. Oxford: Oxford University Press.

Sampson, H., Messinger, S. L., & Towne, R. D. (1964). *Schizophrenic women: Studies in Marital Crisis*. New York: Atherton.

Srole, L. (1985). *Program notes on the Midtown I-II study design*. Unpublished.

Srole, L., & Fischer, A. K. (1984). The Midtown Manhattan longitudinal study versus the mental paradise lost doctrine: A controversy joined. In S. A. Mednick, M. Harway, & K. M. Finello (Eds.), *Handbook of longitudinal research* (Vol. 2). New York: Praeger.

Srole, L., Fischer, A. K., & Biel, R. (1985). *Midtowners lost and found: Search and assessment tactics and results*. Unpublished.

Srole, L., Langner, T., Michael, S., Opler, M., & Rennie, T. (1962). *Mental health in the metropolis: The Midtown Manhattan study* (Vol. 1). New York: McGraw-Hill.

Stampfer, M. J., Willett, W. C., Speizer, F. E., Dysert, D. C., Lipnick, R., Rosner, B., & Hennekens, C. H. (1984). Test of the National Death Index. *American Journal of Epidemiology, 119*(5), 837-839.

Stanley, B., & Stanley, M. (1982). Testing competency in psychiatric patients. *IRB, 4*(8), 1-6.

Steel, L., Wise, L., & Abeles, R. P. (1984). Project TALENT: A longitudinal study of the development and utilization of individuals' capabilities. In S. A. Mednick, M. Harway, & K. M. Finello (Eds.), *Handbook of longitudinal research* (Vol. 2). New York: Praeger.

Stephens, J. H. (1978). Long-term prognosis and followup in schizophrenia. *Schizophrenia Bulletin, 4*(1), 25–47.

Stone, M. H. (1987). Psychotherapy of borderline patients in light of long-term follow-up. *Bulletin of the Menninger Clinic, 51*(3), 231–247.

Stone, M. H. (1988). *Tracing patients for long-term follow-up.* Unpublished manuscript, presented at the N.Y. State Psychiatric Institute, Feb. 24, 1989.

Stone, M. H. (in press). *The PI 500.* New York: Guilford.

Stone, M. H., Stone, D. K., & Hurt, S. W. (1987). Natural history of borderline patients treated by intensive hospitalization. *Psychiatric Clinics of North America, 10*(2), 185–206.

Strauss, J. S., & Carpenter, W. T. (1972). The prediction of outcome in schizophrenia, 1: Characteristics of outcome. *Archives of General Psychiatry, 27*, 739–746.

Strauss, J. S., & Carpenter, W. T. (1974). The prediction of outcome in schizophrenia, 2: Relationships between predictor and outcome variables: A report from the WHO International Pilot Study of Schizophrenia. *Archives of General Psychiatry, 31*, 37–42.

Strauss, J. S., & Carpenter, W. T. (1977). Prediction of outcome in schizophrenia, 3: Five-year outcome and its predictors. *Archives of General Psychiatry, 34*, 159–163.

Strauss, J. S., & Carpenter, W. T. (1978). The prognosis of schizophrenia: Rationale for a multidimensional concept. *Schizophrenia Bulletin, 4*(1), 56–67.

Strauss, J. S., Kokes, R. F., Carpenter, W. T., & Ritzler, B. A. (1978). The course of schizophrenia as a developmental process. In L. C. Wynne, R. L. Cromwell, & S. Matthysse (Eds.), *The nature of schizophrenia: New approaches to research and treatment.* New York: Wiley.

Taub, H. A. (1986). Comprehension of informed consent for research: Issues and directions for future study. *IRB, 8*(6), 7–10.

Toner, J., Gurland, B., & Leung, M. (in press). Chronic mental illness and functional communication disorders in the elderly. *American Speech-Language-Hearing Association Reports.*

Tsuang, M. T. (1984). Long-term follow-up of the major psychoses. In S. A. Mednick, M. Harway, & K. M. Finello (Eds.), *Handbook of longitudinal research* (Vol. 2). New York: Praeger.

Tsuang, M. T. (1986). Predictors of poor and good outcome in schizophrenia. In L. Erlenmeyer-Kimling and N. E. Miller (Eds.), *Life-span research on the prediction of psychopathology.* Hillsdale, NJ: Lawrence Erlbaum.

Tsuang, M. T., & Dempsey, G. M. (1979). Long-term outcome of major psychoses, 2: Schizoaffective disorder compared with schizophrenia, affective disorders, and a surgical control group. *Archives of General Psychiatry, 36*, 1302–1304.

Tsuang, M. T., & Fleming, J. A. (1987). Long-term outcome of schizophrenia and other psychoses. In H. Hafner, W. F. Gattaz, & W. Janzarik (Eds.), *Search for the cause of schizophrenia.* Berlin: Springer-Verlag.

Tsuang, M. T., & Winokur, G. (1975). The Iowa 500: Field work in a 35-year follow-up of depression, mania, and schizophrenia. *Canadian Psychiatric Association Journal, 20*, 359–365.

Tsuang, M. T., & Woolson, R. F. (1978). Excess mortality in schizophrenia and affective disorders. *Archives of General Psychiatry, 35,* 1181–1185.

Tsuang, M. T., Woolson, R. F., & Fleming, J. A. (1979). Long-term outcome of major psychoses, 1: Schizophrenia and affective disorders compared with psychiatrically symptom-free surgical conditions. *Archives of General Psychiatry, 36,* 1295–1301.

Tsuang, M. T., Woolson, R. F., & Fleming, J. A. (1980). Causes of death in schizophrenia and manic-depression. *British Journal of Psychiatry, 136,* 239–242.

Tsuang, M. T., Woolson, R. F., & Simpson, J. C. (1980). The Iowa structured psychiatric interview: Rationale, reliability, and validity. *Acta Psychiatrica Scandinavica,* Supplementum 283, 62.

Tsuang, M. T., Woolson, R. F., & Simpson, J. C. (1981). An evaluation of the Feighner criteria for schizophrenia and affective disorders using long-term outcome data. *Psychological Medicine, 11,* 281–287.

Tsuang, M. T., Woolson, R. F., Winokur, G., & Crowe, R. R. (1981). Stability of psychiatric diagnosis. *Archives of General Psychiatry, 38,* 535–539.

Vaillant, G. E. (1978). A 10-year follow-up of remitting schizophrenics. *Schizophrenia Bulletin, 4*(1), 78–85.

Walker, A. M., Velema, J. P., & Robins, J. M. (1988). Analysis of case-control data derived in part from proxy respondents. *American Journal of Epidemiology, 127*(5), 905–914.

Wentworth, D. N., Neaton, J. D., & Rasmussen, W. L. (1983). An evaluation of Social Security Administration master beneficiary record file and the National Death Index in the ascertainment of vital status. *American Journal of Public Health, 73*(11), 1270–1274.

Westermeyer, J. F., & Harrow, M. (1988). Course and outcome of schizophrenia. In M. T. Tsuang & J. C. Simpson (Eds.), *Handbook of schizophrenia* (Vol. 3): *Nosology, epidemiology and genetics.* New York: Elsevier.

17

Statistical Methods for Research in Chronically Mentally Ill Elderly

Lou Ann McAdams, Dilip V. Jeste

It is possible to pose a research question for which there is no appropriate statistical method available to answer it. But commonly the researcher's problem is not the absence of suitable statistical methods but either unfamiliarity with what statistical procedures are available and reasonably near at hand or unfamiliarity with the criteria for selecting an available technique. The aim of this chapter will be to review some of the many statistical procedures available and to illustrate situations in which their application would be appropriate. In keeping with the goal of this book, we have generally tried to cite examples pertaining to studies of the chronically mentally ill elderly, although the usefulness of the statistical procedures discussed is obviously not limited to that field. Because of obvious space limitations, this chapter is not intended to be a comprehensive discussion of various statistical approaches but is primarily conceptualized as a "triaging" of the more common types of investigations to appropriate statistical techniques.

CLASSIFICATION OF VARIABLES

Unless the study has only a descriptive purpose (e.g., the aim of estimating means, standard deviations, correlations, etc.), early in the planning stage there will be a logical division betwen variables that are potentially to be the predictors—the explanatory, manipulated, experimental, or independent variables—and variables that are to be predicted, explained, or accounted for—the outcome, response, or dependent variable(s). The level of measurement achieved in each variable and the numbers of predictor and outcome variables are some of the most important factors in the selection of statistical technique. Variables may be classified according to the level of measurement, into categorical (e.g., gender-category: male and female) and continuous (e.g., blood pressure measured in mm Hg). There is a third type of variable with a different level of measurement—the ordered variable. Here the outcome variable is quantified but does not have equal intervals or, at any rate, we are not certain that it has (e.g., many nonstandardized tests have scales with ordered response categories, such as 1 through 7, which we cannot be sure are of equal length, e.g., whether the distance from 4 to 5 is the same as that from 5 to 6), or the other assumptions of normality and homogeneity of variance cannot be or are not presumed to be met.

HYPOTHESES AND ERRORS

In the planning stages of the research program, the researcher's research hypothesis is recast or translated into a statistical hypothesis, the *alternative hypothesis*, and its opposite or negation is identified as the *null hypothesis*. The probability of falsely rejecting the null hypothesis—finding a significant difference spuriously (Type I error)—is controlled by the adoption of a significance level for its rejection by means of the statistical test selected. The probability of falsely rejecting the alternative hypothesis (Type II error—not finding a significant difference when it does, in fact, exist) and hence *power* (i.e., 1 minus Type II error) is then determined by Type I error, sample size, and the size of the actual effects (free of scale of measurement) under investigation. The determination of power and/or sample size (power analysis) may be facilitated by use of the tables in books such as that by Cohen (1988).

STATISTICAL METHODS

Statistical techniques described below are grouped according to purpose and according to the level of measurement achieved in the predictor and the outcome variables when the purpose is prediction. For the first several types, the purpose is prediction.

We will discuss nine different types of situations, of which the first five are listed according to the type of predictor and outcome variables:

Predictor Variables	Outcome Variables
1. Categorical	Continuous
2. Categorical	Categorical
3. Categorical	Ordered
4. Continuous	Continuous
5. Continuous	Categorical

Next, we will discuss statistical techniques for special situations:

6. Predicting a change in status in a long-term follow-up study when there are dropouts and/or the follow-up period is variable
7. Studying cyclic phenomena
8. Grouping variables into relevant clusters
9. Classifying subjects into subtypes

STATISTICAL ANALYSIS WHEN THE PREDICTOR VARIABLE IS CATEGORICAL AND THE OUTCOME VARIABLE IS CONTINUOUS

Analysis of Variance

The experimental designs and the techniques developed for experimental research in general (and particularly for agricultural research) are applicable as well to experimental research with the chronically mentally ill elderly. There is a variety of experimental designs available, and the designs are readily extended to survey research. Each design pattern calls for a particular pattern of analysis of variance or ANOVA (Kirk, 1982; Winer, 1971). For example, subjects randomly assigned to three separate groups and exposed to three separate treatments (e.g., one group each to one of three anxiolytics A, B, and C) will necessitate a between-groups or between-subjects ANOVA. In contrast, a single group exposed to three different treatments (e.g., three anxiolytics A, B, and C), with suitable washout periods and suitable random assignment of each subject to a treatment sequence (e.g., A, B, C; B, A, C; C, B, A, etc.), will necessitate a repeated-measures or within-subjects ANOVA (with or without a between-subjects order or sequence effect).

Requisite Assumptions

In the case of the between-subjects design, the requisite assumptions include normality of values within each treatment group and homogeneity of the variance in different treatment groups. In the case of the within-groups design, the requisite assumptions include normality of the orthogonal contrasts of the dataset, and symmetry of the variance-covariance matrix of the orthogonal contrasts of the dataset. For a given design, the appropriate assumptions should be tested before proceeding with the planned analysis (Kirk, 1982; Winer, 1971). Alterations in plans should be made if the assumptions are found to be untenable. For example, if the variances are found to be heterogeneous, a transformation may be applied to the data to obtain homogeneous data. Kirk (1982) and Winer (1971) describe which transformations are likely to accomplish homogeneity under specific circumstances, and the manual for the BMDP statistical packages (Dixon, 1983) also has a graphic procedure for selecting the appropriate transformation. If no such transformation can be found to accomplish the homogeneity, a nonparametric test may be employed (see Woolson, 1987; Siegel, 1956, for alternative statistical tests). Implicit in the assumption of normality is the assumption of continuity of the scale and equal intervals. However, equal intervals will suffice.

Experimental Manipulation and Naturalistic Survey

Study design influences interpretation of statistical analysis as well as the choice of statistical procedure. An investigator may manipulate the predictor variable (e.g., using different doses of an antidepressant to achieve specific blood levels and then studying their effects on improvement in depression) or may use a naturalistic design (e.g., associating antidepressant blood levels and improvement in depression among patients being treated by their respective clinicians in different settings without a fixed treatment protocol). If the researcher has experimentally manipulated the predictor variable or variables, then the level of inference is much stronger than if the predictor variables were merely sampled along with the outcome variables (Susser, 1973). Nonetheless, the experimental approach and the naturalistic survey are both useful approaches. The naturalistic study will sometimes uncover associations that can then be tested experimentally. Without the naturalistic approach to suggest variables for experimental manipulation and/or strong theoretical development, the experimental approach may lack sufficient focus.

More Complex Designs

We can remain in the ANOVA framework and plan simpler studies, or we may design more complex studies than the three-sample investigations mentioned above. If we reduce the experimental manipulations (or number of categories surveyed) to two, we have the familiar unrelated-samples t-test or, if the manipulations are in the same group, the related-samples paired t-test. If we reduce still further the categories to one sample to be compared with some known population mean, we have the familiar one sample t-test (if we know only the population mean) or one-sample z-test (if we also know the population variance). On the other hand, if we increase the number of independent variables to two or more, we have a factorial design that calls for a multiway ANOVA. This analysis must take account of whether each factor is random or fixed in addition to whether each factor is a between-subjects or a within-subjects factor, and there is the possibility of testing hypotheses about one or more interaction (synergistic) effects among factors on the outcome variable.

If there are multiple outcome variables, we can employ the multivariate analogue of the t-test, Hotelling's T^2, or one of several multivariate analogs of ANOVA (MANOVA): Wilk's lambda likelihood ratio statistic, Roy's largest root statistic, etc. (Harris, 1985; Morrison, 1976). Even though there may be only one outcome variable if one or more predictor variables are repeated-measures (within-subjects) factors, it may be desirable to use MANOVA for the repeated-measures factor. This is to be recommended if there is evidence of asymmetry in the variance-covariance matrix for the repeated-measures outcome variable and adequate sample size.

An example of the planned use of the techniques in this category is our current study of late-onset schizophrenia. This is a naturalistic study having a group of late-onset schizophrenia patients and a comparable control group. The outcome measures (e.g., scores on selected neuropsychological tests and computerized values for specific abnormalities on MRI scan such as areas of signal hyperintensity) are quantitative and may be considered continuous. There are many outcome variables making MANOVA, specifically Hotelling's T^2, the omnibus test of differences between groups on subsets of baseline variables. A significant MANOVA (Hotelling's T^2) omnibus test will be followed by univariate ANOVAS (t-tests) on each individual response variable in the subset. Type I error will be controlled for each subset of variables by using Bonferroni corrections (Morrison, 1976). Power analysis was performed to ensure sufficient sample size for univariate test of anticipated effects of the more important outcome variables (Cohen, 1988). Another example is that of Jeste, Kleinman, Potkin, Luchins, and Weinberger (1982).

STATISTICAL ANALYSIS WHEN BOTH PREDICTOR AND OUTCOME VARIABLES ARE CATEGORICAL

The simplest design in this category is the 2 X 2 design: two levels of the predictor variable and two levels of the outcome variable. An example is a study to evaluate male gender as a risk factor for the development of neuroleptic malignant syndrome. Here the predictor variable is gender (male versus female) and the outcome variable is neuroleptic malignant syndrome (present versus absent). (Obviously, we assume that other relevant predictor variables such as amount of neuroleptics are taken into account). The statistical technique for two independent groups is the familiar X^2 test (or Fisher's exact probability test for small samples), while the technique for two related samples is McNemar's test (Marascuilo & McSweeney, 1977; Siegel, 1956).

Of course, the design may have more than two categories in either the predictor variable (e.g., race: caucasian, black, others) or the outcome variable (e.g., mood disorder: bipolar, unipolar, neither), in which case the X^2 test is still appropriate. Sometimes, however, there are more than one predictor variable and or more than one outcome variable. When there are more than two categorical variables altogether, the more recently available methods of cross-classification analysis are appropriate. Probably the most familiar among these are the log-linear models analysis procedure (Bishop, Fienberg, & Holland, 1975; Everitt, 1977; Fienberg, 1980; Knoke & Burke, 1980) and the WLS (weighted least squares) or GSK (Grizzle-Starmer-Koch) approach (Forthofer & Lehnen, 1981; Grizzle, Starmer, & Koch, 1969). Less well-known and less available is the information-theoretic approach (Kullback, 1959). For information about power analysis, see Cohen (1988) and Milligan (1980).

Log-linear modeling is similar to the ANOVA modeling, except that in log-linear models with a single outcome variable, first-order interactions involving that variable have their counterpart in main effects in ANOVA, while second-order interactions involving that variable have their counterpart in first-order interactions in ANOVA; for example, if variable C is the outcome variable, an AC effect is the effect of A on C and the ABC effect is the joint effect of A and B, above and beyond the single effects of A and B upon C. A special measure of agreement between two or more sets of categorical or ordered measures is Cohen's kappa (1960) or generalized kappa statistic (Fleiss, 1981).

STATISTICAL TECHNIQUES FOR CATEGORICAL PREDICTORS AND ORDERED OUTCOMES

An example of this type of situation is a study comparing the effects of milieu therapy, psychotherapy, and pharmacotherapy on overall functioning judged on a scale that uses a 0–3 rating, with 0 = no improvement, 1 = mild improvement, 2 = moderate improvement, and 3 = marked improvement. Here the researcher has available techniques more powerful than those for categorical data but less powerful (efficient) than those of equal-interval continuous (or at least equal-interval discrete) variables.

For the between-groups design, the Kruskal-Wallis one-way ANOVA may be used (Siegel, 1956). For the repeated-measures design, one may employ the Friedman's two-way (subject by independent factor) ANOVA (Siegel, 1956).

STATISTICAL TECHNIQUES WHEN BOTH THE PREDICTOR AND THE OUTCOME VARIABLES ARE CONTINUOUS

These may be experiments but are more typically cross-sectional studies or surveys. An example of such a study is one looking at the relationship between aging and loss of neurons in the brain, determined with quantitative techniques (e.g., Mani, Lohr, & Jeste, 1986). Both the age (predictor variable) and the number of neurons (outcome variable) are continuous variables. In this situation when there are only two variables under consideration—one predictor and one outcome variable— either correlation or simple linear regression is the statistical procedure of choice. In the case of correlation, the assumption made is that both variables are bivariate, normally distributed. However, in the case of linear regression, only the outcome variable, or rather the residual variable—the deviation of the outcome variable from the regression line is assumed to be normally distributed for each value of the predictor variable. The Pearson product-moment correlation coefficient is commonly used in studies of validity or test-retest reliability. Values of 0.8 or better are considered to be good evidence of validity or reliability (Cronbach, 1970). In other applications, values considerably smaller may be considered useful. Cohen (1988) designates $\pm.1$ as small, $\pm.3$ as medium, and $\pm.5$ as large.

Suppose we let x stand for the value of a potential predictor variable and y stand for the value of an outcome variable, and let $hat\text{-}y$ stand for the predicted value of y. The aim of linear regression is to estimate the parameters alpha and beta, the intercept and regression (slope) coefficients, respectively, in the equation $y = alpha + beta \times x + e$ by the estimates a and b, respectively; e is the random error of the model. Prediction of outcome variable from predictor variable from an equation

$$hat\text{-}y = a + bx \text{ (note: residual} = y - hat\text{-}y)$$

may be useful in any clinical situation when it is necessary to anticipate y and it is possible to do so with an assessment of x.

When more than two continuous variables are under consideration and only one of them is the outcome variable, multiple linear regression techniques are employed (Draper and Smith, 1981). These techniques include the so-called direct solution and several stepwise procedures for predicting the outcome from an entire set of variables or from a "best" subset of the available predictors. A multiple correlation may also be calculated. When there are also multiple outcome variables, one or more functions of one set of variables (the predictor set) may be employed to predict the same number of functions of a second set of variables (the outcome set). And a canonical correlation may be employed to assess the strength and significance of each of the orthogonal associations between the two sets of variables (Harris, 1985). Again, see Cohen (1988) for assistance with power analysis. When two variables are ordered and continuous, but one or perhaps both are not known to have equal intervals, the Spearman rank (order) correlation coefficient may be employed to assess the relationship between the two (Siegel, 1956).

Special laboratory procedures, Scatchard plots, etc. are discussed by Finney (1978) and Odell and Daughaday (1971).

STATISTICAL ANALYSIS WHEN MOST OR ALL OF THE PREDICTOR VARIABLES ARE CONTINUOUS AND THE OUTCOME VARIABLE IS CATEGORICAL

An example of such a situation is trying to subtype schizophrenia into type I and type II (Crow, 1980) using predictor variables such as the degree of ventricular enlargement on CT scan or the degree of reduction in psychotic symptoms with a standardized neuroleptic treatment protocol. Until recently, the combination of discriminant analysis and classification analysis, frequently referred to as discriminant function analysis, was employed in this situation. Depending on the number of groups, the number of predictor variables and the relationships among the predictor variables, one or more functions of the predictor variables were used to separate the groups and then classification functions were used to classify cases into groups (Harris, 1985; Klecka, 1980; Lachenbruch, 1975). The limitation of this still widely used technique is that in a strict sense, it can be applied only when all the predictors are continuous. More recently, logistic regression has been used to predict group membership (Fleiss, Williams, & Dubro, 1986). This technique allows for both categorical and continuous predictors, and until recently was available for only two categories of the outcome variable. Now, however, the technique is available in BMDP for several categories of the outcome variable (Dixon, Brown, Engelman, & Jennrich, 1990; Hosmer & Lemeshow, 1989).

The techniques discussed so far are those best employed for experimental, cross-sectional, retrospective, or short-term follow-up research studies. We will now focus on methods best employed for long-term follow-up studies with their attendant risk of loss-to-follow-up and risk of events that compete with or preclude the outcome of interest.

STATISTICAL TECHNIQUES FOR PREDICTING A CHANGE IN STATUS IN THE PRESENCE OF DROPOUTS FROM STUDY AND/OR VARIABLE FOLLOW-UP PERIOD

This type of situation is illustrated by prospective long-term follow-up studies of incidence of and risk factors for tardive dyskinesia in patients starting treatment with neuroleptics. We recently began such a study in patients over age 45. Kane, Woerner, and Lieberman (1988) have been conducting this work for several years. In these seminaturalistic investigations, different patients enter the study at different time points and have variable periods of follow-up with a certain dropout rate. The question may be originally posed as, on average, how long (after starting neuroleptics) is the period before the change (development of tardive dyskinesia) occurs. But if so, the question may be converted to what is the risk of the change occurring. Or the question may be originally posed as what factors determine *how long* until the change occurs. In the latter case, the question may be converted to what factors determine the risk of the change occurring.

Both the *product-limit estimator* (Kaplan & Meier, 1958), for ungrouped data, and the *life table method* (Cutler & Ederer, 1958), for data grouped into time intervals will assess the risk of change (i.e., incidence), taking into account dropouts and risks other than the one being studied. Both the Log Rank Test and the Gehan Test Statistic compare two *survival curves*. The Cox regression or proportional-hazards method will identify, in stepwise fashion, factors influencing the risk of the event of interest, taking account of dropouts and risks other than the one being studied (Cox and Oakes, 1984; Kalbfleisch and Prentice, 1980). A pertinent example of the latter is the Woolson, Tsuang, and Fleming paper (1980) on longevity of psychotic patients.

STATISTICAL METHODS FOR STUDYING CYCLIC (OR PULSATILE) PHENOMENA

Some behavioral and physiological responses (e.g., sleep-wakefulness cycle, menstrual cycle, seasonality of births of schizophrenic patients) occur in a predictable cyclic pattern—daily, monthly or seasonal. To identify these patterns, one needs frequent measurements taken over the course of several cycles (days, months, years). With data for one or more groups, the pattern may be discerned with the aid of several time-series analysis techniques. In the case of two or more groups, the patterns may be compared (Box & Jenkins, 1976; Chatfield, 1984; Fuller, 1976).

However, some cyclical or pulsatile phenomena are not so regular (e.g., hormone secretions). Automated peak detection programs have been developed in an attempt to provide objective measures of these peaks. CLUSTER (Veldhuis & Johnson, 1986) and DETECT (Oerter, Guardabasso, & Rodbard, 1986) are two of the more recent computer programs now available for studying patterns of peripheral hormone concentrations. As these tools are still being refined, it remains to be seen how useful they will be in specific applications. For an application and a review of contemporary methods, see Urban et al. (1988).

STATISTICAL METHODS TO REDUCE THE NUMBER OF VARIABLES CARRYING THE RELEVANT INFORMATION

An illustration of this kind of work is an investigation to determine which symptoms of schizophrenia respond to neuroleptics and which do not. Using a rating scale such as the Brief Psychiatric Rating Scale or BPRS (Overall & Gorham, 1962) and a standardized treatment protocol, we may find that say 10 symptoms (e.g., delusions, hallucinations) improve more than 50%, while 14 symptoms (e.g., affective blunting) do not. It would be useful to try to cluster the 10 neuroleptic-responsive symptoms into say three relevant groups (e.g., positive symptoms, depression symptoms, etc.). The major statistical techniques, collectively called *factor analysis*, differ in mathematical underpinnings. In applications, one should evaluate assumptions about the number of factors to be extracted, the definition of commonality, and whether or not factors are or even should be allowed to be correlated. Harmon's (1967) book remains a classic reference, and Kim and Mueller (1978) make the essentials accessible. Test construction is one practical application of these techniques, and here, especially, theoretical constructs strongly influence which items are included in the test battery. These techniques are, however, more often employed to reduce the number of variables to a more manageable number. But to use these techniques, one needs to have several-fold more subjects than variables to obtain a stable factor structure solution. Also, researchers often complain that factors identified have less clear meaning than the individual variables that contributed to their extraction and identification. The factor analytic technique may appropriately be employed to provide a new measuring stick for further research, or it may be appropriately employed as a first step in the analysis stage of a research project. Kim and Mueller (1978) point out that the use of factor scores (based on original measures and coefficients derived from the factor analysis) in a subsequent stage of analysis may lead to different conclusions than using the original measures in that stage of analysis.

STATISTICAL METHODS TO CLASSIFY SUBJECTS INTO SUBTYPES

Cluster analysis (there are several types) may be used to group individuals whose response patterns are similar. This approach may produce subtypes of a disorder (Everitt, 1980). A previously mentioned example of subtyping schizophrenic patients into type I and type II on the basis of CT-scan abnormalities and neuroleptic-responsiveness applies here too.

Factor analysis can also be used to cluster subjects into subtypes rather than to cluster test items into factor scales. But here there should be several-fold more items than subjects to obtain a stable factor structure solution (i.e., syndromes) (Guilford, 1954).

SUMMARY

In this chapter we have associated a number of statistical techniques with both the purpose and the particular level of measurement achieved in the predictor and outcome variables of a study. The techniques mentioned do not constitute an exhaustive list but rather serve to illustrate that the choice of a statistical technique is related to the research question, number of variables, the level of measurement achieved in each of the variables, as well as other attributes of the variables (normality, homogeneity, independence) and the constancy or inconstancy of the observation period. In most instances, references have been supplied for both the technique and a particular application of the technique. Increased familiarity with techniques discussed in this chapter will enable the reader not only to plan studies better and analyze data generated by their programs of research more appropriately but also to make them better users of the psychiatric literature in general (Hokanson et al., 1986).

ACKNOWLEDGEMENT

This work was supported, in part, by NIMH grant #1-R01-MH43693-01, and by the Veterans Administration.

REFERENCES

Bishop, Y. M. M., Fienberg, S. E., & Holland, P. W. (1975). *Discrete multivariate analysis: Theory and practice*. Cambridge, MA: Massachusetts Institute of Technology Press.

Box, G. E. P., & Jenkins, G. M. (1976). *Time series analysis: Forecasting and control* (rev. ed). San Francisco: Holden-Day.

Chatfield, C. (1984). *The analysis of time series: An introduction* (3rd ed.). New York: Chapman and Hall.

Cohen, J. (1960). A coefficient of agreement for nominal scales. *Educational and Psychological Measurement, 20*, 37–46.

Cohen, J. (1988). *Statistical power analysis for the behavioral sciences* (2nd ed.). Hillsdale, NJ: Lawrence Erlbaum.

Cox, D. R., & Oakes, D. (1984). *Analysis of survival data*. London: Chapman and Hall.

Cronbach, L. J. (1970). *Essentials of psychological testing* (3rd ed.). New York: Harper & Row.

Crow, T. L. (1980). Molecular pathology of schizophrenia: More than one disease process? *British Medical Journal, 280*, 66–68.

Cutler, S. J., & Ederer, F. (1958). Maximum utilization of the life-table method in analyzing survival. *Journal of Chronic Diseases, 8,* 699–713.

Dixon, W. J., Brown, M. B., Engelman, L., & Jennrich, R. I. (1990). *BMDP statistical software manual,* Vols. 1 and 2. Berkeley: University of California Press.

Draper, N. R., & Smith, H. (1981). *Applied regression analysis* (2nd ed.). New York: Wiley.

Everitt, B. S. (1977). *The analysis of contingency tables.* London: Chapman & Hall.

Everitt, B. (1980). *Cluster analysis* (2nd ed.). New York: Halsted Press.

Fienberg, S. E. (1980). *The analysis of cross-classified categorical data* (2nd ed.). Cambridge, MA: MIT Press.

Finney, D. J. (1978). *Statistical method in biological assay* (3rd ed.). London: Griffin.

Fleiss, J. L. (1981). *Statistical methods for rates and proportions* (2nd ed.). New York: Wiley.

Fleiss, J. L., Williams, J. B. W., & Dubro, A. F. (1986). The logistic regression analysis of psychiatric data. *Journal of Psychiatric Research, 20,* 195–209.

Forthofer, R. N., & Lehnen, R. G. (1981). *Public program analysis: A new categorical data approach.* Belmont, CA: Lifetime Learning Publications.

Fuller, W. A. (1976). *Introduction to statistical time series.* New York: Wiley.

Grizzle, J. E., Starmer, C. F., & Koch, G. G. (1969). Analysis of categorical data by linear models. *Biometrics, 25,* 489–504.

Guilford, J. P. (1954). *Psychometric methods* (2nd ed.). New York: McGraw-Hill.

Harmon, H. H. (1967). *Modern factor analysis* (2nd ed.). Chicago: University of Chicago Press.

Harris, R. J. (1985). *A primer of multivariate statistics* (2nd ed.). New York: Academic Press.

Hokanson, J. A., Bryant, S. F., Gardner, R., Jr., Luttman, D. J., Brock, G. G., & Brenkowski, A. C. (1986). Spectrum and frequency of use of statistical techniques in psychiatric journals. *American Journal of Psychiatry, 143,* 1118–1125.

Hosmer, D. W., Jr., & Lemeshow, S. (1989). *Applied logistic regression.* New York: Wiley.

Jeste, D. V., Kleinman, J. E., Potkin, S. G., Luchins, D. J., & Weinberger, D. R. (1982). Ex uno multi: Subtyping the schizophrenia syndrome. *Biological Psychiatry, 17,* 199–222.

Kalbfleisch, J. D., & Prentice, R. L. (1980). *The statistical analysis of failure time data.* New York: Wiley.

Kane, J. M., Woerner, M., & Lieberman, J. (1988). Tardive dyskinesia: Prevalence, incidence and risk factors. *Journal of Clinical Psychopharmacology, 8*(suppl.), 52S–56S.

Kaplan, E. L., & Meier, P. (1958). Nonparametric estimation from incomplete observations. *Journal of the American Statistical Association, 53,* 457–481.

Kim, J., & Mueller, C. W. (1978). *Factor analysis: Statistical methods and practical issues.* Beverly Hills: Sage.

Kirk, R. E. (1982). *Experimental design: Procedures for the behavioral sciences* (2nd ed.). Monterey, CA: Brooks/Cole.

Klecka, W. R. (1980). *Discriminant analysis.* Beverly Hills: Sage.

Knoke, D., & Burke, P. J. (1980). *Log-linear models.* Beverly Hills: Sage.

Kullback, S. (1968). *Information theory and statistics.* New York: Dover.

Lachenbruch, P. A. (1975). *Discriminant analysis.* New York: Hafner Press.

Mani, R. B., Lohr, J. B., & Jeste, D. V. (1986). Hippocampal pyramidal cells and aging in the human: A quantitative study of neuronal loss in sectors CAl-CA4. *Experimental Neurology, 94,* 29–40.

Marascuilo, L. A., & McSweeney, M. (1977). *Nonparametric and distribution-free methods for the social sciences.* Monterey, CA: Brooks/Cole.

Milligan, G. W. (1980). Factors that affect type I and type II error rates in the analysis of multidimensional contingency tables. *Psychological Bulletin, 87*, 238–244.

Morrison, D. F. (1976). *Multivariate statistical methods* (2nd ed.). New York: McGraw-Hill.

Odell, W. D., & Daughaday, W. H. (1971). *Principles of competitive protein-binding assays.* Philadelphia: Lippincott.

Oerter, K. E., Guardabasso, V., & Rodbard, D. (1986). Detection and characterization of peaks and estimation of instantaneous secretory rate of episodic pulsatile hormone secretion. *Computers and Biomedical Research, 19*, 170–191.

Overall, J. E., & Gorham, D. R. (1962). The brief psychiatric rating scale. *Psychological Reports, 10*, 799–812.

Siegel, S. (1956). *Nonparametric statistics for the behavioral sciences.* New York: McGraw-Hill.

Susser, M. (1973). *Causal thinking in the health sciences: Concepts and strategies of epidemiology.* London: Oxford University Press.

Urban, R. J., Evans, W. S., Rogal, A. D., Kaiser, D. L., Johnson, M. L., & Veldhuis, J. D. (1988). Contemporary aspects of discrete peak detection algorithms. I. The paradigm of the luteinizing hormone pulse signal in men. *Endocrine Reviews, 9*, 3–37.

Veldhuis, J. D., & Johnson, M. L. (1986). Cluster analysis: A simple, versatile, and robust algorithm for endocrine pulse detection. *American Journal of Physiology, 250*, E486–E493.

Winer, B. J. (1971). *Statistical principles in experimental design* (2nd ed.). New York: McGraw-Hill.

Woolson, R. F. (1987). *Statistical methods for the analysis of biomedical data.* New York: Wiley.

Woolson, R. F., Tsuang, M. T., & Fleming, J. A. (1980). Utility of the proportional hazards model for survival analysis of psychiatric data. *Journal of Chronic Diseases, 33*, 183–195.

18

Measuring Mental Health, Health, Function, and Coping in the Chronically Mentally Ill Elderly

Richard Schulz, Paul Visintainer

A prerequisite to the measurement of health status in any population is some knowledge of the object of measurement. We need at least some ballpark notion of size, shape, and function of the thing we wish to measure. The fact that we are able to derive some descriptive and predictive accounts of chronic mental illness presumes the existence of some measurement tools. Our goal here is to identify and address issues of measurement in chronically mentally ill (CMI) elderly populations.

This discussion is divided into three parts, corresponding to the major questions one might ask about measuring health in the CMI elderly. First, we will address the question *what are the goals of measurement?* Next, we will fix our attention on issues concerning the *who and what of measurement.* This will be followed by a discussion on the *measurement of change.* Finally, we will make some concluding comments and recommendations.

GOALS OF MEASUREMENT

The choice of measures is closely linked to the goals of any data collection effort. Kane and Kane (1983) describe a number of functions that data collection might serve, each with its own requisites regarding measurement tools.

Clinical assessments are usually carried out in secondary and tertiary prevention contexts, and typically involve a detailed examination of an individual with the goal of reaching a diagnostic conclusion and assignment to treatment or intervention. Assessment tools must therefore be able to delineate functioning in small units, cover a broad range to minimize error, and above all yield accurate diagnoses—that is, minimize both false positives and false negatives. *Population assessments*, on the other hand, are aimed at providing descriptive data on the distribution, determinants, and modifiers of disease. The basic tool in population assessments is the screening instrument, which must be efficient, simple, flexible, portable, have practical significance, and be valid—e.g., have high levels of sensitivity and specificity. In general, issues of reliability and validity of measurement are paramount in population studies. Frequently such data are collected by epidemiologists and used as baseline indicators in intervention studies.

Monitoring involves the repeated measurement over time and requires instrumentation that is sensitive to change and at the same time reliable and valid. A final goal of measurement is *prediction*. Most clinical intervention is based on the prediction that a given treatment will result in a particular desired outcome. Thus, all clinical treatment can be viewed as involving prediction. More commonly, though, prediction is a central feature of experimental research, controlled clinical trials, and program evaluations. The goal in these research efforts is to relate antecedent conditions and a planned intervention to particular outcomes, hopefully in a way that allows the researcher to make valid causal conclusions. Demonstrating effects in this context requires measures that are both very reliable and valid.

In any given study or practice context, the investigator or clinician needs to be clear about the goals of measurement. Each of the functions described above has associated with it its own set of measurement tools as well as criterion set points regarding issues of validity and reliability. In addition, the costs of making mistakes can vary substantially. A false positive psychiatric diagnosis can be extremely costly for the patient, family, and the health-care system, while the primary cost of measurement errors made in predictive studies is to increase error variance and yield inconclusive results.

Economic Evaluation as a Goal

Assessing the cost of care for the chronically mentally ill has been a major interest of both researchers and policy makers for several decades, although the research in this area has generated more controversy than consensus. Such analyses are useful in planning the allocation of health-care resources for the community as a whole and to a lesser extent in making decisions on behalf of the individual patient. The typical economic analysis of health care involves the computation of a number of inputs such as (1) direct health-care costs to the system, patient, and family; (2) indirect costs (e.g., production losses) resulting from the patients' inability to be part of the work force; as well as (3) a number of intangible costs such as pain and suffering. These inputs are measured in relation to a set of outputs which might include (1) number of patients treated, (2) a health effect such as the functional status attained by the patient, (3) number of years of life gained, and (4) improvements in the quality of life.

Advocates of *cost-benefit analyses* focus on the problem of translating all health effects into measurable monetary units, while *cost-effectiveness* devotees are more interested in identifying the net cost for achieving a net change in health. A third approach is advocated by Drummond (1987) which he calls *cost-utility analysis*. This is a type of cost-effectiveness analysis in which the denominator of the ratio is expressed in terms of quality-adjusted life-years, a measure of life extension gained, which is adjusted by a series of utility weights reflecting the relative value of one health state compared to another. For example, interventions that add years to life with little or no residual disability would be viewed as more cost-effective and be more highly valued than interventions which add years but leave the patient in a severely disabled condition.

Economic analyses of health care present difficult but important challenges in that they place a premium on objective and easily quantifiable measures that ideally can be converted into monetary units. Paradoxically, such analyses also require measures that reflect extremely subjective judgments about the value and meaning of life. Economic considerations frequently reside in the background of clinical trials, psychosocial intervention research, and demonstration projects. It would be useful to bring them to the foreground in studies of the chronically mentally ill elderly since these factors are likely to play a major role in policy decisions regarding the care provided this population.

WHAT AND WHOM DO WE MEASURE?

It would be a mistake to talk about the mental health of the CMI Elderly without at the same time considering their physical health and functional status. Few researchers would disagree with the notion that physical and mental health and functioning can be differentiated at least at a conceptual level and that for most purposes, it is essential to assess all three areas of functioning. However, there is likely to be considerable disagreement among us when it comes to identifying specific instruments and assessment techniques to be used to achieve this goal.

There are hundreds of individual instruments designed to measure various aspects of mental and physical health and functioning as well as dozens of multidimensional instruments designed to assess all three. Many of these instruments were originally developed for younger populations and therefore may not be appropriate for the elderly, but more and more such instruments have been developed or adapted for the elderly. The availability of a growing number of anthologies or compendia of measurement instruments for middle-aged and elderly adults speaks to the widespread availability of measurement tools (e.g., Kane & Kane, 1983; Karoly, 1985; Mangen & Peterson, 1982; McDowell & Newell, 1987).

It would be both too time-consuming and tedious to review in detail the advantages and disadvantages of specific measurement tools. Instead, we will focus on the common content areas any adequate measurement instrument would need to cover, as well as some unique areas of measurement needed for CMI elderly populations.

In general, we endorse the consensus reached at the recent Portugal Conference on the Measurement of Quality of Life (Katz, 1987) that the health status of any individual requires the assessment of five distinct dimensions: physical health, mental health, everyday functioning in social and role activities, and general perceptions of well-being (Ware, 1987). Assessment in the first four categories is often carried out with behavior-based scales while the fifth category is based on individual self-perceptions of health. The latter category is important because behavior measures do not capture the underlying differences such as pain, degree of difficulty, level of effort required, or worry or concern about health. Generic measures applicable to all populations and clinical groups should capture important differences in adult populations, including those suffering from specific diseases.

The measurement of quality of life at this generic level has a long history going back to the development of the Karnofsky scale, the work of Gurin, Veroff, and Field on Americans' view of their mental health (1960); Bradburn on the structure of psychological well-being (1969); Andrews and Withey on social indicators of well-being (1976); Campbell, Converse, and Rodgers on the quality of American life (1976); and many others, including Katz, Ford, Moskowitz, Jackson, and Jaffee (1963) and Spitzer et al. (1981). Given the widespread availability of large numbers of global well-being measures, it is regrettable that many investigators continue to assume that completely different generic scales need to be designed each time a new population is studied or a new hypothesis is being tested (Spitzer, 1987). Indeed, one of the advantages of using existing scales is the ability to make comparisons between groups and across time.

For most studies such a generic measure of quality of life should serve as a minimal requirement. In addition, given the nature of the CMI elderly population, it would be useful to include measures that capture unique characteristics such as their ability to "reintegrate to normal living (Wood-Dauphinee & Williams, 1987). The importance of this concept is that it distinguishes between absolute levels of functioning from relative levels. It recognizes that being able to do what one has to do or wants to do does not necessarily mean being free from all disease or disability. This view emphasizes that quality of life is an intrapersonal subjective experience based on an individual's tolerance, priorities, expectations, and satisfaction with what has already been accomplished (p. 493). When disease or disability is permanent, the mode of adjustment involves acceptance and perhaps lowered life expectations on the part of the patient. This relativist perspective is reflected in the construction of the items such as "I move around my living quarters as I feel is necessary" or "I feel that I can deal with life events as they happen."

The reintegration perspective also raises a more basic issue regarding standards of functioning for the CMI elderly. Should we have minimal standards for normal living based on societal expectations or clinical judgment, or should normal living be based on context specific assessments of what is possible and appropriate? How one answers this question has important implications for measurement.

In addition to these generic measures, specific measurement tools are often needed to assess the effects of particular diseases and treatments or to test a specific hypotheses. Such measures may be broad or specific, depending upon the question being addressed. For example, in the recently published results of the Vermont Longitudinal Study of Persons with Severe Mental Illness, two relatively generic outcome measures designed specifically for psychiatric populations were used to assess patient status. The Global Assessment Scale (Harding, Brooks, Ashikaga, Strauss, & Breir, 1987) was used to "provide a single score that would capture the essence of the subjects' psychological and social functioning" (p. 722). This instrument classifies individuals based on the extent to which they exhibit symptoms and are able to function. The second instrument, the Strauss-Carpenter Levels of Functioning Scale was used to classify subjects from "poor to best" on nine items of interest, such as having a close friend, being employed in the past year, displaying symptoms.

Other examples of hypothesis-testing studies requiring specific focused instrumentation include the studies of intelligence and abstract thinking in elderly psychotics (Harrow, Marengo, Pogue-Geile, & Pawelski, 1987), the physical and social environment of the patient (Cohen, 1987), information-processing patterns in schizophrenics (Niederehe & Rusin, 1987) or lateral cerebral ventricular size in schizophrenics (Pearlson, Garbacz, Tompkins, Ahn, & Rabins, 1987). For most of the areas identified in these studies—intelligence, abstract thinking, information processing, or ventricular size—extensive methods of measurement are available, and the researcher would be doomed to fail were he to ignore existing measurement tools and methods.

However, there are some areas that could benefit from further development. For example, our ability to meaningfully characterize the social environment of the community-residing CMI elderly patient is very limited. A number of comprehensive scales are currently available for assessing institutional environments, but we have few tools that would capture the important aspects of the social and physical environments and their role in facilitating or disrupting functioning in the chronically mentally ill. One approach to this problem might be to assess environments in terms of their triggering potential for pathological episodes among certain types of psychiatric patients. Alternatively, one might develop systems for matching patient functioning or potential functioning with the amount of autonomy or control a particular environment provides.

Finally, it is important not to overlook the obvious. Basic descriptive epidemiologic data such as morbidity and cause of mortality should be an essential component of the measurement tools for the CMI elderly. Researchers frequently note that CMI elderly have higher rates of physical illnesses and higher rates of mortality when compared to nondisabled age-matched comparison groups. But we are rarely told what those physical illnesses were and what the cause of mortality was for those individuals who were lost to mortality in long-term follow-up studies (e.g., Harding et al., 1987). Such information is likely to be at least as important in gaining an understanding of the life history of the CMI elderly as data regarding the mental health status of the patient.

Data Sources

For most purposes the source of the data one wishes to collect is self-evident. If the goal is to carry out a clinical diagnosis, then the primary data source will be the patient. On the other hand, if we wish to assess the impact of patient disability on family functioning, it is essential that data be obtained from both family members and patient. Not uncommonly, though, the researcher or clinician must rely on proxy sources for information about the patient. Because of cognitive deficits, the patient is no longer able to provide reliable self-report data; as a result, a family member or primary informant may be asked to provide needed information. However, such data should be cautiously interpreted. A growing body of literature indicates that evaluative data provided by relatives of the patient may be systematically biased, particularly in areas pertaining to patient affect (Schulz, Tompkins, Wood, & Decker, 1987; Schulz & Williamson, 1990).

MEASUREMENT OF CHANGE

Assessing change over time, particularly long periods of time, requires that we have adequate base-rate information about a population against which deviations can be identified. Two types of base-rate information are needed in order to understand the CMI elderly. First, we need to know something about the normative course of adult development for the general population. Second, we need to know something about the life history of the chronically mentally ill.

While we know little about the natural history of chronic mental illness, it is useful to examine the normative life course for clues as to what to look for in enhancing our understanding of chronic mental illness.

One of the fundamental characteristics of human society is that roles, relationships, and behaviors change with age. Contemporaneous with these changes are subtle and profound changes in health status. At the most basic level, the life course can be defined as the major life events and transitions an individual experiences between birth and death. Some theorists have claimed there is an underlying structure to adult life within which the personal biographies of individuals are enacted, while others have taken their cues from Homes and Rahe and the Dohrenwends and have partitioned the life course into critical or significant life events such as marriage, having a child, leaving home, and retirement (cf. Schulz & Rau, 1984). Because the empirical base for the latter approach is better developed, particularly with respect to the areas of health and social support, the discussion of the life course will be guided by the earlier work of Danish, Smyer, and Nowak (1980), Brim and Ryff (1980), Hultsch and Plemons (1979), Cohler and Ferrono (1987), and Schulz and Tompkins (1990).

A number of researchers have developed a conceptual system for classifying life-course events and transitions based on temporal normativity—the notion that there are strong expectations within our culture that certain events should happen at a particular time in the life course. People should go to college in their early twenties, have babies in their twenties and thirties, retire in their sixties, and so on. We feel that this typology should be expanded to include the notion of statistical normativity. Events are defined as statistically normative when they happen to most individuals in a cultural group, and they are temporally normative when they occur within a predictable limited age range, because of biological constraints and/or because of cultural norms. If we cross-tabulate these two variables, we obtain a four-celled classification table in which two of the four cells classify events that are both statistically and temporally normative or neither statistically nor temporally normative; the remaining two cells would include events that are either statistically or temporally normative, but not both. For example, marriage in the twenties, birth of first child in twenties or thirties, retirement at age 65 would be considered both statistically and temporally normative, while experiencing a natural disaster or winning the lottery are neither temporally nor statistically normative. Entering college at middle age or becoming widowed at a young age would be considered temporally nonnormative but statistically normative. Finally, events such as spinal-cord injury, stroke, or winning a prestigious professional award are statistically nonnormative but temporally normative.

This classification system is helpful because it enables us to see some broad structural relationships among the triad of life-course events, social relationships, and health. Those life transitions that are experienced by most people and that occur within narrow expected age ranges are not likely to be particularly troublesome because they are predictable—and as a result our culture ensures wide-spread anticipatory socialization of both the individual experiencing the event and the potential support system—but also because the social network has the ability, knowledge, and motivation to provide support. Ability and knowledge are acquired through socialization. The motivation to act has its source in societal sanctions regarding interpersonal exchanges within and across generations: parents are supposed to help their college-aged children, husbands are supposed to be supportive of their wives during pregnancy and the birth of a child, children are supposed to help care for their frail parents, and so forth. Finally, to the extent that a culture judges an event to be both common and potentially stressful, it is likely to establish both formal and informal support systems to help the individual cope with the event.

Life-course events that are unexpected either because they occur off-time or are statistically infrequent are likely to be more problematic. Because the individual often does not have the opportunity to prepare for them, they are likely to be inherently more stressful. Moreover, members of the support network are less likely to have the appropriate abilities or knowledge to provide support even if they have the motivation. As a result, a society frequently trains professional helpers and develops specialized programs to help individuals cope with these events.

The CMI elderly patient clearly falls into our statistically nonnormative category but may vary considerably in the extent to which his current patient status was preceded by a normative or nonnormative life course. Cohler and Ferrono (1987) have written about the adult life course of the schizophrenic and point out, as others have, that it is important to identify the patterns of episode and recovery of those individuals whose first episode occurs in young adulthood from those whose initial episode occurred in middle or late life. For either type of patient it seems plausible to assume that psychiatric symptoms and hospitalization "may cause time relationships to become dislocated and time disordered" (p. 192), although the magnitude of asynchronies created may vary with time of onset for the first episode. For example, Clausen (1986) found in his 15- to 20-year follow-up of married adult psychiatric patients that a favorable prognosis was strongly associated with the acquisition of social competence prior to an incapacitating breakdown.

The impact of psychiatric episodes are also likely to extend to the informal support system. For example, Anderson, Hogarty, Bayer, and Needleman (1984) found that the social networks of parents of schizophrenic patients are smaller than those of parents of normal offspring and that network size was smaller, the longer the length of illness. These data suggest that while the burden of providing support is increasing with the age of the patient, the number of support persons among whom the burden can be distributed is decreasing. Moreover, the ability of the parents to provide support is also decreasing because of their own aging. The extent to which the community-residing CMI elderly patient is dependent on the caregiving of relatives paints a bleak picture of patient prognosis.

The major point of this lengthy discussion is that we need to know a great deal more about the life history of the CMI elderly and the contexts in which they are played out. Case histories of the CMI elderly are one valuable source of data for this, but more importantly, we need to ask questions concerning the social networks, support systems, stressors, and coping strategies used by psychiatric patients at different points in the life course. We have available a number of well-developed conceptual systems and measurement tools useful in describing stress-coping phenomena for individuals at different points in the life course. One approach to understanding the CMI elderly would be to ask how relevant existing models are to this special population.

Regarding the measurement of change, we not only need to know *what* we want to measure, but we must also address issues concerning (1) the equivalence of measures over time and (2) the possibility of changes in distributions and norms (Labovie, 1986). One of the most basic measurement issues facing the researcher interested in psychopathology over the life course concerns the functional equivalence of measures in relation to their underlying concepts. In other words, how do we know whether a given measure is assessing the same construct in individuals of different ages or cohorts, and how do we know whether formally different measures are related to the same construct either in the same population measured at different points in time or in different populations? With respect to diagnosing psychopathologies, this issue becomes even more complex because both concepts and their formal measures change over time. As a result, researchers are sometimes faced with the herculean task of diagnosing patients by applying current diagnostic criteria using data collected more than 30 years earlier for another purpose. One generally accepted method for addressing this concern is to use multiple sets of measures for each concept being investigated in order to establish systematic patterns of convergent and discriminant validity. Another approach might be to examine the covariance structures of measures used in longitudinal studies.

A second measurement issue concerns the use of age- and cohort-specific norms in the description and measurement of psychopathology. A given behavioral event may be interpreted as either a high-frequency or low-frequency event, depending on the normative distribution being used as reference point. Bias is a potential problem anytime age and cohort norms for one group are applied to another. Perhaps the best way of addressing this issue is to be sensitive to possible criterion shifts over time.

SUMMARY AND RECOMMENDATIONS

It is noteworthy that the mentally ill were not included as a target population in the recently convened Portugal Conference on Measuring Quality of Life and

Functional Status in Clinical and Epidemiological Research (Katz, 1987). Whether this was a case of benign neglect or intentional omission is not known to us, but it would be valuable to engage in a similar detailed examination of the current status of measurement of the CMI elderly. We can learn a great deal from the work that has already been carried out on the measurement of other chronically ill populations, but at the same time it is essential to identify (a) unique measurement tools for the CMI elderly and assess their adequacy; (b) existing measures that are appropriate and/or could be adapted for this population; and (c) new measures that need to be developed.

We have identified a number of measurement issues that might serve as focal points for such an effort. First, it is important to keep in mind that measurement serves multiple purposes and the criterion for choosing measures and translating measurement results into decisions will vary substantially as a function of the goals of the researcher or clinician. We all know this to be true, but it would be useful to clearly articulate some guidelines for making those choices in the context of assessing the CMI elderly and their environments.

Second, the adequacy of existing measurement instruments needs to be closely examined. In particular we need to (a) know whether existing instruments are sensitive enough to assess the range of functioning typically found among the CMI elderly; (b) assess the extent to which they tell us about relative or context specific levels of functioning as opposed to absolute levels of functioning; and (c) place more emphasis on the inclusion of measures that will facilitate economic evaluations of treatment programs for the CMI elderly. It may also be desirable to develop new measures such as instruments that will enable us to characterize the physical and social environments of this population. However, we endorse the views expressed by others that the development of new measures should be approached cautiously and reluctantly. It would be useful to set minimal standards, as others have (e.g., Spitzer, 1987), for the development of new measures. We are particularly concerned about past failures to address the issues of discriminant validity in the development of new measures.

Third, since assessment of the CMI elderly often involves the measurement of change, we must first recognize that it is very difficult to do this well and then make sure we use the best methods, tools, and analytic strategies available for this task. Given the nature of the population of interest, it is particularly important that we address issues concerning the equivalence of measures over time and across cohorts, as well as cohort- and time-related criterion shifts. An important prerequisite for achieving this goal is a better understanding of the life history of chronic mental illness. In sum, all of these recommendations boil down to carefully taking stock of what we have done in this area thus far, assessing how well we have done it, and then figuring out how to improve future endeavors.

ACKNOWLEDGMENTS

This manuscript was prepared for presentation at a National Institute of Mental Health sponsored meeting on The Chronically Mentally Ill Elderly, Orlando, Fla., December 9, 1987. Preparation of this manuscript was supported by the Mental Disorders of the Aging Research Branch, National Institute of Mental Health.

REFERENCES

Anderson, C. M., Hogarty, G., Bayer, T., & Needleman, R. (1984). Expressed emotion and social networks of parents of schizophrenic patients. *American Journal of Psychiatry*, *144*, 247–255.

Andrews, F. M., & Withey, S. B. (1976). *Social indicators of well-being*. New York: Plenum Press.

Bradburn, N. M. (1969). *The structure of psychological well-being*. Chicago: University of Chicago Press.

Brim, O. G., Jr., & Ryff, C. D. (1980). On the properties of life events. In P. B. Baltes & O. G. Brim Jr. (Eds.), *Life-span development and behavior* (Vol. 3, pp. 368–387). New York: Academic Press.

Campbell, A., Converse, P. E., & Rodgers, W. L. (1976). *The quality of American life*. New York: Russell Sage Foundation.

Clausen, J. A. (1986). A 15- to 20-year follow-up of married adult psychiatric patients. In L. Erlenmeyer-Kimling & N. E. Miller (Eds.), *Life-span research on the prediction of psychopathology*. Hillsdale, NJ: Lawrence Erlbaum.

Cohen, C. (1987). Elderly schizophrenics and paranoics living in single-room occupancy hotels. In N. E. Miller & G. D. Cohen (Eds.), *Schizophrenia and aging*. New York: Guilford Press.

Cohler, B. J., & Ferrono, C. L. (1987). Schizophrenia and the adult life-course. In N. E. Miller & G. D. Cohen (Eds.), *Schizophrenia and aging*. New York: Guilford Press.

Danish, S. J., Smyer, M. A., & Nowak, C. A. (1980). Developmental intervention: Enhancing life-event processes. In P. B. Baltes & O. G. Brim, Jr. (Eds.), *Life-span development and behavior*. New York: Academic Press.

Drummond, M. F. (1987). Resource allocation decisions in health care: A role for quality of life assessments? *Journal of Chronic Disease*, *40* (6), 505–592.

Gurin, G., Veroff, J., & Field, S. (1960). *Americans view their mental health*. New York: Basic Books.

Harding, C. M., Brooks, G. W., Ashikaga, T., Strauss, J. S., & Breier, A. (1987). The Vermont Longitudinal Study of persons with severe mental illness, I: Methodology, study sample, and overall status 32 years later. *American Journal of Psychiatry*, *144*, 718–726.

Harrow, M., Marengo, J., Pogue-Geile, M., & Pawelski, T. J. (1987). Schizophrenic deficits in intelligence and abstract thinking: Influence of aging and long-term institutionalization. In N. E. Miller & G. D. Cohen (Eds.), *Schizophrenia and aging*. New York: Guilford Press.

Hultsch, D. F., & Plemons, J. K. (1979). Life events and life span development. In P. B.

Baltes & O. G. Brim, Jr. (Eds.), *Life-span development and behavior* (pp. 1–31). New York: Academic Press.

Kane, R. A., & Kane, R. L. (1983). *Assessing the elderly*. Lexington, MA.: D.C. Heath.

Karoly P. (Ed.). (1985). *Measurement strategies in health psychology*. New York: Wiley.

Katz, S. (Ed.). (1987). The Portugal conference: Measuring quality of life and functional status in clinical and epidemiological research. *Journal of Chronic Disease, 40* (6), 459–645.

Katz, S., Ford, A. B., Moskowitz, R. W., Jackson, B. A., & Jaffee, M. W. (1963). Studies of illness in the aged. The Index of ADL: A standardized measure of biological and psychosocial function. *Journal of the American Psychological Association, 185,* 94ff.

Labovie, E. W. (1986). Methodological issues in the prediction of psychopathology: A life-span perspective. In L. Erlenmeyer-Kimling & N. E. Miller (Eds.), *Life-span research on the prediction of psychopathology*. Hillsdale, NJ: Lawrence Erlbaum.

Mangen, D. J., & Peterson, W. A. (Eds.). (1982). *Research instruments in social gerontology, Vol. 1: Clinical and social psychology*. Minneapolis: University of Minnesota Press.

McDowell, I., & Newell, C. (1987). *Measuring health: A guide to rating scales and questionnaires*. New York: Oxford University Press.

Niederehe, JG., & Rusin, M. J. (1987). Schizophrenia and aging: Information processing patterns. In N. E. Miller & G. D. Cohen (Eds.), *Schizophrenia and aging*. New York: Guilford Press.

Pearlson, G. D., Garbacz, D., Tompkins, R. H., Ahn, H. S., & Rabins, P. V. (1987). Lateral cerebral ventricular size in late onset schizophrenia. In N. E. Miller & G. D. Cohen (Eds.), *Schizophrenia and aging*. New York: Guilford Press.

Schulz, R., & Rau, M. T. (1984). Social support through the life course. In S. Cohen & L. Syme (Eds.), *Social support and health*. New York: Academic Press.

Schulz, R., & Tompkins, C. A. (1990). Life events and changes in social relationships: Examples, mechanisms, and measurement. *Journal of Social and Clinical Psychology, 9,* 69–77.

Schulz, R., Tompkins, C. A., Wood, D., & Decker, S. (1987). The social psychology of caregiving: Physical and psychological costs of providing support to the disabled. *Journal of Applied Social Psychology, 17,* 401–428.

Schulz, R., & Williamson, G. M. (1990). Biases in family assessments of depression in Alzheimer's disease. *American Journal of Psychiatry, 147,* 377–378.

Sisk, E. (1987). Discussion: Drummond's "Resource allocation decisions in health care: A role for quality of life assessment?" *Journal of Chronic Disease, 40* (6), 617–620.

Spitzer, W. O. (1987). State of science 1986: Quality of life and functional status as target variables for research. *Journal of Chronic Disease, 40* (6), 465–471.

Spitzer, W. O., Dobson, A. J., Hall, J., Chesterman, E., Levi, J., Shepherd, R., Battista, R. N., & Catchlove, B. R. (1981). Measuring the quality of life of cancer patients. A concise QL-index for use by physicians. *Journal of Chronic Disease, 34,* 585–597.

Ware, J. E., Jr. (1987). Standards for validating health measures: Definition and content. *Journal of Chronic Disease, 40* (6), 473–480.

Wood-Dauphinee, S., & Williams, J. I. (1987). Reintegration to normal living as a proxy to quality of life. *Journal of Chronic Disease, 40* (6), 491–500.

19

Research Resources: Developing Trained Researchers

Steven H. Zarit

The development of a systematic body of knowledge on the chronically mentally ill aged depends in part on training a cadre of skilled researchers who will pursue theoretically important and policy-relevant lines of inquiry. The number of researchers trained in the area of mental health and aging is limited, with only a minority interested in the specific problems of the chronically mentally ill. A concerted effort is needed to bring both experienced and new researchers into this field.

A variety of incentives can be used to encourage researchers to focus on problems of chronic mentally ill elderly, including research training grants and specific research initiatives. A corresponding effort is needed for development of a framework that generates intellectual excitement by highlighting important clinical research and policy issues. Certainly, the chapters in this volume contribute toward that goal.

The problem of the chronically mentally ill has for too long been given too little attention. These patients have been given low priority because they represent our treatment failures and because their personal and social characteristics often make them undesirable as clients or research subjects. A research program on this group is important for its own sake, as it can lead to improved treatment and other changes that will increase overall quality of life for chronic patients. The implications for theory and practice in the mental health field, however, will often touch on broad central issues. As an example, by concentrating on mental illness only in its early manifestations, we may miss some important characteristics that may illuminate key aspects of these disorders. Differentiating courses of disorders can contribute to diagnostic classification and may lead to identification of more homogeneous groups for trials of new treatments. Similarly, the study of illness characteristics is typically undertaken using one time of measurement, but since the major disorders tend to be fluctuating and episodic, studies of how features of the disorder change over time might illuminate etiology or at least suggest better ways of treating recurrent episodes. Another important issue is the provision of long-term care, including how to maximize independent functioning, involve families without excessive burden or burnout, and develop effective systems of social and medical care.

Research on the chronically mentally ill elderly requires knowledge and skills from several domains. Traditional discipline-based training can provide a foundation, but a multidisciplinary approach is needed to deal with the scope and complexity of research questions in this field. By cutting across various disciplines, a multidisciplinary approach also encourages creative integration of theory and methods. In the following sections, a training curriculum will be presented, followed by a discussion of methods of training and recruitment of trainees.

A TRAINING CURRICULUM

While a training program cannot cover everything that the student might potentially want or need to know about chronic mental illness, five areas seem especially pertinent: (1) psychopathology; (2) a lifespan developmental perspective on adulthood and aging; (3) clinical issues in later life; (4) pertinent substantive areas of research; and (5) values. The contributions of these areas to a training curriculum are described below.

Psychopathology

Knowledge of the epidemiology, etiology, treatment, and course of psychopathology is a basic part of a curriculum on chronic mental illness. The focus should be on those disorders which continue to have a high prevalence in middle and later life. Affective disorders and schizophrenia are the most prominent, but other problems warrant attention.

Two chronic problems that are prevalent in the elderly, but which are frequently overlooked, are alcoholism and personality disorders. There is a tendency to underdiagnose alcoholism in the elderly, attributing cognitive effects to dementia or aging (Zimberg, 1987). Two patterns of alcoholism in later life have been described: (1) cases of relatively recent onset, often in reaction to losses, and (2) people with long-standing histories of abuse, often dating back to early adulthood (Mishara & Kastenbaum, 1980; Zimberg, 1987). Alcohol abuse has immediate and practical implications for older people's functioning, and can complicate treatment of other medical and mental health problems.

The problem of personality disorders in old age is also relatively unexplored. Clinical examples suggest both persistence and change in personality disorders from adulthood to old age. Some people may become better adapted as they age, while others become dramatically more symptomatic, as in the examples of an individual with a schizoid pattern who develops paranoid symptoms in later life (Post, 1980, 1987). Research on personality disorders has been limited by the lack of reliable diagnostic tools. Recent investigations suggest possible adaptations of screening measures with older populations (Hyer & Harrison, 1986; Thompson, Gallagher, & Czirr, 1988).

The study of psychopathology should also include a critical evaluation of treatment approaches and historical trends in treatment. Among the issues in the treatment literature, attention should be given to the possible effects of long-term use of neuroleptics (see chapters by Jeste and Fogel in this volume). A historical perspective is useful because mental health care has gone through numerous changes during the lifetime of the older chronic patient. A major emphasis has been deinstitutionalization. A historical perspective is also useful for understanding patients' attitudes toward treatment. Their willingness to participate in new treatment programs or to receive other mental health services may in part depend on ideas they have about mental health practices that are no longer employed. Additionally, the older literature sometimes addresses mental health problems that are quite contemporary. Articles about effects of institutional care in mental hospitals, for example, provide timely observations on how the environment of nursing homes may affect residents.

A Lifespan Developmental Perspective

The combination of knowledge of major types of psychopathology with a lifespan developmental perspective provides a strong foundation for studying the chronically mentally ill elderly. Several features of the life span approach are particularly important when considering aging and older people (see Baltes, 1987).

The lifespan developmental perspective emphasizes normal development. Normative patterns of development can serve as a baseline for comparison of characteristics of the chronic patient, so that we do not mistakenly attribute the effects of chronic problems to age and vice versa.

A major feature of the lifespan approach is that development is viewed as continuous through the life course. Change is multidirectional, that is, there can be both continued growth and decline. There can also be both intra- and interindividual differences in the timing and rates of growth and decline. Some abilities will be more differentially affected by aging (for instance, speed of response), while some older people will demonstrate compensation for specific types of decline.

Another feature of the lifespan perspective is attention to the methodologies needed for studying change. In particular, it is critical to understand the limitations of generalizing about development from cross-sectional data, both for viewing normal development and for assessing how psychopathology might change over time. Longitudinal and sequential designs are potentially powerful tools for studying the course of psychopathology, though some technical problems such as subject attrition are likely to be even greater than in normal populations. There should also be attention to cohort and historical events which have been found to influence behavior and cognition across the adult years (see Schaie & Willis, 1986, for a review). Beliefs, attitudes, and behaviors of the older chronic patient are likely to have been influenced by the events of that person's historical time.

A lifespan developmental perspective also stresses the need for multidisciplinary and multivariate investigations. These approaches are especially important for mental health research, which has relied too much perhaps on single variables and univariate statistics. Rigorous training in methodology would be an important element in a training program.

Application of a life-course perspective to chronic mental illness would also suggest identifying the developmental course of disorders and how these disorders affect, and in turn are affected by, normal developmental change. The multiple influences on development should be identified and considered for their impact on the course of mental disorders. Focusing specifically on the developmental course of chronic problems, we need to identify ages at risk for first onset of disorders and probabilities for future episodes. These ages of risk will be associated with particular normative and nonnormative events. Further, current problems of the chronically mentally ill older person may relate specifically to how earlier developmental issues were addressed. As an example, an irregular work history earlier in life has implications for financial status in old age.

Baltes (1987) recently proposed a developmental framework for conducting intervention research. Interventions which "test the limits" can indicate the potential for growth and change as well as indicating limitations imposed by aging or other factors. As an example, he cites the use of method of loci for improving short-term memory. Results of studies on this approach suggest older people are able to learn supraspan lists of numbers (e.g., strings of 60–70 digits), though at slower rates than younger people. Thus, this intervention demonstrates both plasticity and limitations of older subjects.

Clinical Issues in Later Life

A third part of a curriculum should be attention to the specific clinical issues of later life. Training needs to emphasize the unique clinical issues of aging. Special considerations affect every aspect of clinical practice, including assessment, treatment approaches, treatment settings and personnel, and public policy.

While assessment is an important part of every type of clinical practice and research, it can be argued that accurate assessment has even greater implications for older people. Many clinical questions revolve around differential assessment of memory complaints and memory problems. The chronic patient's current functioning can be compromised further by the presence of age-associated problems such as dementia, delirium, or depression. As with older people, the chronic patient should be evaluated for these age-related disorders, with an emphasis on identifying potentially treatable components. As an example, an older person with a long-term schizophrenic disorder may develop dementia, which puts different strains on that patient's support system, but there may also be depressive symptoms which can be treated (Teri & Gallagher, in press).

A major challenge is determining if mild cognitive changes are early manifestations of dementia or have some other cause. This problem is quite complex under usual circumstances but may be even more difficult when assessing a chronic patient. Differentiation of mild cognitive changes associated with early dementia from long-standing deficits is a particular problem. Indeed, research that has operationalized the construct of pseudodementia suggests that many such patients may have chronic mental health problems (Caine, 1981). Identification and treatment of treatable components of these age-associated disorders will enhance functioning of the chronic patient.

In addition to contributing to differential diagnosis, assessment plays a key role in establishing baselines of functioning and identifying strengths as well as weaknesses. Because of the predominantly negative stereotypes associated with aging, accurate assessment can serve to distinguish between overly pessimistic expectations or attributions, as when a person assumes that forgetting a name means he has Alzheimer's disease, and actual deficits. Identification of strengths and assets will contribute to development of a treatment plan as well as to counter negative expectations for outcome.

Another assessment issue which arises frequently in cases of older people is determining who the client is. In many instances, family or friends may decide that the older person needs assistance, but the designated patient may or may not concur. Assessment can distinguish the extent to which treatment should focus on the older person or on family. Identification of resources and deficits in the patient's support system will also play a critical role in development of a treatment plan.

Assessments may also, on occasions, address clinical problems that require interface with the legal system, including competency, the possibility of elder abuse, and suicidal and/or homicidal risk.

The assessment process should be structured in ways that take into account limitations likely to be found in an older population. Steps such as breaking up the evaluation if the patient becomes fatigued, evaluating whether hearing and vision deficits affect perception of test stimuli, and allowing the older person adequate time to respond can lead to more accurate assessments. Age-appropriate tests and age norms should be used whenever available.

Treatment issues focus on both the age of the patient and the age of the therapist. How the patient's age affects treatment is a central theme in the literature. While empirical studies are still quite limited, initial reports suggest optimistic findings for response to psychotherapy, with the major difference that older persons take somewhat longer to respond (Smyer, Zarit, & Qualls, 1990). How these findings might generalize to treatment of the chronic patient is not known. On the other hand, attention should be given to the age of the therapist. Knight (1986) provides an excellent discussion of how the age difference between therapist and client may lead to distorted beliefs toward each other that adversely affect the treatment process.

Knight (1986) also suggests some common topics and themes which emerge in psychotherapy with older persons. Major topics in psychotherapy include chronic illness and disability; death and dying; love, marriage, and sexuality; and interpreting aging. Major themes are empowerment of the older person; identifying and engaging in enjoyable activities, and life review. These topics and themes are likely to be salient for many chronic patients. As Knight and others (e.g., Wilber & Zarit, 1987) have cautioned, however, the patient's age does not determine that a particular set of psychological issues will be raised; rather, age increases the likelihood that the patient might focus on these concerns. A too-literal interpretation of psychological constructions of aging, for instance, Erikson's (1963) dichotomy of integrity-despair, can blind the therapist to the real concerns a person might be raising.

Another issue affecting clinical practice with older persons is the treatment settings and personnel who provide treatment (Smyer et al., 1990). Older people are underrepresented in some settings; for example, community mental health centers and private practice. In turn, older people with mental health problems are found in considerable numbers in nursing homes and board-and-care homes, even though these settings often have very limited resources for mental health assessment and treatment (Smyer, Cohn, & Brannon, 1988). Responsibility for care of these patients typically falls on those with the least training (LPNs, aides), while professional staff with specific mental health training are rare. Nursing homes and personal-care (or board-and-care) homes are likely residences for many chronic mental patients.

Policy issues affecting mental health delivery, including the role of Medicare and Medicaid and state policies, should be considered. The type of treatment provided and likelihood that the patient will receive treatment at all depend on these policies. Effects of current policies are to limit the amount of treatment that is reimbursed and to shift responsibility for care of the older chronic patient from mental health to aging services (e.g., board and care homes, case-management programs) that do not necessarily have adequate skills or resources.

Pertinent Substantive Areas of Research

Several related areas of research seem especially pertinent to the study of older chronic patients. These areas include social support, family caregiving, stress and coping, and the influence of race, ethnicity, and gender.

The availability of social support is an important issue for any older person with a mental health problem, but particularly for the chronic patient whose support network may be diminished because of the continued strain of interpersonal conflict or excessive demands. The disrupted life history of many chronic mental patients may result in no kin being available to provide assistance, or responsibility may fall upon siblings or other relatives rather than children. Appreciation of the multidimensionality of social support, the potential for both support and conflict in relationships with significant others, and the ways interventions can mobilize supportive persons are all relevant. Study of the support systems of chronic patients will also provide a good test of the generalizability of current theoretical models of social support.

Related to social support is the issue of family caregiving. As Cohler, Pickett, and Cook (this volume) have indicated, we know little about family involvement with this population. Consideration of models of family functioning and stress, the specific disruptions and benefits associated with caregiving, and the interface of the family with the service system are all relevant to understanding the caregiving family.

Third, there needs to be consideration of theories of stress and coping, from the perspective of both the chronic patient and his support system. As Cohler et al. (this volume) suggest, the chronic mentally ill person may have a special vulnerability to stressful life events. Issues such as the measurement and timing of stressful events are especially important. Attention to daily hassles and events may be a particularly promising approach for studying vulnerability to stress and adaptive processes (Kinney & Stephens, 1989).

The outcome of stressful events may depend on behavioral and cognitive coping strategies the chronic patient uses. Measurement of coping is a complex issue. While some general measurement strategies have been developed, conceptualizations of coping suggest that responses may be specific to different domains or problems (see Pearlin & Schooler, 1978). Indeed, the researcher looking at a chronic patient or her family will be interested in responses to some specific set of situations or stressors. This type of focus is likely to require instrument construction as well as conceptualization of adequate and inadequate coping responses.

Another important substantive area is the influence of factors such as race, ethnicity and gender on the manifestation, identification, treatment, and course of mental illness and on associated factors that affect patient outcome, such as the availability of family support. Variability in the course and outcome of disorders among different groups in the population might also be suggestive of new treatment approaches.

Values

Many important decisions about the development of interventions or research on the chronically mentally ill older person involve values. While the conduct of research should be value-free—that is, the methods and procedures should not bias the results—the choice of research questions reflects values and beliefs about the phenomena to be studied. In areas such as aging and chronic mental illness which are associated with strong stereotypical beliefs, examination of values is essential.

There is no set of "appropriate" values for a researcher in this field. Within the diversity of values which might be espoused, however, several beliefs warrant consideration. First is the belief in the possibility of change. While the amount of change that might occur in any situation is an empirical question, the belief that change can occur will motivate investigations which look at innovative interventions.

A related belief is that older people should be empowered to make decisions about their own lifestyle. Particularly with a chronic mental patient, the tendency is to assume that other people such as family or service providers may be better able to anticipate needs and set goals. In fact, because of the nature of chronic mental health problems, many individuals will not consistently make decisions that are in their best interest. Nonetheless, the person's right to make his own decisions must be respected, except in instances when the person is not legally competent to do so.

A basic value is that people should have the opportunity to reside in the least restrictive environment commensurate with their ability to care for themselves. There are obvious advantages to more restrictive protected settings, including the greater assurance that physical needs of people will be adequately met. Yet institutional settings necessarily impose restrictions that diminish independence. The need to have patients conform to institutional procedures and routines can result in negative effects. Everyone familiar with nursing homes has witnessed the downward spiral that occurs for patients who are resistant or disruptive. These patients will typically be treated with medication and/or restraints, which can further compromise their functioning.

The choice, then, between more and less restrictive settings should include an evaluation of the relative risks of each setting. The choice of which risks to accept is a matter of values. Some individuals will willingly give up some independence for the security of a controlled environment. Others, however, will fiercely maintain their independence. Acceptable levels of risk, in which there is no imminent danger to self or others, need to be tolerated so that the opportunity for minimal restriction can be provided. Additionally, institutional settings need to make the effort to maximize personal control and minimize the intrusiveness of routines and personnel into everyday life.

METHODS OF TRAINING

A training program for research on older people with chronic mental health problems should have four main components: (1) classroom instruction, (2) research apprenticeship, (3) practicum experience, and (4) professional socialization. The need for classroom instruction in relevant substantive and methodological domains is obvious, so comments will focus on the other three areas.

Hands-on experience as part of a research team is excellent training for a young researcher. This apprenticeship provides a link between classroom studies and the practical problems that researchers face in implementing a study. When used as part of predoctoral training, an apprenticeship should include at least two different experiences so that trainees have broad exposure to methods and procedures of research. While postdoctoral training often emphasizes development of independent research efforts, trainees may also benefit from being part of ongoing teams on other projects, providing opportunities to improve their research skills and learn about the functioning of teams.

A practicum experience in clinical settings provides the trainee with firsthand knowledge of the people and organizations that are the focus of her program of research. Some trainees may want supervised clinical practice which can enrich their understanding of the chronically mentally ill. For others, however, it would be sufficient to gain interviewing or other experiences that build an understanding of the people they will research or the settings. Indeed, the practice of some researchers of conducting in-depth interviews or focus groups before developing research questions and instruments is a trend that should be encouraged. As our analytical methods become more sophisticated, there is increasing risk of applying elegant models to banal or irrelevant questions. The researcher who looks only at datasets may lose sight of important processes or dimensions that have yet to be evaluated. By grounding research in the context and phenomenology of experience, the investigator is more likely to engage in a dialectical process of ideas and experience that will lead to better and more innovative studies.

Finally, there needs to be consideration of professional socialization, including preparing research for presentation and publication, attending meetings of relevant professional societies, and interacting with researchers conducting work on similar topics. Some teaching experience may also be relevant for trainees who want an academic career.

RECRUITMENT

A variety of strategies can be used to recruit new researchers to the study of older people with chronic mental health problems. There are obvious approaches (e.g., training fellowships, availability of research funds), which should not be overlooked. Four other strategies may also contribute to recruitment. First, studies of the extent of the problem of chronic mental illness and need for trained reseachers can indicate to students the potential for career development in this area. Second, inclusion of material on the chronically mentally ill within standard textbooks and introductory courses can create interest among students. For a long time, a goal of the gerontology field was to include information about aging and older people in basic undergraduate courses, such as introductory sociology, psychology, or abnormal psychology. While units on aging in the courses are not universal, there has certainly been some progress. We might ask colleagues writing textbooks on mental illness or aging to include information about the population of chronically mentally ill.

A third approach would be to assist current research training programs by developing a list of speakers who might be invited as part of a colloquium series. Fourth, a limited amount of funding might be made available for students to participate in national conferences that focus on this topic. Thus, students not on training grants could receive travel support to present papers or attend conferences. Particular attention might be given to including graduate students in smaller invited conferences that highlight current trends or methodological issues in research on the chronically mentally ill.

CONCLUSIONS

Creation of a group of committed researchers concerned with problems of the chronically mentally ill elderly depends in part on demonstration of need and creating intellectual excitement about the potential contributions to theory and practice. As with many other issues in aging, a broad multidisciplinary knowledge base can serve as the foundation of training. This base would be augmented by specific clinical research and professional experiences.

REFERENCES

Baltes, P. B. (1987). Theoretical propositions of life-span development psychology: On the dynamics between growth and decline. *Developmental Psychology, 23*(5), 611–626.

Caine, E. D. (1981). Pseudodementia: Current concepts and future directions. *Archives of General Psychiatry, 38*, 1359–1364.

Erikson, E. (1963). *Childhood and society* (2nd ed.). New York: Norton.

Hyer, L., & Harrison, W. R. (1986). Later life personality model: Diagnoses and treatment. *Clinical Gerontologist, 5*, 399–416.

Kinney, J. M., & Stephens, M. A. P. (1989). Hassles and uplifts of giving care to a family member with dementia. *Psychology and Aging, 4*, 402–408.

Knight, B. (1986). Therapists' attitudes as explanation of underservice of elderly in mental health: Testing an old hypothesis. *International Journal of Aging and Human Development, 22*, 261–269.

Mishara, B. L., & Kastenbaum, R. (1980). *Alcohol and old age*. New York: Grune & Stratton.

Pearlin, L. I., & Schooler, C. (1978). The structure of coping. *Journal of Health and Social Behavior, 19*, 2–21.

Post, F. (1980). Paranoid, schizophrenia-like, and schizophrenic states in the aged. In J. E. Birren & R. B. Sloane (Eds.), *Handbook of mental health and aging* (pp. 591–615). Englewood Cliffs, NJ: Prentice-Hall.

Post, F. (1987). Paranoid and schizophrenic disorders among the aging. In L. L. Carstensen & B. A. Edelstein (Eds.), *Handbook of clinical gerontology* (pp. 43–56). New York: Pergamon Press.

Schaie, K. W., & Willis, S. (1986). *Adult development and aging* (2nd ed.). Boston: Little Brown.

Smyer, M. A., Cohn, M. D., & Brannon, D. (1988). *Mental health consultation in nursing homes*. New York: New York University Press.

Smyer, M. A., Zarit, S. H., & Qualls, S. H. (1990). Psychological intervention with the aging individual. In J. E. Birren & K. W. Schaie (Eds.), *Handbook of the psychology of aging* (pp. 375–404). New York: Academic Press.

Teri, L., & Gallagher, D. (in press). Cognitive behavioral interventions for depressed patients with dementia of the Alzheimer's type. In T. Sunderlund (Ed.), *Treatment of the Alzheimer's patient*. New York: Grune & Stratton.

Thompson, L. W., Gallagher, D., & Czirr, R. (1988). Personality disorder and outcome in the treatment of later-life depression. *Journal of Geriatric Psychiatry, 21*(2), 133–146.

Wilber, K. H., & Zarit, S. H. (1987). Practicum training in gerontological counseling. *Educational Gerontology, 13*, 15–32.

Zimberg, S. (1987). Alcohol abuse among the elderly. In L. L. Carstensen & B. A. Edelstein (Eds.), *Handbook of clinical gerontology* (pp. 57–65). New York: Pergamon Press.

Index